Reke

Dysphagia
Diagnosis and Management
Second Edition

Edited by
Michael E. Groher

With 13 Contributors

Butterworth–Heinemann
Boston   London   Oxford   Singapore   Sydney   Toronto   Wellington

Every effort has been made to ensure that the drug dosage schedules within this text are accurate and conform to standards accepted at time of publication. However, as treatment recommendations vary in the light of continuing research and clinical experience, the reader is advised to verify drug dosage schedules herein with information found on product information sheets. This is especially true in cases of new or infrequently used drugs.

Recognizing the importance of preserving what has been written, it is the policy of Butterworth-Heinemann to have the books it publishes printed on acid-free paper, and we exert our best efforts to that end.

Library of Congress Cataloging-in-Publication Data

Dysphagia : diagnosis and management / edited by Michael E. Groher ;
 with 13 contributors. —2nd ed.
    p.   cm.
 Includes bibliographical references and index.
 ISBN 0-7506-9078-X
 1. Deglutition disorders.   I. Groher, Michael E.
 [DNLM: 1. Deglutition Disorders—diagnosis.   2. Deglutition
Disorder—therapy.   WI 250 D998]
 RC815.2.D87   1992
 616.3'1—dc20
 DNLM/DLC
 for Library of Congress   92-20110
                                                                CIP

British Library Cataloguing-in-Publication Data.

A catalogue record for this book is available from the British Library.

Butterworth–Heinemann
80 Montvale Avenue
Stoneham, MA 02180

10   9   8   7   6   5   4   3   2   1

Printed in the United States of America

Contents

Contributors

Wendy Avery-Smith, MS, OTR
Senior Occupational Therapist
Department of Rehabilitation Medicine
The New York Hospital
New York, New York

Norman H. Bass, MD
Professor of Neurology and Rehabilitation Medicine
University of Pittsburgh
Senior Vice President, Medical Affairs and Chief Medical Officer
Harmarville Rehabilitation Center
Pittsburgh, Pennsylvania

James F. Bosma, MD
Research Professor, Department of Pediatrics and Dentistry for Children
Clinical Professor, Department of Neurology: Rehabilitation
University of Maryland Schools of Medicine and Dentistry
Baltimore, Maryland

Jean E. Curran, MS, RD
Clinical Dietitian and Geriatric Neurology Specialist
Department of Veterans Affairs Medical Center
New York, New York

Olle Ekberg, MD, PhD
Department of Radiology
University of Lund
Malmö General Hospital
Malmö, Sweden

Elizabeth Enderle Gonzalez, MS, CCC
Staff Speech Pathologist
Presbyterian/St. Luke's Medical Center
Denver, Colorado

Susan M. Fleming, PhD
Adjunct, Assistant Professor of Otolaryngology
Wayne State University
Associate Chief, Swallowing and Voice Pathology
Harper Hospital
Detroit, Michigan

Barbara A. Griggs, RN, MA
Manager of Market Development
Corpak/Thermedics, Inc.
Wheeling, Illinois

Michael E. Groher, PhD
Chief of Audiology
Speech Pathology Service
James A. Haley Veterans Hospital
Adjunct Professor
Department of Communication Sciences
University of South Florida
Tampa, Florida

Gregory F. Hulka, MD
Resident, Division of Otolaryngology—Head and Neck Surgery
University of North Carolina Hospitals
Chapel Hill, North Carolina

Robert M. Miller, PhD
Clinical Assistant Professor
Department of Speech and Hearing Sciences Rehabilitation Medicine and
    Otolaryngology—Head and Neck Surgery
University of Washington
Chief, Audiology and Speech Pathology
Seattle Veterans Administration Medical Center
Seattle, Washington

Roger M. Morrell, MD, PhD
Professor of Neurology
Michigan State University
East Lansing, Michigan
Heritage Hospital
Taylor, Michigan

Harold C. Pillsbury, III, MD, PhD
Professor and Chief
Department of Surgery—Division of Otolaryngology—Head and Neck Surgery
University of North Carolina at Chapel Hill School of Medicine
Attending Physician
University of North Carolina Hospitals
Chapel Hill, North Carolina

William J. Ravich, MD
Associate Professor of Medicine
Division of Gastroenterology
The Johns Hopkins School of Medicine
Director, The GI Endoscopy and GI Diagnostic Laboratory Unit
Clinical Director, The Johns Hopkins Swallowing Center
Baltimore, Maryland

Preface

Health care providers agree that good nutrition is a prerequisite for maintaining and improving health and that receiving this nutrition orally is most expedient and psychologically pleasurable. It is surprising then that only in the past decade have we begun in earnest systematically to evaluate and treat patients with swallowing disorders in an effort to provide quality nutritional care. Documentation of these efforts resulted in the first edition of *Dysphagia: Diagnosis and Management*. Since its publication, dysphagia diagnosis and management has become a recognized subspecialty of care. This edition provides the clinician with a review of the explosion of information that has improved the management of patients with dysphagia within the past decade. In an effort to provide the clinician with the immense range of medical disciplines that have contributed to the care of dysphagic patients, additional sections in pediatrics, gastroenterology, and radiology have been included.

Prior to the early 1970s, patients incapable of swallowing were managed by feeding gastrostomy or by nasogastric tube feedings. Return to oral feeding was a primary goal, but attempts to move in this direction were half-hearted, partly from ignorance, partly from lack of time. To complicate matters, no one person had direct responsibility for monitoring patients' feeding and swallowing.

Health care professionals have discovered that active intervention with dysphagic patients, including carefully planned diagnostic evaluations and subsequent management and rehabilitative techniques, often assists a patient's return to normal feeding and swallowing, a result that speeds recovery and enhances the quality of life. Demonstrations of this improvement in care are now documented in the literature.

It is apparent to me that our efforts to provide this care require close cooperation of a professional, multidisciplinary staff, wherein each member possesses particular expertise. It is the combined expertise that links diagnosis and treatment. A diagnosis is established through cooperation between the physician with primary care responsibility and consultants in neurology, radiology, gastroenterology, surgery, and psychiatry. Further evaluation by the nurse and speech/language pathologist is critical to measure the level of function and to follow the rate of improvement during treatment sessions. The dietitian and therapist must join forces to ensure adherence to dietary requirements and appropriateness of food formula and consistency. The speech/language pathologist, physical therapist, and occupational therapist must design and implement a program of rehabilitation tailored to each individual, always in cooperation with the nursing staff, who are responsible for daily management of the patient.

Because dysphagia management involves multiple disciplines, our basic core of knowledge is dispersed among many different journals, making it difficult for the beginning clinician to read about and understand the current state of the art. Since the publication of the first edition of this volume, the emergence of the journal *Dysphagia* has helped to provide both multidisciplinary and international contributions, bridging the gap that previously existed among disciplines concerned with the dysphagic patient. This second edition is an extension of the development of the subspeciality of dysphagia, combining each discipline's perspective toward a common goal and allowing an understanding of how each affects the care of dysphagic patients.

We know that disorders of the swallowing mechanism can result from a broad spectrum of disabilities and that each stage of swallow has potential interactions with another, as facilitators in the normal process and as contributors to disability. These disorders range from minimal difficulty swallowing foods and liquids to inability to swallow without a high risk of aspiration in a patient who may require gastrostoma or a feeding tube for nutritional maintenance. At one extreme the disability is severe, the cause usually clear, and the therapy urgent. At the other are patients with mild-to-moderate dysphagia, no clear diagnosis, but a significant disability that may become life-threatening. This book is written with both groups of patients in mind.

While the focus is the adult population, an additional chapter on pediatric issues has been added in an effort to detail disorders specific to the first years of life. Those working with this population also will benefit from the chapters on diagnosis, evaluation, and program development. Some discussions of management and rehabilitative techniques will not directly apply to newborns and infants, but cetain conceptual frameworks will, e.g., the importance of a thorough physical and laboratory evaluation, and the use of diet modifications to circumvent disability.

Throughout the text, the distinction between neurologic and mechanical disorders of the swallowing mechanism is maintained. This is done for several reasons. Diagnostically, the two categories often are mutually exclusive, and attempts to classify the more subtle disorders should be made with this separation in mind. The distinction is also valid in therapy, since some of the techniques and the level of patient cooperation may differ between those with mechanical disorders and those with neurologic mechanisms of impairment. From the outset, the careful clinician must have the differential diagnosis of dysphagia clearly in mind and must not stop after the first few common disorders have been ruled out. To leave the patient with no diagnosis or to conclude that the origin is psychiatric when persistent investigation would uncover a treatable cause is the pitfall that we hope this resource will help clinicians avoid.

It is my firm conviction that resorting immediately to tube or gastrostomy feedings in cases with dysphagia is a mistake, particularly if the condition has not been adequately diagnosed and other therapeutic measures have not been tried. The limitations and the compromise of quality of life to the patient are unacceptable.

Not all patients will respond to our rehabilitative efforts; however, improved management of their swallowing dysfunction short of total rehabilitation should not be underestimated. The importance of delivering adequate nutrition to hospitalized patients, particularly those who cannot receive nourishment by mouth, should be clear to all who invest their time with this patient group. More rapid wound healing, a briefer hospital stay, less morbidity and mortality, and an improved psychological outlook for the patient are important dividends.

Techniques used in establishing a clear diagnosis followed by the development of creative and realistic treatment protocols require in-depth didactic preparation and clinical exposure. They require a well-trained staff for implementation, cooperation on the part of the patient and family, considerable time and patience, and most important, a team approach.

Michael E. Groher
Tampa, Florida

Dysphagia
Diagnosis and Management
Second Edition

1

The Neurology of Swallowing

Norman H. Bass
Roger M. Morrell

Normal swallowing includes an integrated interdependent group of complex feeding behaviors emerging from interacting cranial nerves of the brain stem and governed by neural regulatory mechanisms in the medulla, as well as in sensorimotor and limbic cortical systems. Such sensory-guided discriminatory feeding and sensory-cued stereotyped swallowing behaviors may be, for purposes of simplification, divided into three stages: (1) the oral stage is the transfer of material from the mouth to the oropharynx; (2) the pharyngeal stage is the highly coordinated transport of material away from the oropharynx, around an occluded laryngeal vestibule, and through a relaxed cricopharyngeus muscle into the upper esophagus; and (3) the esophageal stage is the transport of material along the esophagus into the gastric cardia (Figure 1.1). It is important to remember that the anatomic arrangement mediating the pharyngeal stage of swallowing involves complex behavioral interactions of the hypopharynx and larynx, where neurologic dysfunction can result in life-threatening aspiration (Ardran and Kemp 1951, 1952). Hence, the anatomic and physiologic aspects of this interdependent group of voluntary and involuntary behaviors requires detailed understanding if we are to rehabilitate persons with dysphagia caused by a wide array of neurologic impairments, resulting from injury and/or disease affecting the central nervous system, cranial nerves, and muscles.

The oral cavity extends from the lips anteriorly to the nasopharynx posteriorly and contains the tongue, gums, and teeth (Figure 1.2). The oral cavity is separated from the nasal cavity by the bony palate and muscular palate. It is composed of a highly mobile lower jaw or mandible, consisting of a U-shaped body containing important ridges for muscle attachments. The upper jaw or maxilla meets the zygomatic or cheek bone and is adjoined by the L-shaped palatine bones, lying posterior to the nasal cavity. The perpendicular part of the palatines forms the back of the nasal cavity, whereas the horizontal part forms the back of the bony palate. The muscular palate and posterior nasopharyngeal wall seal and open communication between the nasal and oral cavities during swallowing and respiratory behaviors, respectively. The nasopharynx lies above the muscular palate, and the oropharynx lies posterior to the mouth. The pharynx extends below to the esophagus; its inferior portion is called the hypopharynx

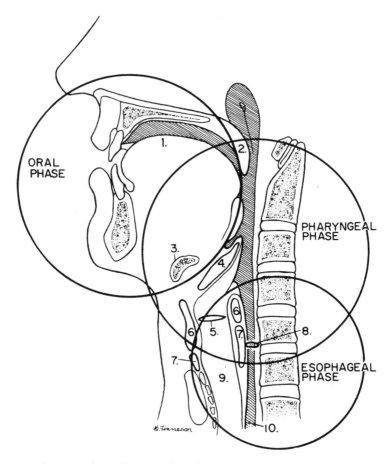

Figure 1.1 The normal swallow involves three separate stages that are interdependent and highly coordinated: (1) tongue, (2) soft palate, (3) hyoid bone, (4) epiglottis, (5) vocal folds, (6) thyroid cartilage, (7) cricoid cartilage, (8) pharyngoesophageal sphincter, (9) trachea, and (10) esophagus. (Reprinted by permission of the publisher and the author, from Schultz et al., 1979.)

and is separated from the esophagus by the cricopharyngeus muscle. The cartilaginous larynx lies anterior to the hypopharynx at the upper end of the trachea, suspended by muscles attached to the hyoid bone (Brown 1971). The cricoid cartilage lies above the trachea, with the thyroid cartilage above it. Both are suspended from muscles attached to the hyoid bone, which in itself is suspended between the jaw, tongue, and sternum by suprahyoid and infrahyoid musculature. The respiratory system is protected during pharyngeal swallow by occlusive muscular constriction of the vestibule and downward displacement of the epiglottis. The true vocal cords are at the inferior margin of the laryngeal ventricle and are attached anteriorly at the thyroid cartilage and posteriorly at the aryte-

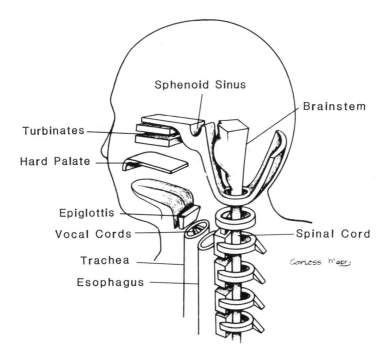

Figure 1.2 Relationship between bony and muscular structures associated with normal swallowing.

noid cartilages. The false vocal folds separate the ventricle and vestibule. The epiglottis extends from the base of the tongue into the pharyngeal cavity.

The valleculae are lateral recesses at the base of the tongue on each side of the epiglottis (Figure 1.3). The piriform sinuses are lateral recesses between the larynx and the anterior hypopharyngeal wall. These recesses serve as important anatomic landmarks in videoradiographic assessment of pharyngeal swallow.

MUSCULOSKELETAL ACTIONS

Oral Stage

The mandibular branch of the trigeminal nerve (cranial nerve V) innervates the principal muscles for chewing behaviors. The primary muscles of chewing are the masseters, temporalis, and pterygoid muscles, which attach to the sphenoid wing of the temporal bone (Table 1.1). The masseter closes the jaw while the temporalis moves it up, forward, or backward. The medial pterygoid muscles work bilaterally to elevate the mandible while unilaterally they shift the jaw to the opposite side. The lateral pterygoid muscles work together, pulling down or

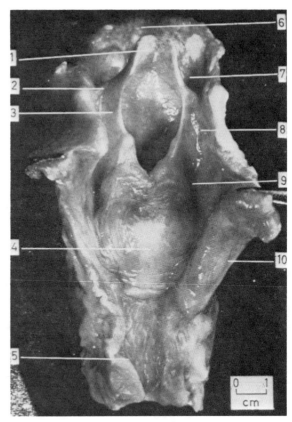

Figure 1.3 The vallecular (7) and piriform spaces (8, 9) are potential sites for abnormal retention of food and liquid. Note their relationship to other laryngeal structures: (1) epiglottis; (2) pharyngoepiglottic fold; (3) aryepiglottic fold; (4) postcricoid region; (5) cervical esophagus; (6) base of tongue; (10) posterolateral pharyngeal wall. (Reprinted by permission of the publisher, from Ballantyne and Groves, 1971.)

forward while unilaterally moving the jaw or chin to the opposite side. Both sets of pterygoid muscles cooperate to grind in mastication.

The facial nerve (cranial nerve VII) innervates lower facial muscles attached to the maxillae and mandible of the skull (Table 1.2). These include the buccinator muscles, which compress the lips and flatten the cheeks in the movement of food across the teeth. The buccinator fibers blend with those of the orbicularis oris—the sphincter of the lips.

The hypoglossal nerve (cranial nerve XII) innervates the tongue, which contains four separate intrinsic muscle masses that have different effects on the shape, contour, and function of the tongue.

Pharyngeal Stage

The pharyngeal cavity of the neck, which is suspended from the base of the skull and anchored to the top of the sternum, is formed by 26 pairs of striated muscles innervated by six cranial and four cervical nerves. The horseshoe-

Table 1.1 Muscles of Mastication

Muscle	Origin	Insertion	Nerve	Action
Temporalis	Temporal fossa of skull	Ramus and coronoid process of mandible	Trigeminal	Elevates or closes mandible, retracts mandible
Masseter	Zygomatic arch	Ramus of mandible	Trigeminal	Elevates or closes mandible
Medial pterygoid	Palatine bone, lateral pterygoid plate, tuberosity of maxilla	Ramus of mandible	Trigeminal	Elevates or closes mandible
Lateral pterygoid	Great wing of sphenoid and lateral pterygoid plate	Neck of condyle of mandible	Trigeminal	Depressor or opener of mandible, protrudes mandible, permits side-to-side movement of mandible

shaped hyoid bone in the neck serves as a bony fulcrum that provides a mechanical advantage for pharyngeal musculature associated with swallowing behaviors of the posterior tongue, pharynx, and larynx.

In the nasopharynx, five muscles related to the muscular palate adjust its position with respect to the food bolus (Table 1.3). These are the palatoglossal and levator veli palatini muscles (pharyngeal plexus and accessory nerve), which elevate the soft palate and seal the nasopharynx, and the tensor veli palatini (mandibular branch of the trigeminal nerve), which tenses the palate and dilates the orifice of the eustachian tube. The palatopharyngeus muscle (pharyngeal plexus and spinal accessory nerve) depresses the soft palate, approximates the palate or pharyngeal folds, and constricts the pharynx. The muscularis uvula (spinal accessory nerve) shortens the soft palate.

The hypoglossal (cranial nerve XII), trigeminal (V), and facial (VII) nerves innervate the suprahyoid group of muscles (Table 1.4). The hypoglossal nerve supplies the geniohyoid, which draws the hyoid bone up and forward, depressing the jaw, and the trigeminal nerve supplies the mylohyoid, which elevates the hyoid bone and tongue and depresses the jaw. The digastric muscles contain anterior and posterior bellies. The anterior belly is innervated by the mandibular branch

Table 1.2 Muscles of the Face

Muscle	Origin	Insertion	Nerve	Action
Orbicularis oris	Neighboring muscles, mostly buccinator; has many layers of tissue around the lips	Skin around lips and angles of the mouth	Facial	Closes, opens, protrudes, inverts, and twists lips
Zygomaticus minor	Zygomatic bone	Orbicularis oris in upper lip	Facial	Draws upper lip upward and outward
Levator labii superioris	Below infraorbital foramen in maxilla	Orbicularis oris in upper lip	Facial	Pulls up or elevates upper lip
Levator labii superioris alaeque nasi	Process of maxilla	Skin at mouth angle, orbicularis oris	Facial	Raises angle of the mouth
Zygomaticus major	Zygomatic bone	Fibers of the orbicularis oris, angle of the mouth	Facial	Draws upper lip upward, draws angle of mouth upward and backward; the smiling muscle
Levator anguli oris (caninus)	Canine fossa of maxilla	Lower lip near angle of the mouth	Facial	Pulls down corners of mouth
Depressor anguli oris	Outer surface and above lower border of mandible	Skin of cheek, corner of mouth, lower border of mandible	Facial	Draws lower lip down, draws angle of mouth down and inward
Depressor labii inferioris	Lower border of the mandible	Skin of lower lip, orbicularis oris	Facial	Depresses lower lip
Mentalis	Incisor fossa of mandible	Skin of chin	Facial	Pushes up lower lip, raises chin

Table 1.2 Muscles of the Face *(continued)*

Muscle	Origin	Insertion	Nerve	Action
Risorius	Platysma, fascia over the masseter skin	Angle of mouth, orbicularis oris	Facial	Draws corners or angle of mouth outward, causes dimples, gives expression of strain to face
Buccinator	Alveolar process of maxilla, buccinator ridge of mandible	Angle of mouth, orbicularis oris	Facial	Flattens cheek, holds food in contact with teeth, retracts angles of the mouth.

Table 1.3 Muscles of the Palate

Muscle	Origin	Insertion	Nerve	Action
Levator veli palatini	Apex of temporal bone	Palatine aponeurosis of soft palate	Vagus and accessory	Raises soft palate
Tensor veli palatini	Fossa of sphenoid bone	Palatine aponeurosis of soft palate	Trigeminal	Stretches soft palate
Palatoglossus	Undersurface of soft palate	Side of tongue	Vagus and accessory	Raises back of tongue during the first stage of swallowing
Palatopharyngeus	Soft palate	Pharyngeal wall	Vagus and accessory	Shuts off nasopharynx during second stage of swallowing
Uvular	Posterior nasal spine and palatine aponeurosis	Into uvula to form its chief bulk or content	Vagus and accessory	Shortens and raises uvula

Table 1.4 Suprahyoid Muscles

Muscle	Origin	Insertion	Nerve	Action
Mylohyoid (anterior belly digastric)	Inner surface of mandible	Upper border of hyoid bone	Trigeminal	Elevates tongue and floor of mouth, depresses jaw when hyoid bone is in fixed position
Digastric (anterior belly)	Intermediate tendon by loop of fascia to hyoid bone	Lower border of mandible	Trigeminal	Raises hyoid bone if jaw is in fixed position, depresses jaw if hyoid bone is in fixed position
Geniohyoid	Mental spine of mandible	Hyoid bone	Cervical (C1 and C2) through hypoglossal	Draws hyoid bone forward, depresses mandible when hyoid bone is in fixed position
Stylohyoid	Styloid process of temporal bone	Body of hyoid at greater cornu	Facial	Elevates hyoid and tongue base
Hyoglossus	Greater cornu of hyoid	Into tongue sides	Hypoglossal	Tongue depression
Genioglossus	Upper genial tubercle of mandible	Hyoid, inferior tongue, and tip	Hypoglossal	Protrusion and depression
Styloglossus	Anterior border of styloid process	Into side of tongue	Hypoglossal	Elevates up and back
Palatoglossus	Anterior surface of soft palate	Dorsum and side of tongue	Glossopharyngeal, vagus, and accessory	Narrows fauces and elevates posterior tongue

Table 1.5   Muscles of the Pharynx

Muscle	Origin	Insertion	Nerve	Action
Palatopha-ryngeus	Extends from soft palate to pharyngeal wall	Posterior border of thyroid cartilage and pharyngeal aponeurosis	Pharyngeal plexus and accessory	Narrows oropharynx, elevates pharynx, shuts off nasopharynx
Stylopharyngeus	Medial side of root of styloid process	Superior and inferior borders of thyroid cartilage	Glossopharyngeal	Raises and dilates pharynx
Salpingo-pharyngeus	Pharyngeal end of auditory tube	Blends with palatopharyngeus	Pharyngeal plexus and accessory	Raises nasopharynx, draws lateral pharyngeal walls up.

of the trigeminal nerve and depresses the jaw or raises the hyoid, whereas the posterior portion is innervated by the facial nerve (VII) and elevates or retracts the hyoid. The hypoglossal nerve (XII) innervates the stylohyoid muscle, which elevates the hyoid bone during swallowing. In addition, the hyoglossus and the genioglossus serve as laryngeal elevators, as well as extrinsic tongue muscles, and are designed to depress the tongue or help to elevate the hyoid bone when the tongue is fixed. The accessory nerve (cranial nerve XI), in association with the hypoglossal (XII) nerve, innervates the styloglossus, which draws the tongue up and back during swallowing, and in association with the palatoglossus, raises the back of the tongue and lowers the sides of the soft palate.

The vagus nerve (cranial nerve X) and the spinal accessory nerve (XI) innervate the muscular pharynx, whose superior, middle, and inferior constrictor muscles constitute its external circular layer and work together to strip a bolus of food toward the esophagus during swallowing. Three other muscles constitute the internal longitudinal layer of the pharynx: the palatopharyngeus, stylopharyngeus, and salpingopharyngeus. The stylopharyngeus (glossopharyngeal nerve) elevates the pharynx and to some extent the larynx during swallowing, while the salpingopharyngeus (accessory nerve and pharyngeal plexus) draws the lateral walls of the pharynx up (Table 1.5).

The cricopharyngeus muscle is an important single muscle that lies at the transition level between pharynx and esophagus. Functionally, it is separate from both the pharynx and esophagus and acts as a sphincter, relaxing during passage of the bolus from the pharynx into the esophagus. It has been shown to be innervated by both pharyngeal branches of the vagus and sympathetic fibers from the middle and inferior cervical ganglia.

BEHAVIORAL SEQUENCE OF NORMAL SWALLOWING

Healthy persons simultaneously perform many acts involving the sequential steps of chewing and swallowing that depend on highly intricate coordination. Thus, a single bolus of varying texture and size can be chewed and swallowed while the person carries on a conversation, and at the same time a beverage may be imbibed while one holds various portions of the more solid food in the mouth. With relaxation, a sword can be passed from the pharynx through the crico-pharyngeus, and with effort, one can swallow solids while standing on one's head.

Food introduced into the mouth cannot be prepared for swallowing by being formed into a bolus unless it is mixed with saliva contributed from three pairs of salivary glands. The parotid gland receives parasympathetic nerve supply by way of the glossopharyngeal nerve from the inferior salivary nucleus, located in the lower brain stem. The submandibular and sublingual glands are innervated by parasympathetic fibers of the facial nerve. Each gland has single or multiple excretory ducts opening into the mouth.

The usual conditions associated with normal swallowing are a moist cavity, open nostrils, and a closed mouth. The steps involved are illustrated in Figure 1.4. As a bolus is masticated, the tongue tip is elevated to occlude the anterior oral cavity at the alveolar ridge, and the bolus is compressed against the hard palate. This is a preparatory position in which the posterior portion of the tongue has maneuvered the bolus into position. As pharyngeal swallowing begins, the anterior portion of the tongue is retracted and depressed, mastication then ceases, and respiration is inhibited. Retraction of the tongue and elevation against the hard palate force the bolus into the upper part of the pharynx. The palatopha-ryngeal folds are pulled medially to form a slit through which properly masticated food can pass. The levator and tensor veli palatini muscles help to elevate the soft palate and block the nasopharyngeal opening. The tongue moves posteriorly to drive the bolus into the pharynx while the entire larynx is pulled upward and forward. This action causes the epiglottis at the back of the tongue to depress and protect the airway. Food is directed to either side of the epiglottis. Further airway protection is provided when respiration has ceased, allowing the apposed vocal cords to close off the trachea (Doty and Bosma 1956; Donner et al. 1985). In preparation for propulsion of food toward the esophagus, the cricopharyngeus relaxes and the bolus is propelled into the esophagus. In the esophagus, the bolus is carried toward the stomach by gravity and peristalsis.

The following five sequential steps of pharyngeal swallow are outlined in Figure 1.5: (1) tongue movements that initiate the act of swallowing require concomitant contraction of mylohyoid, geniohyoid, and digastric muscles in the floor of the mouth; (2) the styloglossus and hyoglossus muscles force the root of the tongue against the soft palate and posterior pharyngeal wall; (3) the levator and tensor veli palatini muscles elevate the muscular palate, with addi-

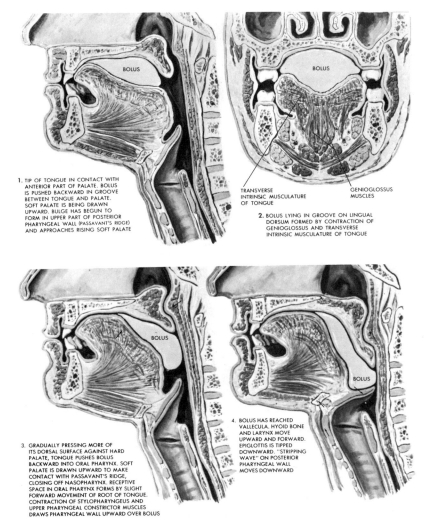

Figure 1.4 Sequential presentation of the steps involved in the normal swallow. © Copyright 1959, CIBA Pharmaceutical Company, Division of CIBA-GEIGY Corporation. Reprinted with permission, from THE CIBA COLLECTION OF MEDICAL ILLUSTRATIONS, illustrated by Frank H. Netter, M.D. All rights reserved.

tional shortening and dorsal thickening, until approximation against the posterior pharyngeal muscle prevents nasopharyngeal regurgitation; (4) the middle and inferior pharyngeal constrictor muscles narrow the hypopharynx and contribute to the peristaltic movements involving the posterior pharyngeal wall, which generally are located between the level of Passavant's cushion and the

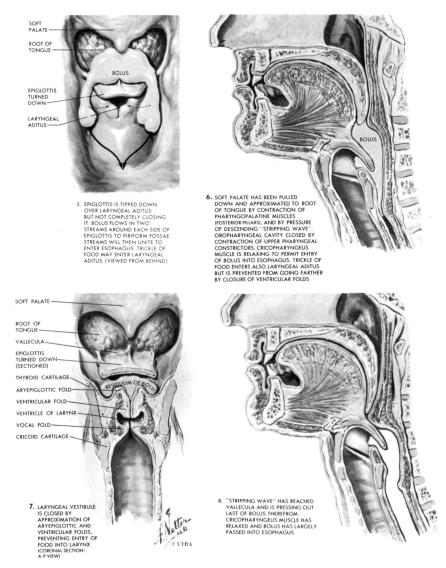

SOFT
PALATE

ROOT OF
TONGUE

BOLUS

EPIGLOTTIS
TURNED
DOWN

LARYNGEAL
ADITUS

5. EPIGLOTTIS IS TIPPED DOWN
OVER LARYNGEAL ADITUS
BUT NOT COMPLETELY CLOSING
IT. BOLUS FLOWS IN TWO
STREAMS AROUND EACH SIDE OF
EPIGLOTTIS TO PIRIFORM FOSSAE
STREAMS WILL THEN UNITE TO
ENTER ESOPHAGUS. TRICKLE OF
FOOD MAY ENTER LARYNGEAL
ADITUS (VIEWED FROM BEHIND)

6. SOFT PALATE HAS BEEN PULLED
DOWN AND APPROXIMATED TO ROOT
OF TONGUE BY CONTRACTION OF
PHARYNGOPALATINE MUSCLES
(POSTERIOR PILLARS), AND BY PRESSURE
OF DESCENDING "STRIPPING WAVE".
OROPHARYNGEAL CAVITY CLOSED BY
CONTRACTION OF UPPER PHARYNGEAL
CONSTRICTORS. CRICOPHARYNGEUS
MUSCLE IS RELAXING TO PERMIT ENTRY
OF BOLUS INTO ESOPHAGUS. TRICKLE OF
FOOD ENTERS ALSO LARYNGEAL ADITUS
BUT IS PREVENTED FROM GOING FARTHER
BY CLOSURE OF VENTRICULAR FOLDS

BOLUS

SOFT PALATE

ROOT OF
TONGUE

VALLECULA

EPIGLOTTIS
TURNED DOWN
(SECTIONED)

THYROID CARTILAGE

ARYEPIGLOTTIC FOLD

VENTRICULAR FOLD

VENTRICLE OF LARYNX

VOCAL FOLD

CRICOID CARTILAGE

RESIDUUM OF BOLUS

7. LARYNGEAL VESTIBULE
IS CLOSED BY
APPROXIMATION OF
ARYEPIGLOTTIC AND
VENTRICULAR FOLDS,
PREVENTING ENTRY OF
FOOD INTO LARYNX
(CORONAL SECTION:
A-P VIEW)

8. "STRIPPING WAVE" HAS REACHED
VALLECULA AND IS PRESSING OUT
LAST OF BOLUS THEREFROM.
CRICOPHARYNGEUS MUSCLE HAS
RELAXED AND BOLUS HAS LARGELY
PASSED INTO ESOPHAGUS

Figure 1.4 *(continued)*

cricopharyngeal sphincter; and (5) dorsal and downward tilting of the epiglottis is brought about by the muscular elevation of the larynx and contraction of the floor of the mouth, with concomitant elevation and posterior movement of the hyoid bone (Donner and Siegel 1965).

The food bolus is prevented from passing through the laryngeal vestibule by contraction of intrinsic laryngeal muscles that shorten and widen the aryepiglottic folds and vocal and vestibular folds, producing an airtight soft stopper

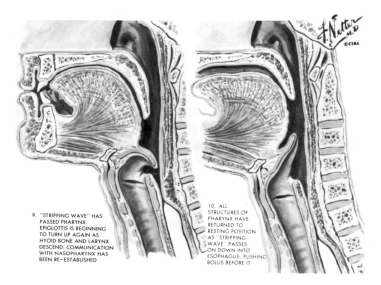

9. "STRIPPING WAVE" HAS PASSED PHARYNX. EPIGLOTTIS IS BEGINNING TO TURN UP AGAIN AS HYOID BONE AND LARYNX DESCEND. COMMUNICATION WITH NASOPHARYNX HAS BEEN RE–ESTABLISHED

10. ALL STRUCTURES OF PHARYNX HAVE RETURNED TO RESTING POSITION AS "STRIPPING WAVE" PASSES ON DOWN INTO ESOPHAGUS, PUSHING BOLUS BEFORE IT

Figure 1.4 *(continued)*

for the subglottic region. The laryngeal ventricles probably are obliterated at this point, while the epiglottis moves downward and backward as a result of approximation of the thyroid cartilage to the hyoid bone. Epiglottic depression does not completely close the laryngeal aditus, which results in the insertion of small particles of the bolus into that opening for a short distance.

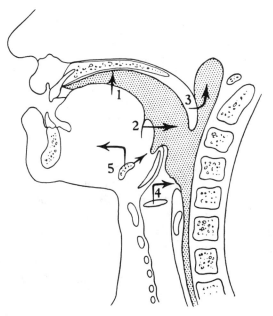

Figure 1.5 Summary of the five important physiologic events involved in the normal swallow. (Reprinted by permission of the publisher from Donner, *American Journal of Roentgenology,* vol. 94, © 1965.)

A liquid bolus is usually split by the epiglottis, traveling on each side of the larynx through the piriform recesses to rejoin behind the cricoid cartilage (see Figure 1.3). The epiglottis acts as a ledge, checking the descent of the bolus and obviating early closure of the larynx. Protection of the larynx during swallowing is effected by closure of the vocal folds and contraction of the sphincteric girdle of muscle that surrounds the laryngeal vestibule. This occurs without elevation of the larynx. The larynx may be closed at any stage during swallowing, but is always closed when the last of the bolus leaves the pharynx, at which point material entering the vestibule of the larynx is squeezed out. The hood formed by the epiglottis bending downward over the entrance to the larynx prevents the deposition of bolus residue, and negative pharyngeal pressure associated with reinflation of the airway carries any residue upward, trapping it in the valleculae.

Esophageal tasks require an ordered pattern of function that depends on coordinated activities in three distinct zones: esophageal inlet, esophageal outlet, and body of the esophagus. The inlet consists of visceral striated muscle that maintains the lumen in a closed position and is integrated with the tongue and hypopharynx. In the esophageal outlet, the lumen is closed by specialized muscle that is distinguished from the body of the esophagus and separates it from the stomach. Swallowing initiates a moving contraction that is ring-like and sweeps rapidly through the upper striated portion and less rapidly through the lower smooth muscle portion (Dodds 1976; Castell 1980).

FUNCTIONAL ASSESSMENT OF NEUROGENIC DYSPHAGIA

Patients with neurogenic dysphagia involving the oral stage of feeding may present with complaints of oral spill at the lips (drooling), difficulty chewing, and difficulty in initiating swallow. Patients may complain of excess saliva volume, when actually its volume is normal or diminished. Bolus preparation may be impaired by deficient salivations, and patients may also report having a dry mouth, with the implication of deficiency of saliva or increase in its viscosity. Some of these persons have diminution in neurosecretory function, which can be demonstrated by quantitative assessment of salivary secretions, with and without pharmacologic stimulation. If muscles of lingual manipulation are weak or excessively fatigable, patients may report arduous efforts with the bolus in the oral cavity, or often mistakenly complain of poorly fitting dentures and pay numerous visits to the dentist. Patients may restrict their diet to pureed food or may be noted to be exerting excessive effort at vigorous chewing in order to conform with the time constraints implicit in social dining. Frequent small meals associated with avoidance of certain foods that cannot readily be particulated for pharyngeal swallowing may make feeding easier, but may fail to maintain daily nutritional requirements. Although weight loss is common, it is not always found with dysphagia, based on the fact that some patients consume excessive quantities of high-calorie swallow-ready foods, such as ice cream.

Family, friends, or care persons may observe voluntary compensation measures for oral dysphagia. These may include craniocervical flexion, followed by slow extension of the neck to control the transfer of the food bolus at the junction of the mouth and pharynx. Occasionally, patients may use fingers to push the food bolus toward the pharynx. They also use fingers to place the bolus on the molar teeth when muscles of the tongue are weakened and exhibit vertical as opposed to rotary chewing. Some patients prefer to drink liquids through a straw, thereby using suckle feeding to overcome impairments associated with the oral stage of dysphagia. However, such compensation measures may become inadequate with increasing nuclear or supranuclear weakness of the facial nerve, which may result in difficulty with straw feeding, as well as in drooling and loss of food out of the mouth, as a result of impaired lip closure. Patients with abnormal face and tongue performance may report retention of food in the buccal area, referred to clinically as "squirreling" behavior. Finally, we must mention those neurologic patients with cognitive dysfunction who simply do not know what to do with the food placed in front of them, or even with food placed in their mouth. In such cases, patients are unlikely to report symptoms of dysphagia, and care givers must be relied on to provide pertinent feeding history. Milder forms of cognitive dysfunction may lead to improper bolus sizing and inappropriate speaking and/or breathing during feeding.

Neurogenic dysphagia involving the pharyngeal stage of swallowing can be more hazardous if the swallow fails to empty the pharynx of the bolus, with or without subsequent bolus penetration into the larynx. Fortunately, in many patients with this disability, there is effective physiologic compensation for pharyngeal dysphagia. This compensation may mask the clinical abnormality so that it can be detected only by videoradiography. Repeat swallowing may be used to clear retained material in the pharyngeal recesses. Tilting the head forward or to the side may facilitate swallowing, and some patients discover that manual pressure against one side of the neck helps them to swallow, particularly in the case of asymmetric pharyngeal weakness. However, even after careful history taking in patients with neurogenic pharyngeal dysphagia, the clinician may fail to identify patients who have adapted their feeding style to neuromuscular compensations within the pharynx. In such cases, it will be the radiologist who informs the clinician that a patient has neurogenic dysphagia that requires further neurologic evaluation (Robbins et al. 1987). Why should the clinician be concerned about patients with compensated neurogenic dysphagia (Buchholz et al. 1985)? The information is more than academic, for decompensation may occur abruptly. For example, patients who have compensated neurogenic dysphagia, who then suffer a second lesion on the contralateral side, as in stroke or metastatic tumor, or progression of their neurologic lesions, as in amyotrophic lateral sclerosis, may become acutely symptomatic and at risk for bronchopulmonary complications.

Symptoms of decompensation from neurogenic pharyngeal dysphagia are alarming to both patient and clinician. The passage of solids through the pharynx may be delayed, with retention of the food bolus in the pharyngeal recesses and subsequent leakage into the laryngeal vestibule, which may lead to frequent throat clearing and a wet-sounding voice (Curtis and Crain 1987). Nasal regurgitation of liquids may be noted, especially in compromising positions such as bending over to drink from a water fountain. The liquids may be retained in the pharynx or aspirated, resulting in coughing or choking episodes, laryngospasm, or pneumonia. Like ingested liquids, oral and pharyngeal secretions are retained in the valleculae and piriform recesses (Curtis 1986; Curtis et al. 1989). Patients sense an accumulation of phlegm or mucus, as if there were an overproduction of secretions, although the real problem is a swallowing impairment. Laryngeal penetration may cause coughing, choking, stridor, and pneumonia. Sensory impairment of the larynx and airways may result in a life-threatening situation in which airway penetration occurs without respiratory response, leading to recurrent pneumonia (Kaplan 1960). Symptoms of retained secretions during sleep include drooling onto the pillow and awakening with choking. Persons known to have compensated neurogenic dysphagia who show changes in feeding habits or difficulty handling secretions during sleep should be seriously considered for reexamination by videofluoroscopy. In addition, such perosns should have endoscopic evaluation to observe intrinsic motor disorders of the larynx, pharynx, or esophagus, such as vocal fold paresis, transverse shift (curtain movement) of the pharyngeal constrictor wall, and structural deficits such as a web, inflammation, or neoplasm of the esophagus. Such structural abnormalities of the lower pharynx or esophagus can become quite extensive without clinical symptoms and can secondarily complicate the course of neurogenic dysphagia. (See Chapter 6 for discussion of the clinical evaluation.)

STEREOTYPED PHARYNGEAL SWALLOW BEHAVIORS: MEDULLA OF THE BRAIN STEM

Pharyngeal swallow is initiated by sensory impulses transmitted as a result of stimulation of receptors on the fauces, tonsils, soft palate, base of the tongue, and posterior pharyngeal wall. These sensory impulses reach the medulla primarily through the seventh, ninth, and tenth cranial nerves, while the efferent function is mediated through the ninth, tenth, and twelfth cranial nerves (see Table 1.6, Table 1.7, and Figure 1.6). Cricopharyngeal sphincter relaxation occurs at the time when the bolus reaches the posterior pharyngeal wall prior to reaching this sphincter (Schultz et al. 1979; Palmer 1976). There is some controversy over the origin of the cricopharyngeal resting tone, which may not rely solely on the sympathetic nervous system, but may be more heavily dependent on vagal input, both for contraction and relaxation. Reference is made in the literature to a swallowing center in the medulla at the level of the obex of the

Table 1.6 Afferent Controls Involved in Swallowing

Sensory Function	Innervation
General sensation, anterior two-thirds of tongue	Lingual nerve, trigeminal (V)
Taste, anterior two-thirds tongue	Chorda tympani, facial (VII)
Taste and general sensation, posterior one-third of the tongue	Glossopharyngeal (IX)
Mucosa of valleculae	Internal branch of SLN (vagus)
Primary afferent	
Secondary afferent	Glossopharyngeal (IX)
Tonsils, pharynx, soft palate	Pharyngeal branch of vagus (X)
Pharynx, larynx, viscera	Glossopharyngeal (IX) Vagus (X)

fourth ventricle (Figure 1.7.). This is probably an oversimplification. Based on presently available evidence, it is more likely that modulation of oral and pharyngeal swallowing and its voluntary and involuntary behaviors receive major contributions from neural activity in supramedullary structures, of pons, mesencephalon, cerebral cortex, and limbic cortical systems.

The brain stem coordinates efferent impulse flow by way of the trigeminal, vagus, and hypoglossal cranial nerves to the muscles of the oropharynx by way of the tenth cranial nerve to the muscles of the hypopharynx by way of the fifth and twelfth cranial nerves to the extrinsic muscles of the larynx, and by way of the tenth cranial nerve to the intrinsic muscles of the larynx and esophagus. The cervical esophagus may receive two vagal efferent supplies from nerves within the neck: one from the recurrent laryngeal and another from the pharyngoesophageal nerve that rises proximal to the nodose ganglion, or from an esophageal branch of the superior laryngeal nerve (SLN). Such double innervation of the cervical esophagus in humans has not been proved, but might provide a margin of safety to prevent esophageal distension and reflux.

Table 1.7 Efferent Controls Involved in Swallowing

Efferent/Stage	Innervation
Oral	
Masticatory, buccinator, floor of mouth	Trigeminal (V)
Lip sphincter	Facial (VII)
Tongue	Hypoglossal (XII)
Pharyngeal	
Constrictors and stylopharyngeus	Glossopharyngeal (IX)
Palate, pharynx, larynx	Vagus (X)
Tongue	Hypoglossal (XIII)
Esophageal	
Esophagus	Vagus (X)

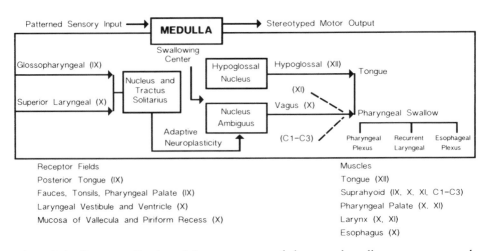

Figure 1.6 Conceptualization of the components of pharyngeal swallow as sensory-cued, stereotyped behaviors.

Sequentially timed discharges from the medulla result in movement of a bolus through successive levels of the esophageal musculature. Esophageal smooth muscle contractions have a sequential behavior by which proximal activity inhibits the next most distal portion of the esophagus successively (Sanchez et al. 1953; Donner 1974; Ekberg and Nylander, 1982). Esophageal distention is signaled on visceral afferent nerves passing in the upper five or six thoracic sympathetic roots, presumably to the thalamus and inferior postcentral gyrus, where they may give rise to symptoms described as pressure, burning, gas, aching, and the like. When such symptoms are described as pain, the referral patterns are based on sensory impulses from tissues innervated by somatic nerves that cross the corresponding spinal levels.

Fibers originating in the nucleus ambiguus innervate the pharyngeal, laryngeal, and upper esophageal striated muscles. It also innervates the heart, lungs, and gastrointestinal tract smooth muscle (Rontal and Rontal 1977). It carries afferents for taste, pharyngeal sensation, and sensation from some regions of skin around the external ear. Rootlets emerging from the medulla form the peripheral vagus, which exits the skull through the jugular foramen. Above the nodose ganglion, the vagus nerve sends branches to the pharyngeal plexus, which supplies the mucosa and musculature of the pharynx, larynx, and upper esophagus.

The very important branch of the vagus, the superior laryngeal (SLN) is sensory to the laryngeal mucosa and motor to the cricothyroid muscle. The vagus terminates as the recurrent laryngeal nerve that loops around the aorta and returns to the larynx and hypopharynx (see Figure 1.8). The recurrent laryngeal nerve supplies muscles intrinsic to the larynx and is thought not to supply the

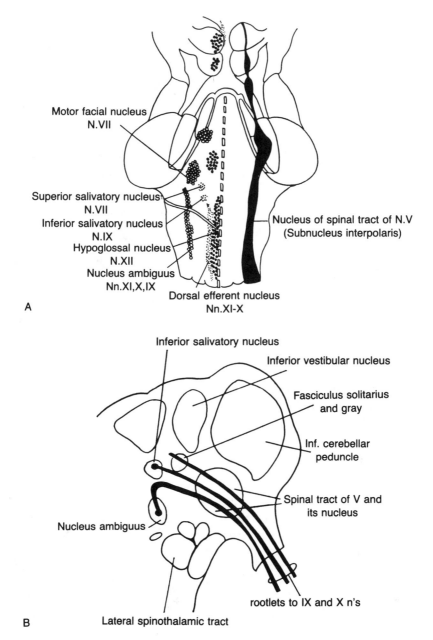

Figure 1.7 (A) Longitudinal section through the medulla showing relationships of the vagus nerve to the surrounding structures (after Crosby). (B) Cross-section at the level of the medulla showing relationship of the vagus nerve to the surrounding structures (after Crosby). (Reprinted by permission of the publisher, from Rontal and Rontal. *Laryngoscope,* vol. 87, no. 1, January 1977.)

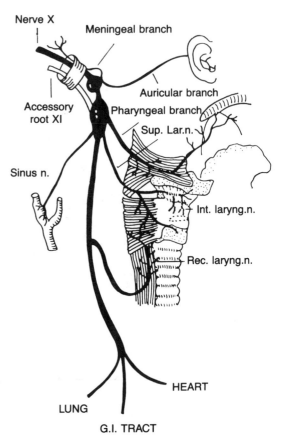

Nerve X

Meningeal branch

Auricular branch

Accessory
root XI

Pharyngeal branch

Sup. Lar.n.

Sinus n.

Int. laryng.n.

Rec. laryng.n.

HEART

LUNG

G.I. TRACT

Figure 1.8 Course of the peripheral vagus nerve on exit from the jugular foramen. Reprinted by permission of the publisher, from Rontal and Rontal, *Laryngoscope,* vol. 87, no. 1, January 1977.

cricopharyngeus, which apparently derives its innervation from the pharyngeal plexus.

The neural control systems that subserve pharyngeal swallow are initiated by the action of cranial nerve afferents, but isolated central activation is not possible even though voluntary components exist. It appears that afferent impulses competent to initiate swallowing must conform to highly codified stimulus patterns that enter the nucleus solitarious of the brain stem by way of its fasciculus and are relayed into the reticular formation where connections exist to motoneurons lying in the nuclei of the fifth, seventh, and twelfth cranial nerves and the nucleus ambiguus. These neurons are interesting in that they lack recurrent collaterals or monosynaptic connections with cranial nerve efferents.

The motoneurons of interest in the neuroregulation of the pharyngeal swallow and speech include the salivatory nuclei on either side of the genu of the seventh cranial nerve and the dorsal motor nucleus of the vagus, which may innervate the esophageal smooth muscle in humans. Experiments to date show that sectioning of the tenth cranial nerve distal to the recurrent laryngeal branch produces degeneration in the nucleus ambiguus as well as in the dorsal motor nucleus. Many neurons in the nucleus of the twelfth cranial nerve participate in swallowing and speech. Histologic studies in patients with bulbar poliomyelitis revealed loss of neurons in rostral nucleus ambiguus in those who had pharyngeal dysphagia, whereas those with laryngeal dysarthria were found to have cell loss in the caudal portions (Baker et al. 1950; Bosma 1976). These effects would be explained by representation of palatopharyngeal and esophageal musculature in the rostral magnocellular part of the nucleus. Comparative studies have revealed great adaptability of human palatopharyngeal and laryngeal musculature, reflecting progressive evolutionary refinement of the controlling interneuronal network.

The neuroregulatory brain stem mechanisms for pharyngeal swallow exist within the medullary reticular formation, 1.5 mm from the midline on either side of the obex of the fourth ventricle (Figure 1.7). On each side of the midline a site exists that communicates with the opposite side through cross-connections running behind the obex. As a result, bilateral symmetry of pharyngeal swallow is achieved. Each half-center exerts ipsilateral inhibition on appropriate motoneurons, although excitatory action may also be strictly ipsilateral, with the exception of excitation to the lower constrictor muscles, which are strictly contralateral.

Pharyngeal swallow involves a sequence of excitation and inhibition produced by several motoneuronal pools on each side of the brain stem (Baker et al. 1950). Through chronologic synergy that can be reproduced electrically by stimulation of the internal branch of the SLN, the esophageal and gastroesophageal components follow. From an electrophysiologic standpoint, pharyngeal swallow is probably the most complex behavioral pattern that can be evoked by electrical stimulation of a sensory branch of a cranial nerve. Since pharyngeal swallow occurs in humans, who congenitally have no brain tissue rostral to the mesencephalon (anencephaly), and in experimental animals, whose brain is intact, at least caudally from the motor nucleus of the tenth cranial nerve, its control appears not to depend unequivocally on cerebral structures or on the cerebellum (Bosma 1963). It appears also that some form of bolus is necessary to sustain repetitive swallowing, a fact that highlights the importance of peripheral afferent stimuli.

Experimental unilateral destruction of the medulla eliminates swallowing in the ipsilateral musculature, except for the crossed constrictor pathway previously described. The responsiveness of the contralateral side to afferent input for the side of the lesion is still normal, however. For example, destruction of the left lateral medulla does not prevent right-sided swallowing if the left SLN is stimulated. This has immediate clinical relevance, especially in the case of unilateral destructive lesions to the brain stem (Doty et al. 1967). As previously outlined, voluntary efforts in the absence of reflex initiation from peripheral stimuli will not result in swallowing. The peripheral stimuli include water, light touch, and chemical stimulation. If we were to seek a principal point from which swallowing is most likely to be initiated, it would normally lie in the palatal area innervated by the maxillary branch of the fifth cranial nerve, although this may vary among species. For example, in cat and dog the principal effective area is the upper pharynx, innervated by the ninth cranial nerve.

The neural organization of swallowing has been largely elucidated by recording the electrical activity of involved muscles, beginning with onset of contraction in the mylohyoid and including concurrent activity in muscles innervated by the fifth cranial nerve and those of the posterior tongue, superior constrictor, palatopharyngeus, palatoglossus, stylohyoid, and geniohyoid. These initiators constitute what has been called the leading complex (Doty and Bosma 1956). Because the constrictors form a continuous sheet of striated muscle, an overlapping firing sequence is observed, beginning with the superior constrictor (the principal muscle), the middle constrictor, and the inferior constrictor, with distinct rostral (thyropharyngeus) and caudal (cricopharyngeus) components. The superior constrictor is active at the same time as the leading complex activity. A reconstruction of firing patterns leads to the conclusion that inhibition would probably be found to surround or bracket (in a time sense) the excitation of swallowing (Doty and Bosma 1956).

From the standpoint of peripheral innervation, elicitation of swallowing may occur as a result of activity in the maxillary branch of the trigeminal, glossopharyngeal, or SLN. It has been suggested that small fibers giving rise to a superficial plexus of beaded terminals on the pharyngeal surface of the epiglottis may be the type of nerve ending that is most likely to be activated in the initiation of swallowing. Many complex endings also exist on the oral side of the soft palate or uvula, although anatomic complexity and overlap make it difficult to identify elements specifically at this point. In addition to sensory endings, there are proprioceptors whose relevance to swallowing has not been clarified (Bosma 1957b; Bosma 1976). It is important that there probably are not more than 2,000 motoneurons on both sides to innervate about 12,000 constrictor muscle fibers, and that this low innervation ratio of the pharyngeal musculature implies neural control comparable in precision with that of the ocular muscles.

VOLUNTARY AND STEREOTYPED ORAL FEEDING BEHAVIORS: CEREBRAL CORTEX AND LIMBIC CORTEX SYSTEMS

In order to better understand the supranuclear (rostral to the brain stem) organization of oral feeding behaviors, it is necessary to deal in more detail with the central afferent systems, motoneuron pools, and efferent systems (Figure 1.9).

The convergent afferent systems include the maxillary branch of the fifth cranial nerve and the ninth and tenth cranial nerves. These lead to the descending or spinal trigeminal system and the fasciculus and nucleus solitarius. The ninth and tenth cranial nerves admix considerably in terms of source and modality. The magnocellular part of nucleus solitarious receives input from the sensori-

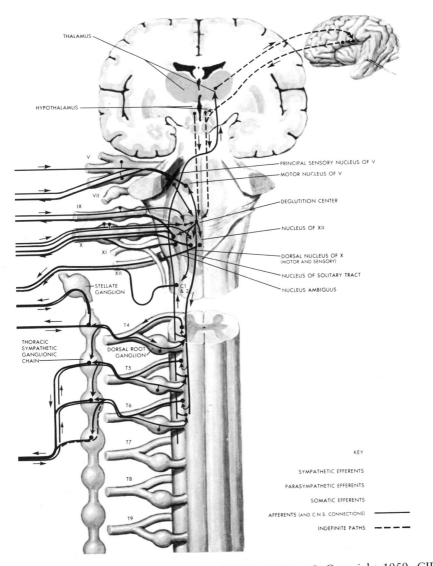

THALAMUS

HYPOTHALAMUS

V

VII

IX

X

XI

XII

STELLATE GANGLION

C1 & 2

T4

THORACIC SYMPATHETIC GANGLIONIC CHAIN

DORSAL ROOT GANGLION

T5

T6

T7

T8

T9

PRINCIPAL SENSORY NUCLEUS OF V

MOTOR NUCLEUS OF V

DEGLUTITION CENTER

NUCLEUS OF XII

DORSAL NUCLEUS OF X (MOTOR AND SENSORY)

NUCLEUS OF SOLITARY TRACT

NUCLEUS AMBIGUUS

KEY

SYMPATHETIC EFFERENTS

PARASYMPATHETIC EFFERENTS

SOMATIC EFFERENTS

AFFERENTS (AND C.N.S. CONNECTIONS) ———

INDEFINITE PATHS ‑ ‑ ‑ ‑

Figure 1.9 Summary of the nervous control of deglutition. © Copyright 1959, CIBA Pharmaceutical Company, Division of CIBA-GEIGY Corporation. Reprinted with permission, from THE CIBA COLLECTION OF MEDICAL ILLUSTRATIONS, illustrated by Frank H. Netter, M.D. All rights reserved.)

motor cortex and the ventromedial thalamus. Some fibers of the ninth and tenth cranial nerves project to the lateral cuneate nucleus (lateral portion of posterior spinal column), serving as a relay to the ventroposteromedial nucleus of the thalamus and limbic cortical system.

The reflexes produced as a result of the afferent, central, and efferent

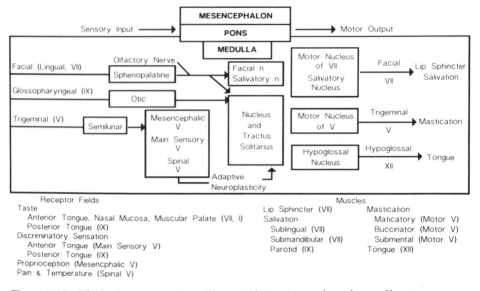

Figure 1.10 The brain stem receives afferent information and produces efferent responses from a number of cranial nerves. This sequence of activity is capable of both sensory-guided discriminatory behaviors and sensory-cued, stereotyped behaviors.

systems for oral feeding behaviors may be divided into brain stem systems (see Figure 1.10), sensory-cued stereotyped (limbic cortical systems) (see Figure 1.11), and sensory-guided discriminatory behaviors (sensorimotor neocortical systems) (see Figure 1.12). As previously mentioned, the neuronal activities resulting in the oral phase of swallow also overlap with those responsible for phonation, coughing, and speech. Normal oral feeding appears to involve not only brain stem reflex initiation by way of several types of peripheral excitation, but a central facilitation of its limbic and cortical sensorimotor pathways.

The highly integrated activities of oral swallow depend on a combination of voluntary and involuntary control of the position of lips, teeth, jaw, cheeks, and tongue, all partly mediated by the fifth cranial nerve-innervated muscles that control both the mandible and the masseter. These muscles are involved in the control of leverage, stabilization, and centering of the movable parts of the buccal cavity. Therefore, mastication depends primarily on the fifth cranial nerve, whereas the muscles of the lips and cheeks depend on motor functions of the seventh cranial nerve. All of the extrinsic muscles of the tongue depend on the motor function of the twelfth cranial nerve, except for the palatoglossus (elevator of the tongue root), which is innervated by the tenth cranial nerve (Stone and Shawker 1988). All of the intrinsic tongue muscles are innervated by the twelfth cranial nerve. All of the muscles of the soft palate are innervated primarily by the tenth cranial nerve, except the tensor veli palatini, which is innervated by the fifth cranial nerve. The stylopharyngeus, a longitudinal muscle, has the

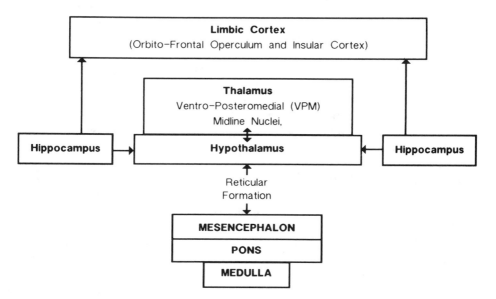

Figure 1.11   Conceptualization of learned components of oral swallow as sensory-cued, stereotyped behaviors from the limbic system.

function of widening the pharynx and is innervated by the ninth cranial nerve, whereas the palatopharyngeus is innervated primarily by the tenth cranial nerve. The maxillary and mandibular sensory divisions of the fifth cranial nerve are primarily involved in providing sensation pertaining to the lips, palate, teeth, inner mouth, and proprioceptive aspects of the muscles of mastication. The gag reflex as well as nasal regurgitation depends on the function or dysfunction of the glossopharyngeal and vagus nerves, whose muscles of innervation have been discussed previously.

The neural structures and organization of oral feeding swallowing behaviors result in more than one basic type of pattern, for example, that found in infancy, and more mature patterns developing later in childhood, adolescence, and adulthood. A fundamental description of the neuroregulation of oral feeding behaviors requires a somewhat artificial isolation of the neural organization. Actually, movements of the palate and oral swallowing are probably closely related to those occurring in speech and respiration. Earlier evolutionary patterns such as swallowing of air by amphibia may be regained by adult humans, for example, victims of poliomyelitis. Such movements require some voluntary control of the inferior constrictor with pumping tongue movements, suggestive of glossopharyngeal breathing (Bosma 1963).

Because of the widespread ramifications and functional significance of the vagus nerve (tenth), lesions in the vagal system may have far-reaching deleterious effects on coughing, swallowing, breathing, and phonation, elements of each of which are interrelated at various vagal levels. Although the details of anatomic and physiologic complexity are beyond the scope of this discussion, it is essential that the reader grasp the major pattern of vagal distribution. The afferent side of swallowing behaviors can be stimulated by voluntary movements of the tongue and larynx. This is subserved to some extent by supranuclear corticobulbar fibers of the sensorimotor neocortical system, some of which provide ipsilateral and others bilateral innervation to the motor outflow of the nucleus ambiguus. It also should be noted that swallowing behaviors associated with phonation or vocal fold adduction can be initiated through pathways associated with the limbic cortical systems.

The voluntary components of sensory-guided discriminatory behaviors of oral swallow probably have their origin in neocortex (inferior precentral and postcentral gyrus) (see Figure 1.12). They operate primarily on striated muscles, but involve the development of "automatisms" that still may be subject to voluntary monitoring and control by mechanisms associated with the limbic cortex (orbitofrontal operculum and insular cortex) (see Figure 1.11). These include the sensory-cued stereotyped motor behaviors or habits of mouth control and chewing, which are largely distinguishable from individual to individual. Many of the neural mechanisms for oral feeding behaviors are dependent on a combination of brain stem and supranuclear pathways, of complex reflexes that have variable expression at different stages of development and evolution. Examples include cough and gag, the rooting and sucking of infancy and the biting reflexes dependent on masseteric stretch. At the limbic cortex, the inferior portion of the precentral gyrus of the insula produces oral and pharyngeal swallowing

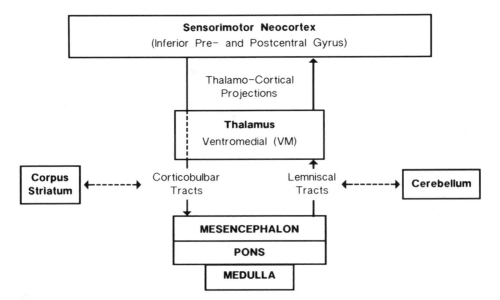

Figure 1.12 Conceptualization of voluntary components of oral swallow as sensory-guided discriminatory behaviors from the neocortex.

on electrical stimulation. These result from efferent connections to the hypo-thalamus and thence to the obex of the fourth ventricle at the caudal medulla.

The sensorimotor neocortex and limbic cortex in primates and many other species produce a combination of chewing and swallowing movements with effects on many structures of the neck, palate, tongue, and pharynx. These behaviors are usually bilaterally represented. It appears that the swallowing elicited by direct stimulation of sensorimotor and limbic systems follows a path through the ventromedial thalamus and hypothalamus, respectively (see Figure 1.11). It is interesting that gagging depends on the spatiotemporal pattern of afferent action integrated at the level of the medulla through the same set of pharyngeal or palatoreceptors that evoke respiration in the limbic and sensori-motor cortical systems. This pluripotential nature of afferent activity is a hall-mark of the complex neural organization under discussion, with special emphasis on the linkage between swallowing and respiration.

SUMMARY

The neuroplasticity of the adult nervous system acknowledges the well-established observation that feeding is a continuously adaptive behavior whose optimal performance can be assessed only in relation to the character, volume, and density of the ingested food, in association with such factors as craniocervical posture (Keogh 1957; Cotman and Nadler 1978; Buchholz et al. 1985). The term adaptive plasticity has been proposed to describe observations that condi-tioned reflexive behaviors, emanating from the pontomedullary area of the brain stem, appear to have the capacity to change over time, when challenged by the environment. For example, if such adaptations occur by finding the appropriate inborn synaptic network, adaptive neuroplasticity will tend to mask clinical symptoms of neurogenic dysphagia. For some patients there is increased liability of sudden decompensation, with progression of neurologic illness and/or by intercurrent nonspecific events such as stress, alcohol, and minor trauma.

Recent investigations have shown that the mature brain is intrinsically labile; that is, although some neural functions such as respiration are reflexive and require minimal learning and experience, others, such as feeding behaviors (oral and pharyngeal swallow), have provided a substrate exquisitely receptive to programming (Bach-y-Rita 1980; Goldberger and Murray 1988). The scien-tific basis for rehabilitation of dysphagia resulting from lesions of the nervous system is based on the hypothesis that the fundamental neuroplastic process responsible for feeding can be reprogrammed through training and environmental change, in order to enhance function. For some behaviors, such as respiration, function may return spontaneously with minimal outside interventions; for others such as feeding, rehabilitation associated with special training routines is usually necessary. However, as we gain a deeper understanding of the fundamental process of neuroplasticity, our ability to predict outcomes, evaluate improvement or regression, and devise new training strategies for dysphagia rehabilitation after nervous system damage is likely to improve (Finger and Stein 1982).

REFERENCES

Ardran GM, Kemp FH. The mechanism of swallowing. Proc R Soc Med 1951; 44: 1038–40.

Ardran GM, Kemp FH. Protection of laryngeal airway during swallowing. Br J Radiol 1952; 25:406–16.

Bach-y-Rita P. Recovery of function: theoretical considerations for brain injury rehabilitation. Baltimore: University Park Press, 1980.

Baker AB, Matzke HA, Brown JR. Poliomyelitis; bulbar poliomyelitis; a study of medullary function. Arch Neurol Psychiatry 1950; 63:257–81.

Bosma JF. Deglutition: pharyngeal stage. Physiol Rev 1957a; 37:275–300.

Bosma JF. Studies of the pharynx. I. Poliomyelitic disabilities of the upper pharynx. Pediatrics 1957b; 19:1053–79.

Bosma JF. Oral and pharyngeal development and function. Physiol Rev 1963; 37: 275–300.

Bosma JF. Sensorimotor examination of the mouth and pharynx. In: Kawamura Y, ed. Frontiers of oral physiology. Basel: Karger 1976; 2:78–107.

Brown, S. In: Ballantyne J, Groves J, eds. Diseases of the ear, nose, and throat. London: Butterworths, 1971.

Buchholz DW, Bosma JF, Donner MW. Adaptation compensation and decompensation of the pharyngeal swallow. Gastrointest Radiol 1985; 10:235–39.

Castell DO. Esophageal manometric studies: a perspective of their physiological and clinical relevance. J Clin Gastroenterol 1980; 2:91–96.

Cotman CW, Nadler JV. Reactive synaptogenesis in the hippocampus. In: Cotman CW, ed. Neuronal plasticity. New York: Raven Press, 1978; 227–71.

Curtis DJ. Radiographic anatomy of the pharynx. Dysphagia 1986; 2:51–62.

Curtis DJ, Crain MC. Aerosol regurgitation as a laryngeal sensitizing event explaining acute laryngospasm. Dysphagia 1987; 2:93–96.

Curtis DJ, Cruess DF, Willgross ER. Abnormal bolus swallowing in the erect position. Dysphagia 1989; 2:46–49.

Dodds WJ. Instrumentation and methods for intraluminal esophageal manometry. Arch Intern Med 1976; 136:515–23.

Donner MW. Swallowing mechanisms and neuromuscular disorders. Semin Roentgenol 1974; 9:273–82.

Donner MW, Bosma JF, Robertson DL. Anatomy and physiology of the pharynx. Gastrointest Radiol 1985; 10:196–212.

Donner M, Siegel C. The evaluation of neuromuscular disorders by cinefluorography. Am J Roentgenol 1965; 94:299–307.

Doty RW, Bosma JF. Electromyographic analysis of reflex deglutition. J Neurophysiol 1956; 19:44–60.

Doty RW, Richmond WH, Storey AT. Effect of medullary lesions on coordination of deglutition. Exp Neurol 1967; 17:91–106.

Ekberg O, Nylander G. Cineradiography of the pharyngeal stage of deglutition in 150 individuals without dysphagia. Br J Radiol 1982; 55:253–57.

Finger S, Stein DG. Brain damage and recovery: research and clinical perspectives. Orlando: Academic Press, 1982.

Goldberger ME, Murray M. Patterns of sprouting and implications for recovery of function. In: Waxman S, ed. Advances in neurology. 1988; 47:361–85.

Kaplan HM. Anatomy and physiology of speech: McGraw-Hill series in speech. New York: McGraw-Hill, 1960.

Keogh CA. The neurology and function of the pharynx and its powers of compensation. Ann Otol Rhinolaryngol 1957; 66:1–23.

Palmer ED. Disorders of the cricopharyngeus muscle: a review. Gastroenterology 1976; 71:510–19.

Robbins JA, Sufit R, Rosenbek J, et al. A modification of the modified barium swallow. Dysphagia 1987; 2:83–86.

Rontal M, Rontal E. Lesions of the vagus nerve: diagnosis, treatment, and rehabilitation. Laryngoscope 1977; 87:72–86.

Sanchez GC, Kramer P, Ingelfinger FJ. Motor mechanisms of the esophagus, particularly its distal portion. Gastroenterology 1953; 25:321–32.

Sasaki C. Paralysis of the larynx and pharynx. Surg Clin North Am 1980; 60:1079–82.

Sasaki CT, Suzuki M, Horiuchi M, et al. The effect of tracheostomy on the laryngeal closure reflex. Laryngoscope 1977; 87:1428–33.

Schultz A, Niemtzow P, Jacobs S, Naso F. Dysphagia associated with cricopharyngeal dysfunction. Arch Phys Med Rehabil 1979; 60:381–86.

Sinclair WJ. The pharyngeal plexus in initiation of swallowing in man. Am J Physiol 1961; 221:1260–63.

Sloan RF, Brummet SW, Westover JL, Ricketts RM, Asjley FL. Recent cinefluorographic advances in palatopharyngeal roentgenography. Am J Roentgenol 1964; 92:977–85.

Splaingard ML, Hutchins B, Sulton LD, Gouri C. Aspiration in rehabilitation patients: videofluoroscopy vs bedside clinical assessment. Arch Phys Med Rehabil 1988; 69: 637–40.

Stone M, Shawker TH. An ultrasound examination of tongue movement during swallowing. Dysphagia 1988; 1:78–83.

2

Neurologic Disorders of Swallowing

Roger M. Morrell

Discussion of the neurologic disorders of swallowing is preceded by some general remarks pertaining to the anatomic regions involved in the swallowing process as described in Chapter 1, and also with regard to the regional and hierarchical arrangement of levels within the nervous system. From the standpoint of the swallowing process itself, the considerations involve the progression from the oral cavity to the distal esophagus and stomach. From the standpoint of the nervous system, the major disorders are divided primarily into those that affect the smooth or striated musculature (myogenic) and those that affect central nervous system (CNS) centers, including the spinal cord and/or peripheral nerves (neurogenic). Finally, consideration is given to the major psychogenic disorders of swallowing.

GENERAL CONSIDERATIONS

The intimate relationship of the last four cranial nerves (ninth through twelfth) results in the possibility of many combinations of nerve lesions that have similar common pathways in terms of symptomatology. Examples include loss of strength of the voice, hoarseness, nasal speech, difficulty in swallowing, and nasal regurgitation or aspiration. Referred or directly mediated painful sensations in the region of the external ear and scalp may draw attention to the ninth and tenth cranial nerves, while weakness and wasting of the sternomastoids, trapezii, and tongue may implicate the eleventh and twelfth cranial nerves.

A neurologic cause of dysphagia is more likely if the anatomy is normal without deformity, although symmetry may be misleading since it may represent bilateral lesions. Deformity may occur in the presence of a sensory deficit, while asymmetry may result from a unilateral problem. Since the larynx is innervated by the tenth cranial nerve, paralysis of one or both vocal cords may be completely separate from neurologic involvement of the palatopharyngeal apparatus. Neurologic involvement of the orobuccal phase of swallowing is related to its volitional nature. Involvement of the reflexly controlled pharynx and the mixed functions of the larynx affect not only swallowing, but speaking and breathing, so that it is important to note associated functions. The symptoms associated with these functions (dysarthria, dysphagia, and dysphonia) may all coexist, as in parkinsonism or other disorders of the basal ganglia. It is difficult to attempt to determine the most likely neurologic localization from symptoms and signs affecting a highly coordinated process such as swallowing. This is apparent when we consider that not only basal ganglia but cerebellum and sensory feedback control are required to coordinate the voluntary as well as reflex muscle movements that permit precise manipulation of the bolus in a normal swallow.

Pathology of the brain stem affecting swallowing frequently takes the form of bulbar palsy, poliomyelitis, trauma, vascular abnormalities such as the Wallenberg's syndrome of the posterior inferior cerebellar artery, and brain stem tumors. The brain stem may also be involved in many congenital degenerative disorders, including hereditary spastic paralysis, familial dysautonomia, amyotrophic lateral sclerosis (ALS), and syringobulbia. A key finding associated with brain stem involvement is failure of the cricopharyngeus muscle to relax during swallowing, with accompanying pharyngeal retention, stasis, and nasal regurgitation (Schultz et al. 1979). As one-half of the brain activates the brain stem nuclei bilaterally, there would be no advantage in having the individual sides of the mouth and throat working separately. Therefore unilateral cerebral lesions often spare the brain stem.

It has been found that lesions of various levels of the CNS, particularly cerebellar, upper motoneuron, lower motoneuron, and extrapyramidal (parkinson-like), produce different and identifiable patterns of lingual, labial, and velar movement as examined cineradiographically (Logemann et al. 1977).

From a diagnostic standpoint, neurologic causes of swallowing disorders are generally identified through such factors as the duration of the swallowing process, difficulties with liquids and solids, nasal regurgitation, and the presence or absence of heartburn. Hoarseness may indicate intrinsic laryngeal disease or relate to carcinoma. It may be accompanied by recurrent laryngeal nerve paralysis complicating such diseases as polymyositis and dermatomyositis (Metheny 1978). Bilateral nuclear involvement of the tenth cranial nerve may be present in both poliomyelitis and polyneuritis. A prominent symptom of dysarthria may be present in ALS, while coughing, especially as a function of the recumbent position, may relate to Zenker's diverticulum, achalasia, or esophageal-tracheal fistula. Hiccup suggests phrenic or diaphragmatic involvement and sometimes accompanies carcinoma and achalasia.

This chapter does not detail the elements of physical examination as it relates to neurologic disorders of swallowing, although certain physical and neurologic signs are reviewed in appropriate sections. It is of interest to itemize conditions related to hypocontractility or lack of contractility of the peripheral region. In this connection, pharyngeal striated muscle may be hypocontractile in the case of poly (dermato) myositis, myasthenia gravis, myotonic dystrophy, diabetic neuropathy, and amyloidosis. Furthermore, syndromes overlap, such as collagen or connective tissue disease and progressive systemic sclerosis, systemic lupus erythematosus (SLE) and polyarteritis nodosa, and progressive systemic sclerosis and SLE. Esophageal smooth muscle may be hypocontractile in scleroderma or progressive systemic sclerosis, in lupus erythematosus, rheumatoid arthritis, periarteritis nodosa, Raynaud's syndrome, diabetic neuropathy, alcoholic neuropathy, and myxedema.

In regional peripheral evaluation, oropharyngeal dysphagia is accompanied by a decreased gag reflex, weakness of cervical or facial muscles, and often a speech disorder. It is a common cause of dysphagia, and if it progresses to pharyngeal paralysis, it may include a number of sensory changes secondary to painful lesions of the mouth or tongue. Such diseases include scarlet fever, mumps, viral infections, herpes, monilia, peritonsillar abscess, carcinoma, or syphilis. Acute thyroiditis also may be a cause. Pharyngeal paralysis eventually often results from poliomyelitis, syringomyelia, multiple sclerosis, cerebrovascular accident involving the brain stem, and diphtheritic neuritis of the ninth and tenth cranial nerves. Muscle weakness leading to pharyngeal involvement is found in myasthenia gravis, myotonic dystrophies, amyloidosis, scleroderma, and dermatomyositis. Other conditions to be considered in the oropharyngeal phase are Plummer-Vinson syndrome, laryngeal fixations secondary to carcinoma, tuberculosis or syphilis, and congenital abnormalities of the tongue and palate. Plummer-Vinson syndrome includes dysphagia, glossitis, hypochromic anemia, and sometimes splenomegaly and achlorhydria (absence of free hydrochloric acid in the stomach). It is often thought to have a dysphagic component that may be due in part to psychic or emotional (hysteria-like) achalasia of the cricopharyngeus muscle. Pharyngeal involvement in such syndromes and others previously mentioned relates to inability of pharyngeal constrictors to initiate peristaltic contraction and empty contents of the pharynx into the esophagus. An isolated pharyngeal palsy may be difficult to evaluate and may result from selective involvement of the nerve supply from the superior branches of the vagus emanating from the cephalic region of the nucleus ambiguus where pharyngeal function is bilateral in terms of motor cortical activity (O'Connor 1976). Furthermore, it has been pointed out in Chapter 1 that lesions of the vagus nerve may produce devastating effects on the functions of swallowing, breathing, and phonation. Sasaki (1980) discussed this in terms of low vagal paralysis (below the nodose ganglion) that rarely affects deglutition, and high vagal paralysis (above the nodose ganglion), which is catastrophic whether unilateral or bilateral. The difference may lie, in part, with the fact that the higher paralysis often is accompanied by widespread involvement of the fifth, seventh, ninth, and twelfth cranial nerves with the overriding threat of aspiration. Most neurologic causes of oropharyngeal dysphagia are chronic or intermittent and need to be analyzed in terms of the foregoing considerations.

Specific causes of laryngeal involvement in the peripheral arrangement of swallowing include herpes zoster (Pahor 1979), mitral valve disease causing paralysis of the left vocal fold and dysphagia (Morgan and Mourant 1980), and intrinsic pathologies such as Crohn's disease with granulomatous changes of larynx and pharynx. Secondary amyloidosis also may produce dysphagia. Since the principal function of the larynx is sphincteric, interruption of reflexes responsible for laryngeal closure result in failure to elevate and close the larynx by contraction of intrinsic laryngeal adductor musculature by way of the sensory limbs of the ninth and tenth cranial nerves. Failure of these mechanisms on a neurologic basis also may include failure to inhibit respiration reflexly or to open the larynx appropriately during inspiration by contraction of the laryngeal abductors. As a result, neurologic disease of the larynx may cause not only aspiration, but stridor and air hunger.

MYOGENIC DISORDERS OF SWALLOWING
Myopathies and Myotonias

For purposes of this discussion, myopathies and myotonias include the dystrophies (i.e., Duchenne's disease) and conditions such as dermatomyositis or polymyositis, which may be harbingers of systemic carcinoma or disease entities in their own right, as listed below:

1. Myopathies and myotonias, dystrophies
2. Dermatomyositis or polymyositis
3. Dysthyroid conditions
4. Myasthenia gravis
5. Neuromuscular esophageal disorders
   a. Scleroderma
   b. Raynaud's disease
   c. Achalasia
   d. Diffuse spasm

The dysphagia and dysphonia of myotonic dystrophy often are accompanied by the pathognomonic features of bilateral facial weakness, temporal balding, cataracts, and extensive peripheral and palatal weakness. Myotonia of the tongue usually is demonstrated by placing a tongue blade flat beneath the tongue and another on edge above the midportion of the tongue. A subsequent impact causes a constrictive band across the top of the tongue. The myopathy of dermatomyositis, acute systemic lupus erythematosus, or oculopharyngeal myopathy involves degenerative or inflammatory changes seen pathologically in muscle. It is demonstrated radiographically by abnormal deglutition, particularly prolongation of muscular activity and weakened or shallow pharyngeal contractions, with retention in pharyngeal recesses with stasis. In myotonia dystrophica, pharyngeal swallow may be only slightly impaired with restricted contraction, or result in complete paralysis leading to nasal and tracheal aspiration. Successive swallows frequently show both improvement in pharyngeal contraction and decreased duration.

Myopathies often are congenital. They usually eventually involve symmetric proximal weakness with patterned wasting depending on the type of myopathy; absence of sensory symptomatology; abnormal electromyography, muscle biopsy, and electrocardiogram; and occasionally, diagnostic patterns of muscle enzyme abnormalities. As an autosomal dominant disorder, myotonic dystrophy may involve the pharynx and esophagus with resultant dysphagia, nasal regurgitation, and aspiration of ingested fluid (Harvey et al. 1965). Symptoms apparently result from abnormal esophageal peristalsis, pooling in the pharynx, inability to propel a normal bolus into the upper esophagus, prominent failure to initiate swallowing of water, and prolongation of contraction and relaxation phases in both upper and lower esophagus. An atonic dilated esophagus may be an additional feature. Aspiration of pharyngeal contents into the larynx and bronchial tree with possible bronchiectasis has been associated with myotonic dystrophy (Ludman 1962). Pierce et al. (1965) described consistent esophageal peristaltic abnormalities in myotonic dystrophy.

Another myogenic disorder known as oculopharyngeal dystrophy is a chronic progressive external ophthalmoplegia occurring in older age groups and characterized by ptosis and dysphagia in an autosomal dominant pattern first described in French-Canadian families. It must be distinguished from such ocular conditions as Graefe's disease, descending ocular myopathy, ophthalmoplegia plus (with retinal pigmentary anomalies, cardiac disorders, etc.), and other heredoataxias. Various *formes frustes* (atypical forms) also complicate the diagnosis, as outlined in the review by Bastiaensen and Schulte (1979). Typically, there are reduced or absent pharyngeal reflexes and weak movements of the soft palate, tongue, and larynx. Cineradiography reveals stagnation in the piriform sinuses, paresis of pharyngeal muscles, and abnormal relaxation of the cricopharyngeal sphincter. The most important cause of dysphagia is absence of reflex relaxation, which requires a rise in pressure in the lower part of the pharynx. Dysphagia results when this pressure rise does not occur due to pharyngeal muscular dystrophy. Diagnosis depends on the involvement of other cranial muscles, myopathic facies, and electromyographic findings characteristic of myopathy. Some patients have increased levels of creatinine phosphokinase (CPK, a blood enzyme) or abnormal immunoglobulins. The disorder must be distinguished from myasthenia gravis and progressive bulbar paralysis; myotonic dystrophy; polymyositis; tumors; inflammation of the brain stem, meninges, and skull base; senile changes with or without organic stenosis of the esophagus; syphilis; and the other ocular dystrophic conditions as mentioned. Bosch et al. (1979) described a patient with secondary inflammatory changes of muscle similar to those of idiopathic polymyositis. Duranceau and associates (1978) drew attention in oculopharyngeal dystrophy to prominent oropharyngeal dysphagia secondary to pharyngo-oral and pharyngonasal regurgitation associated with chronic aspiration and bronchorrhea.

Diagnosis of dysthyroid conditions depends on generalized weakness and reflex abnormality. Often, the examiner finds a pendular quality to reflexes in a setting of documented abnormality of thyroid metabolism based on quantitative hormone determination and, to some extent, response to therapy.

Myasthenia Gravis

Myasthenia gravis is a disorder that should be considered in any healthy adult with laryngeal weakness, varying dysphonia, and dysphagia (Figure 2.1). These manifestations may respond dramatically to a diagnostic injection of intravenous edrophonium (Tensilon). Not all patients with bulbar myasthenia exhibit

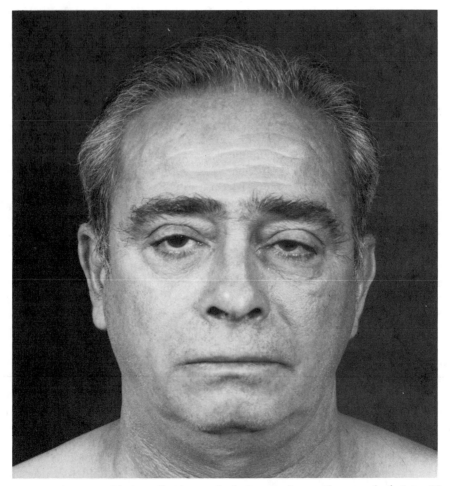

Figure 2.1 Patient with myasthenia gravis demonstrating ocular muscle fatigue. Note ptosis of both eyelids. This patient also had marked facial and tongue weakness, dysphagia, and dysphonia.

ptosis or diplopia, which may be commonly associated with the pharyngeal involvement seen more often in younger patients. Indirect laryngoscopy is indicated, together with fluoroscopic studies of deglutition. Symptoms of myasthenia gravis are similar to those of ordinary fatigue and many psychologic disturbances, especially if pharyngeal or laryngeal involvement is not accompanied by other neurologic signs. Motoneuron disease (ALS) also should be considered in the differential diagnosis, given clinical manifestations of progressive dysarthria, dysphagia, and dysphonia occurring in otherwise healthy patients over 30 years of age.

Myasthenia gravis causes impaired conduction at the myoneural junction of striated muscles. Dysphagia is an early sign and is accompanied by ocular muscle fatigue. Swallowing worsens late in the day and at the end of each meal, but is not accompanied by spasm or hypertrophy of the cricopharyngeal sphincter, a feature that may be seen in brain stem lesions, sideropenic (iron-deficiency) dysphagia, or pharyngoesophageal incoordination. Dysphagia may occur during treatment of myasthenia gravis, due to either cholinergic crisis resulting from relative overdose of anticholinesterases or less commonly, aggressive steroid therapy.

Carpenter et al. (1979) reported that 30 percent of 175 myasthenic patients had oral, pharyngeal, or laryngeal complaints. One-half of the 30 percent had dysphagia, 13 percent dysarthria, and 2 percent had dysphonia. The prominence of these symptoms and signs may give rise to an erroneous diagnosis of primary bulbar involvement. Eaton and Lambert (1957) described a myasthenic syndrome associated with malignant tumors that caused proximal limb weakness and prominent cranial nerve symptomatology, including dry mouth and in some cases reports of impotence. Some patients appear to manifest a cholinergic dysautonomia (Rubenstein et al. 1979). Botulinum intoxication and Sjögren's syndrome are in the differential diagnosis. Although space does not permit a detailed account of the pathophysiology of Eaton-Lambert syndrome, it is due to a defect of acetylcholine release from presynaptic terminals, rather than the highly specific autoimmune receptor defect to which myasthenia gravis is attributed.

Traumatic Myositis

Metheny (1978) has described the vocal and swallowing disorders associated with traumatic myositis. Often present are dysphagia, dysphonia, and weakness of the tongue with radiologic "gaping" or vallecular sign, and defective propulsion of the bolus with altered esophageal motility. This disorder must be differentiated from disseminated lupus erythematosus and scleroderma. Although it is a rare collagen or connective tissue disorder, there is a 50 percent mortality rate within the first two years which may relate to its association with primary carcinoma. There is striking creatinuria, dermatitis, periorbital heliotrope, edema, and proximal symmetrical muscle weakness. Electromyographic and biopsy results are supportive of the diagnosis, with electromyography guiding the area to be biopsied.

Neuromuscular Disorders of the Esophagus

Some general principles may assist in elucidating the problem areas and clinical entities associated with neuromuscular esophageal disorders.

Conditions leading to esophageal dysphagia may affect the upper esophageal sphincter (cricopharyngeal portion) or the lower esophageal sphincter. It may be accompanied by sticking sensations, need to drink liquids to push the bolus, and disproportionate problems with solid foods. In patients in the lower age range (10 to 45 years), common causes include achalasia, scleroderma, constrictive ring, and spasm. Above age 45, carcinoma and peptic esophagitis are more frequent causes.

The scope of this chapter does not allow an exhaustive review of all neuromuscular causes of esophageal motility disorders (see Chapter 4). A useful review is provided by Fischer and associates (1965). They described 42 patients who were divided into broad categories of cerebrovascular disease, Parkinson's disease, ALS, multiple sclerosis (MS), peripheral neuropathy, undiagnosed central nervous system disease, myasthenia gravis, thyrotoxic myopathy, and myotonic dystrophy. The most striking abnormalities were primarily in myopathic disorders such as myasthenia gravis and myotonic dystrophy. Decrease in peristaltic waves with or without spasm could be found in patients with lesions in many locations, central or peripheral. Additionally, patients with ALS exhibited impaired upper sphincter activity. Those with pseudobulbar palsy and Parkinson's disease exhibited decreased peristalsis.

Abnormalities of motility appear to be associated anatomically with vagal involvement at the supranuclear, nuclear, or peripheral levels. Pharyngeal dysphagia may result from disorders associated with nonperistaltic episodes including segmental spasm. These disorders have come to be called high dysphagia. Although the emphasis in this chapter is on neurologic disease, it must be mentioned, especially in connection with the lower esophageal sphincter, that neuropharmacologic effects may be significant. Cholinergic agonists and metoclopramide increase tone, whereas alcohol and anticholinergic substances decrease it.

Intrinsic Esophageal Disorders

A useful introduction to the problems of intrinsic esophageal muscular disorders or conditions of neuromuscular origin is the article by Vantrappen and co-workers (1979). Achalasia predominantly occurs in the third, fourth, and fifth decades. The esophagus is dilated with symptoms of obstruction, regurgitation, and possibly early pain. Achalasia is due to motor failure and is characterized by feeble and incoordinated contractions. It must be distinguished from diffuse spasm, which is less common, usually occurs after age 60 years, is generally accompanied by significant substernal pain during swallowing, and exhibits diffuse spastic narrowing on radiography, with segmental constriction or pseudodiverticulum formation. Simultaneous and repetitive contractions of considerable amplitude occur in the smooth muscle of the esophagus in contrast to the findings in achalasia. Manometry may be necessary to diagnose diffuse spasm. The term vigorous achalasia describes a condition that differs from either of the above by exhibiting simultaneous repetitive contractions after swallowing, but with decreased amplitude and more pain than with achalasia. Achalasia must be differentiated from megaesophagus or Chagas's disease (ganglionic cell fallout), and from cardiospasm or functional obstruction of the esophagus at the level of the hiatus with thoracic esophageal dilatation. Enlargement of the esophagus may occur in esophageal dyssynergia due to failed relaxation of the distal esophagus.

A generalized disease known as scleroderma or progressive systemic sclerosis may involve the esophagus, with abnormal manometric signs appearing before clinical symptoms are noted. Esophageal involvement is more prevalent in patients with associated Raynaud's disease (acrosclerosis: scleroderma of upper extremities). Again, neuromuscular failure of the smooth muscle portion of the esophagus exists with retention of peristalsis in the striated muscle.

It is important to recognize that neuromuscular disorders affecting the esophagus may exhibit similar manometric abnormalities, yet be widely different in terms of etiology or specificity. For example, abnormal manometric patterns with decreased motility or absent peristalsis may be found in myasthenia gravis, myotonic dystrophy, the peripheral neuropathy of diabetes or alcoholism, and Parkinson's disease; whereas MS may reveal changes characteristic of diffuse spasm, which also may occur as a result of cerebrovascular accidents. A fallacious terminology has crept into the literature with the appearance of the term "bulbar palsy" describing abnormal relaxation of the upper esophageal sphincter resulting from pharyngoesophageal involvement. This term should be reserved for conditions that result from pathology affecting the brain stem, its nuclei, and peripheral cranial nerves or their respective branches. Myotonic dystrophy and myasthenia gravis, therefore, are not bulbar palsies, even though the muscles affected are those innervated by the brain stem.

Students of esophageal disorders have subdivided diffuse spasm and achalasia into phases or stages with reference to variations in segmental esophageal differences in neuromuscular tone. Pope (1977) drew attention to the difficulty of classifying esophageal disorders. He stated that diffuse spasm is more rare and may be more difficult to classify. Although myotomies of various kinds have been promoted for the treatment of spasm in numerous segments of the esophagus, their efficacy has not been widely documented by manometric or cineradiographic studies. Latimer (1981) reported the effective use of biofeedback and self-regulation in the treatment of one case of diffuse spasm. Diffuse spasm was reported by Peppercorn et al. (1979) in association with systemic lupus erythematosus. The concept of presbyesophagus has met some resistance in view of the fact that many elderly individuals have decreased amplitude of esophageal propulsive contractions; however, symptomatic disorders of motility or dysphagia imply disease and require specific evaluation and diagnosis. For a complete discussion of dysphagia secondary to esophageal disorders, see Chapter 4.

NEUROGENIC DISORDERS OF SWALLOWING

The principal neurogenic causes of dysphagia are as follows:

1. Riley-Day syndrome
2. Acquired central disorders
   a. Stroke syndromes and vascular disorders
      (1) Capsular infarct

      (2) Lacunar disease
      (3) Pseudobulbar palsy
      (4) Apraxias and agnosias
      (5) Brain stem stroke
      (6) Vasculitis
   b. Movement disorders
      (1) Parkinson's disease
      (2) Dystonias and dyskinesias
      (3) Huntington's disease
      (4) Palatal myoclonus
   c. Poliomyelitis and other systemic infections
      (1) Diphtheria
      (2) Botulism
      (3) Rabies
      (4) Tetanus
   d. Amyotrophic lateral sclerosis
   e. Other causes
      (1) Dementias
      (2) Multiple sclerosis
      (3) Tuberculosis
      (4) Syphilis
      (5) Neoplasms
      (6) Degenerative disorders
3. Acquired peripheral disorders
   a. Recurrent laryngeal neuropathy
   b. Cranial neuropathies
      (1) Diabetes
      (2) Leukemia
      (3) Lymphoma
      (4) Carcinoma
   c. Other neuropathies
4. Neurodevelopmental disorders
   a. Syringomyelia and syringobulbia
   b. Klippel-Feil syndrome
   c. Arnold-Chiari syndrome
   d. Cerebral palsy
   e. Other

Riley-Day Syndrome

Riley-Day syndrome is a congenital and familial dysautonomia of autorecessive genetic pattern that includes feeding problems associated with dysphagia. It is accompanied by different degrees of sensory neuropathy that involve afferent impulses.

Stroke Syndromes

Stroke syndromes are numerous and can be confusing in terms of their effects on swallowing, depending upon whether the predominant features of the syndrome are upper or lower motoneuronal.

Upper Motoneuron Syndromes

The upper motoneuron syndromes include diseases of the cortex, internal capsule, and suprabulbar areas adjacent to the hypothalamus, as well as posterior and descending tracts within the internal capsule beneath the genu. These lesions, regardless of size, may affect both voluntary corticospinal pathways and reflex connections by means of partial or complete interruption of corticobulbar pathways. Bilateral lesions are always more severe since there is bilateral representation in the brain stem, which may be spared functionally by a unilateral hemispheral lesion. Infarctions of the internal capsule often involve hemisensory deficts as well as hemianopia (visual field defect). Lacunar disease eventually may be related to multi-infarct dementia and is usually associated with hypertension. There are no specific or diagnostic swallowing defects associated with these clinically defined entities. Pseudobulbar palsy is due to suprasegmental interruption of cortical influences on the lower bulbar musculature with resultant functional disruption. Bilateral cortical bulbar interruption results in dysarthric speech, dysphagia, drooling, strangling on attempt at drinking, impaired gag reflex, and susceptibility to aspiration. Interpersonal contact or stimulus may sometimes result in laughing or crying without appropriately associated emotional content. Frontal release reflexes such as grasp, snout, or suck may occur as a result of bilateral cerebral infarctions leading to this syndrome. Also, ALS and advanced MS may cause this disorder.

Apraxias and agnosias may result from stroke that affects higher cortical function at the cognitive level. They interfere with coordination of a voluntary movement or a series of movements based on a disconnection between the neural processing required to elaborate it and the motor sequence required to carry it out. Apraxias and agnosias often accompany aphasia with its characteristic cognitive abnormalities of language and thinking. The neuromuscular apparatus for swallowing may be normal, yet the motor concept is not transmitted in a sequential fashion. "Swallowing agnosia" has not been described, but should be acknowledged as a possibility on theoretical grounds.

Brain Stem Stroke

Strokes affecting the brain stem are becoming more common and are extremely important, but may be confusing to the non-neurologist because of the number of eponymic descriptions associated with them. The vascular supply to the brain stem can be considered to be divided into two major subdivisions: the medial one-third and the lateral two-thirds. Vascular occlusions or ischemia occurring in either region will affect the structures within that region, and the resulting functional abnormalities reflect the ischemic deficits of the deprived tissue. Strokes of the brain stem that affect structures involved in the control of swallowing usually affect the cricopharyngeal muscle's ability to relax. Again, it is important to note that one-half of the brain activates brain stem nuclei bilaterally, and therefore unilateral brain lesions spare the brain stem. Some brain stem strokes, however, especially hemorrhages, may cross the midline in the region of the pons, affecting a volume of tissue in the rostrocaudal dimension aside from anatomic partial transection of the brain stem.

A classic brain stem vascular syndrome affecting swallowing is that of Wallenberg; it is secondary to occlusion of a dominant vertebral artery or the posterior inferior cerebral artery, a branch of the vertebral. Typically, the patient has vertigo, nausea, vomiting, prostration with severe ataxia followed by hiccups, nystagmus and gaze abnormalities, and few sensory complaints. Clinical examination reveals an absent ipsilateral corneal reflex and analgesia of the ipsilateral upper face accompanied by ipsilateral Horner's syndrome. There is hoarseness due to paralysis of the ipsilateral vocal fold (incomplete) and paresis of the ipsilateral palate. Further examination reveals diminution of pain and temperature on the opposite side of the body. The ischemia or infarction affects the lateral medulla and vertigo results from involvement of the vestibular complex. Involvement of the descending nucleus and tract of the fifth cranial nerve causes the corneal and facial analgesia, while crossed thermal loss is caused by involvement of the spinothalamic tract and nucleus of the fifth cranial nerve carrying pain and temperature from the opposite side of the body. Examination of a cross-sectional diagram of the medulla reveals that ischemia of the lateral two-thirds produces ipsilateral ataxia due to involvement of the restiform body (Figure 2.2). Palatal and laryngeal weakness, sometimes accompanied by hiccups, reflect involvement of the nucleus ambiguus and may require tracheostomy, although recovery is expected.

Strokes affecting the basilar artery may produce palatal myoclonus, a rhythmic jerking at frequencies of 80 to 120 beats per minute that also may include muscles of the face, neck, larynx, tongue, and eyes. This appears to involve the dentate nucleus of the cerebellum, red nucleus of the basal ganglia, and inferior olive of the brain stem, together with the central tegmental tract connecting the red nucleus and inferior olive in the tegmental pons. Infarction of the paramedian pons as a result of occlusive arterial disease is often signaled by internuclear ophthalmoplegia. This also may be a common finding in MS, but is not limited to it.

Most brain stem strokes that specifically involve structures underlying swallowing affect the medulla and possibly the vagal nuclei or peripheral nerves as they exit. The same brain stem structures that are affected by occlusive arterial disease may also be affected by irritative or inflammatory arterior disease in the form of vasculitis. Vasculitis may be associated with connective tissue disorders or may be idiopathic or immune-related. Just as the diagnosis of arterial occlusive disease depends upon associated risk factors and evidence of arterial disease on

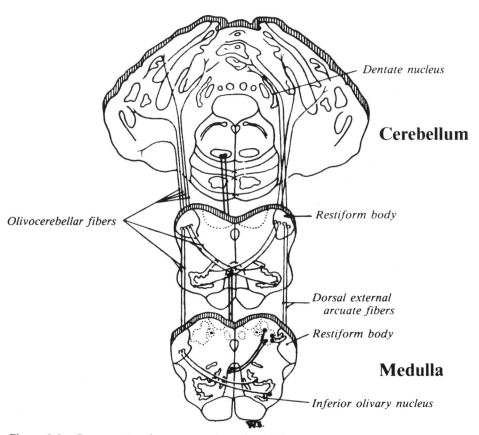

Dentate nucleus

Cerebellum

Olivocerebellar fibers

Restiform body

Dorsal external
arcuate fibers

Restiform body

Medulla

Inferior olivary nucleus

Figure 2.2 Cross-sectional representation of medullar-cerebellar tracts illustrating how ischemic involvement of the lateral medulla can involve the restiform body and its cerebellar connections. Therefore, dysphagia resulting from brain stem stroke may also be accompanied by ataxia. (Adapted and reprinted by permission of the publisher, from Everett, *Functional neuroanatomy*, Philadelphia: Lea & Febiger, 1967.)

angiography, vasculitis occurs in a setting of immunologic abnormalities such as drug abuse, and may require a full angiographic investigation.

Movement Disorders

Of the movement disorders that consistently affect swallowing, Parkinson's disease is of special importance. It is a common neurologic disorder characterized by tremor and/or muscular rigidity, and/or bradykinesia or akinesia with dysarthric speech, a shuffling walk, and an expressionless stare or masklike facies. It is caused by a deficiency of dopamine, which is produced by cells of the substantia nigra that affect basal ganglia function. Disorders of deglutition and esophageal function in Parkinson's disease are relatively common (Pallis 1971). This may include rapid weight loss with dysphagia, leading to a search for primary carcinoma. There may be delay in the initiation of swallow, irregular movement of the epiglottis, and stasis in the piriform fossae and valleculae. Esophageal motility may be reduced, resulting in defects of peristalsis. Autonomic dysfunction may be partially responsible for the dysphagia, together with other autonomic signs, including sialorrhea (drooling), seborrhea, and orthostatic hypotension. Urinary incontinence may also be a feature. Some of these signs are related to pathologic changes in the dorsal vagal nucleus, sympathetic ganglia, locus ceruleus (floor of fourth ventricle), and hypothalamus. These have been summarized by Lieberman and colleagues (1980). The dysphagia has been described by Caine and colleagues (1970), and specific abnormalities in esophageal motility by Bramble et al. (1978). Dystonias and dyskinesias (notably tardive dyskinesia) also may affect elements of deglutition, most commonly, the orobuccal phase. Huntington's disease is an example of a choreiform disorder that may affect the coordination of swallowing, especially in the late stages of disease.

Systemic Infections

Several infections or intoxications result in disorders of swallowing. Bulbar poliomyelitis may do so by direct involvement of neurons of the brain stem comprising the neural control of aspects of swallow described in Chapter 1. A diphtheritic polyneuropathy may affect the swallowing musculature in a completely separate manner from direct diphtheritic extension in the oropharynx. The toxin elaborated in botulism paralyzes the pharyngolaryngeal musculature. In rabies (rare in humans) there may be involvement of brain stem or medullary neurons similar to that of poliomyelitis secondary to the rabies virus. Dysphagia has been described as a primary symptom of tetanus (Weider and Tingwald 1970).

Amyotrophic Lateral Sclerosis

Amyotrophic lateral sclerosis is a disease of insidious onset characterized by degeneration of motor units as a result of involvement of upper and lower motoneurons. It causes spastic and atrophic symptoms in the cranial, spinal, and peripheral musculature. It often affects the motoneurons of the brain stem, resulting in bulbar palsy with prominent slurred speech, hoarseness and breathiness, dysphagia, and dyspnea. The progressive deterioration of speech and swallow have been described by Dworkin and Hartman (1979). Since there is both spasticity and flaccidity as a result of upper and lower motoneuron involvement, there are effects on three levels of the upper airway: articulatory or speech-related, velopharyngeal (palatine pharynx), and phonatory (larynx).

Tongue weakness is apparent and the palate and larynx are affected by disorders in the ninth and tenth cranial nerves. These changes have been detailed by Carpenter et al. (1978) and McGuirt and Blalock (1980). Management issues have been discussed by Delisa and associates (1979), Smith and Norris (1975), and Hillel and Miller (1989). As a result of pharyngeal dysphagia in ALS, there may be concomitant dilatation of the stomach and first part of the duodenum. Cineradiographic disorders of the pharynx in ALS have been described by Bosma and Brodie (1969), while pressure measurements have been detailed by Smith et al. (1957).

In concluding a brief account of acquired central nervous disorders, several diagnoses must be considered with respect to possible effects on deglutition. These include the dementias such as Alzheimer's disease, as well as MS, tuberculosis, syphilis, neoplasms of various types, and so-called degenerative disorders. Some of the neoplasms are of particular interest. For example, in addition to causing cerebellar signs of nausea, vertigo, and veering, certain cerebellar hemangioblastomas may produce hoarseness and strangling on fluids. The palatal weakness and vocal fold paresis are explained by so-called pressure palsies of cranial nerves that are more often associated with cerebellar masses than is commonly recognized. In considering intracranial mass or expanding lesions, abscess and syringobulbia must not be overlooked. The four lowest cranial nerves, especially the first three that exit from the same foramen, may be involved in several malignant diseases including nasopharyngeal carcinoma. From a diagnostic standpoint, neural involvement of swallowing mechanisms by neoplasms is usually progressive.

ACQUIRED PERIPHERAL DISORDERS
Cranial Nerve Neuropathies

The most important peripheral cranial neuropathy is secondary to involvement of the vagus (tenth cranial nerve) or its branches. Remembering that the fifth, seventh, ninth, tenth, and twelfth cranial nerves are involved in the neural control of swallowing, with inclusion of the eleventh for certain functions, it becomes apparent that pathology of one or more of these nerves may result in dysphagia. Specific involvement of these cranial nerves can occur as a result of several conditions that "normally" affect them. For example, a cerebellopontine angle tumor may compress the fifth and seventh cranial nerves, resulting in forms of dysfunction. The most common of these tumors are the acoustic neurinoma or meningioma with early symptoms of deafness, tinnitus, and facial numbness secondary to involvement of the fifth, seventh, and eighth cranial nerves. These may progress to direct compression or distortion of the brain stem, leading to pharyngeal and laryngeal symptomatology. Similarly, the seventh cranial nerve may be affected by Bell's palsy, and may be involved bilaterally, particularly in its motor branches. This is found in postinfectious myeloradiculopathies such as Guillain-Barré syndrome.

A prominent example of involvement of the tenth cranial nerve is paralysis of the vocal fold (usually left) and dysphagia occurring in the course of mitral valve disease (Morgan and Mourant 1980). These may occur separately or in combination, and are thought to result from compression of the recurrent laryngeal nerve as it passes around the aortic arch. Dysphagia also may develop as a result of damage to autonomic nerve plexuses supplying the esophagus. This leads to abnormal peristalsis that may result from external compression by a tense left atrium. The ninth, tenth, eleventh, and twelfth cranial nerves are most commonly coinvolved in jugular venous bulb thrombosis, direct spread of nasopharyngeal carcinoma, or leukemic or lymphomatous infiltration along the base of the skull. The left recurrent laryngeal nerve may be damaged by carcinoma near the hilum of the left lung or by enlargement of several lymph nodes at that site. The right recurrent nerve may be affected by carcinoma at the lung apex or by tuberculosis and vascular abnormalities such as subclavian aneurysm. Although syphilitic aortitis is uncommon, this cardiovascular manifestation of tertiary syphilis may cause or be accompanied by dysphagia resulting from left recurrent laryngeal nerve involvement and connoted clinically by the well-known brassy cough. The nodose ganglion, located within the skull but outside the medulla, is the point of bifurcation of the main trunk of the vagus into the superior laryngeal nerve, which then subdivides peripherally into its motor and sensory branches (see Figure 1.8 [page 20] for anatomic reference). Catastrophic lesions above the nodose ganglion, even though external to the medulla, often result in bilateral total laryngeal paralysis with denervation of the pharynx. Lesions below the nodose ganglion usually are less life threatening, primarily because of diminished probability of aspiration.

Diabetic neuropathies usually only affect the oculomotor cranial nerves, although other cranial nerves may be damaged.

Infectious and peri-infectious involvement of cranial nerves occurs in herpes, diphtheria, and botulism, all of which may produce degrees of dysphonia and dysphagia that require early and drastic emergency measures. Since the conditions themselves may be self-limited, survival and/or reversibility of deficits often are dependent on appropriate and skillful management, particularly nursing care.

Amyloidosis (metabolic disorder marked by accumulation of amyloid deposits) may cause an autonomic neuropathy or directly infiltrate any of the cranial nerves, resulting in disordered deglutition.

Carter (1978) has reviewed postvagotomy dysphagia, and Pahor (1979) has reviewed herpes zoster of the larynx. The latter may accompany or be discrete from aural and facial herpes.

Cranial neuropathies secondary to leukemia, lymphoma, and carcinoma may evidence direct infiltration of cranial nerves with or without expansion and compression against unyielding bone, bony lesions with collapse of periforaminal conduits for cranial nerves, extraneural growth of infiltrating or metastasizing lesions, and enlarged lymphatic structures, or any combination of these disorders.

The cranial nerves may be affected by many disorders that rarely affect peripheral nerves and therefore even though they are peripheral to the central nervous system, they form a special category. Since numerous cranial nerves are involved at a particular site, they can be discussed in terms of site, those involved, usual pathologic cause, and eponymic syndrome.

At the cerebellopontine angle, in addition to involvement of the fifth and seventh cranial nerves, dysphagia may be secondary to possible disease of the ninth cranial nerve. At the jugular foramen, the ninth, tenth, and eleventh cranial nerves may be damaged by tumors or aneurysms (Vernet's syndrome); at the posterior laterocondylar space, cranial nerves nine through twelve, usually caused by tumors of parotid gland, carotid body, and secondary or metastatic tumors (Collet-Sicard syndrome); and at the posterior retroparotid space, cranial nerves nine through twelve with Horner's syndrome, caused by tumors of parotid, carotid body, and lymph node expansions including tuberculous adenitis (lymph gland inflammation). Although brain stem syndromes were previously discussed, it is often the case that certain cranial nerves are affected regularly, together with brain stem syndromes. Those of interest in relation to dysphagia or dysphagia/dysphonia include the following: (1) tegmentum of the medulla—involvement of the tenth cranial nerve, the corticospinal tract, with Horner's syndrome secondary to ischemic necrosis or tumor resulting in paralysis of soft palate, vocal fold, and a contralateral hemiplegia, or Avellis' syndrome; (2) tegmentum of the medulla—tenth and twelfth cranial nerves, corticospinal tract, Avellis' syndrome and ipsilateral tongue paralysis, soft palate and vocal fold paralysis, and contralateral hemiplegia, or Jackson's syndrome; and (3) Wallenberg's syndrome (previously described). The pathologies that may be encountered resulting in Wallenberg's syndrome include meningioma, cholesteatomas, and sarcomas, in addition to neurinoma and carcinoma. Chordomas may affect a succession of lower cranial nerves, giving rise to any of these syndromes. When a motor disorder does not cause atrophy, the question of myasthenia gravis must be raised.

Other Acquired Peripheral Disorders

Other acquired peripheral disorders affecting cranial nerves include neuropathies such as glossopharyngeal neuritis (etiology unknown, possibly analogous to Bell's palsy), and ankylosing vertebral hyperostosis (Leclercq and DeRobbio 1978). The latter condition usually causes dysphagia by direct mechanical protrusion and involvement of the posterior aspect of the pharyngoesophagus. It also may compromise the blood supply to the medulla or associated cranial nerves.

Neurodevelopmental Disorders

Numerous neurodevelopmental disorders may affect the normal swallow. Syringomyelia is a condition of unknown and complex etiology that often occurs early in life. It progresses in the form of an enlarging cystic cavity centrally located in the spinal cord or medulla. When it involves the spinal cord, it is more commonly situated in the region adjacent to the cervical cord. This affects the neural outflow to the upper extremities. Syringomyelia (affecting the spinal cord) is less commonly associated with dysphagia than syringobulbia, which affects the medulla or other regions of the brain stem in a similar process, obliterating structures necessary for normal swallowing.

Klippel-Feil syndrome occurs as a result of fusion of cervical vertebrae during embryonic development with a resultant decrease in the length of the cervical spine. This is expressed as shortening of the neck and is accompanied by paraparesis. There may be direct involvement of the medulla as a result of buckling or compression of the brain stem, and there may be associated syringobulbia.

Dandy-Walker syndrome results from prenatal obstruction to the outflow of cerebrospinal fluid through normal apertures in the fourth ventricle. This is accompanied by the development of a cyst in the posterior fossa and dilation of the fourth ventricle and aqueduct, with upward displacement of some brain stem structures and compression of others. Involvement of neural structures subserving swallow depends on the specific abnormalities in a given patient.

Arnold-Chiari syndrome is a congenital abnormality that displaces the hindbrain downward with alteration of relationships of the pons, medulla, and cerebellum. The abnormality may be accompanied by vascular lesions in the tegmentum of the medulla as a result of changes in the vascular arrangement to the herniated portion of the brain stem as the arteries are stretched. In addition to hemorrhages in the medulla, compression or traction of the vagus and other lower cranial nerves may result. Patients may have respiratory distress, apnea, vocal fold paralysis, or inability to swallow (Papasozomenos and Roessmann 1981).

The term cerebral palsy is used to describe a number of syndromes resulting from defective development of the embryonic brain. The changes usually are not progressive beyond birth, but are the result of teratogenic or other abnormalities occurring during pregnancy. Defects in swallowing often are related to abnormalities in neuromuscular coordination, frank paresis or paralysis of swallowing-related structures, or complex disturbances that may include weakness, incoordination, seizures, and cognitive dysfunction. The predominant abnormalities appear to be motor rather than sensory.

Other neurodevelopmental causes of dysphagia include abnormalities in the growth and resultant angle of the vault of the skull with the cervical spine, called platybasia or basilar invagination. In these disorders, the altered shape and inclination of the skull base with relationship to the foramen magnum and the associated contents results in compression of brain stem structures and subsequent dysphagia.

A malignant form of neurofibromatosis includes many types of recurrent neoplasms of the nervous system, especially neurofibromas (neurinomas), sarcomas, and meningiomas. These may occur in virtually any location, but are of note in relation to swallowing when they involve the brain stem, associated cranial nerves, and/or contiguous bony structures.

PSYCHOGENIC CAUSES OF DEGLUTITION DISORDERS

A number of conditions having primary, predominant, or associated emotional or psychogenic causes may affect swallowing. Since the strict definition of dysphagia requires that "difficulty in swallowing" be encountered during or seconds after the act of swallowing, some of these disorders cannot properly be included under the heading of dysphagia.

Swallowing difficulties that reflect a person's emotional state, coping mechanisms, or responses to life stress may involve other areas of the gastrointestinal tract in a complex fashion. In the case of peptic ulcer or hiatal hernia, a chain of events may result; the dysphagia may be secondary to the effects of stress on the primary disease. In Plummer-Vinson syndrome, several specific abnormalities occur and have been described. In addition to these, achalasia and hiatal hernia may coexist, together with recognizable emotional disturbances that appear to be part of this syndrome. Patients with emotional conversion symptoms who suffer from anxiety may complain of a lump in the throat (globus hystericus), which is extremely uncomfortable but does not appear to interfere with their ability to swallow (Bockus 1944). Less dramatic responses to stress often are accompanied by prolonged esophageal emptying time (Wolfe and Almy 1949). It is important that patients with symptoms referable to swallowing that are accompanied by positive features of psychogenic or emotional origin not be denied an appropriate history and physical examination lest a physical or organic cause be overlooked. The relationship between psychogenic dynamics and organic causes was highlighted by Black (1980), who reported treatment by hypnosis of dysphagia following traumatic pseudobulbar palsy.

SUMMARY

It is apparent that the process of moving a bolus from mouth to stomach takes place in an organized fashion only if the necessary neuromuscular and neuroregulatory controls are intact. Perhaps the inherent complexity of the process predisposes its delicately balanced neural control to potential failure from the myriad of disease entities under discussion. Even as this chapter details the neurologic disorders of swallowing, the clinician may feel overwhelmed when confronted with the process of differentially diagnosing swallowing disorders secondary to neurogenic and myogenic causes. It should be apparent that most swallowing dysfunctions are not without cause, and most often are the result of an underlying disease process. For this reason, patients with dysphagic complaints require diagnostic exploration. Discovery of the disease process may be difficult, especially in its beginning stagtes, as the initial symptoms frequently suggest more than one condition. The difficulty in specifying a particular disease or disorder may not be as important initially as discovering which neuromotor system is involved or at which anatomic level the pathology exists. Although a careful analysis of clinical and laboratory data suggests that this task is immediately feasible, the existence of multiple diagnostic and nosologic entities presenting as apparently identical or similar symptoms constitutes a challenge to clinicians to devise additional reliable tests of the neuromuscular components of swallowing. Completion of such an evaluation should provide the clinician with reasonable assumptions about short- and long-term treatment strategies.

REFERENCES

Bastiaensen LAK, Schulte BPM. Oculopharyngeal dystrophy: diagnostic problems and possibilities. Doc Ophthalmol 1979; 46:391–401.

Black S. Dysphagia of pseudobulbar palsy successfully treated by hypnosis. NZ Med J 1980; 91:212–4.

Bockus HL. Gastroenterology. Philadelphia: W.B. Saunders, 1944.

Bosch EP, Gowans JDC, Munsat T. Oculopharyngeal dystrophy. Muscle Nerve 1979; 2:73–7.

Bosma JF, Brodie DR. Cineradiographic demonstration of pharyngeal area myotonia in myotonic dystrophy patients. Radiology 1969; 92:104–9.

Bramble MG, Cunliffe J, Dellipiani W. Evidence for a change in neurotransmitter affecting esophageal motility in Parkinson's disease. J Neurol Neurosurg Psychiatry 1978; 41:709–12.

Calne DB, Shaw DG, Spiers ASD, Stern GM. Swallowing in Parkinsonism. Br J Radiol 1970; 43:456–7.

Carpenter RJ 3rd, McDonald TJ, Howard FM Jr. The otolaryngologic presentation of amyotrophic lateral sclerosis. Otolaryngology 1978; 86:479–84.

Carter SL. Resolution of postvagal dysphagia. JAMA 1978; 240:2656–57.

Delisa JA, Mikulic MA, Miller RM, Melnick RR. Amyotrophic lateral sclerosis: comprehensive management. Am Fam Physician 1979; 19:137–42.

Duranceau CA, Letendre J, Clermont RJ, Leresque HP, Barbeau A. Oropharyngeal dysphagia in patients with oculopharyngeal muscular dystrophy. Can J Surg 1978; 21: 326–9.

Dworkin JP, Hartman DE. Progressive speech deterioration and dysphagia in amyotrophic lateral sclerosis: case report. Arch Phys Med Rehabil 1979; 60:423–5.

Eaton L, Lambert E. Electromyograph and electrical stimulation of nerves in disease of motor unit: observation on myasthenic syndrome associated with malignant tumors. JAMA 1957; 163:1117–21.

Everett NB. Functional neuroanatomy. Philadelphia: Lea and Febiger, 1965.

Fischer RA, Ellison GW, Thayor WR. Esophageal motility in neuromuscular disorders. Ann Intern Med 1965; 63:229–48.

Harvey JC, Sherbourne DH, Siegel CI. Smooth muscle involvement in myotonic dystrophy. Am J Med 1965; 39:81–90.

Hillel AD, Miller RM. Bulbar amytrophic lateral sclerosis: Patterns of progression and clinical management. Head Neck 1989; Jan-Feb:51–9.

Lambert JR, Tepperman P, Jimenez JJ, Newman A. Cervical spine disease and dysphagia. Am J Gastroenterol 1981; 76:35–40.

Latimer PR. Biofeedback and self–regulation in the treatment of diffuse esophageal spasm: a single case study. Biofeedback Self Regul 1981; 6:181–9.

Leclercq TA, DeRobbio AV. Dysphagia secondary to ankylosing vertebral hyperostosis. RI Med J 1978; 61:347–50.

Lieberman AM, Horowitz L, Redmond P, Pachter L, Lieberman I, Leibowitz M. Dysphagia in Parkinson's disease. Am J Gastroenterol 1980; 74:157–60.

Logemann JA, Boshes B, Blonsky ER. Speech and swallowing evaluation in the differential diagnosis of neurologic disease. Neurologica Neurocirugia Psiquiatria 1977; 18:71–8.

Ludman H. Dysphagia in dystrophia myotonica. J Laryngol 1962; 76:234–6.

McGuirt WF, Blalock D. The otolaryngologist's role in the diagnosis and treatment of amyotrophic lateral sclerosis. Laryngoscope 1980; 90:1496–1501.

Metheny JA. Dermatomyositis: a vocal and swallowing disease entity. Laryngoscope 1978; 88:147–61.

Morgan AA, Mourant AJ. Left vocal cord paralysis and dysphagia in mitral valve disease. Br Heart J 1980; 43:470–3.

O'Connor AFF, Ardran GM. Cinefluorography in the diagnosis of pharyngeal palsies. J Laryngol Otol 1976; 90:1015–19.

Pahor AL. Herpes zoster of the larynx—how common? J Laryngol Otol 1979; 93:93–8.

Pallis CA. Parkinsonism: natural history and clinical futures. Br Med J 1971; 3:683–90.

Papasozomenos S, Roessmann U. Respiratory distress and Arnold-Chiari malformation. Neurology 1981; 31:97–100.

Peppercorn MA, Docken WP, Rosenberg S. Esophageal motor dysfunction in systematic lupus erythematosus. JAMA 1979; 242:1895–6.

Pierce JW, Creamer B, MacDermot V. Abnormalities in swallowing associated with dystrophia myotonica. Gut 1965; 6:392–5.

Pope CE. Motor disorders of the esophagus. Postgrad Med 1977; 61:118–25.

Rubenstein AE, Horowitz SH, Bender AN. Cholinergic dysautonomia and Eaton-Lambert syndrome. Neurology 1979; 29:720–3.

Sasaki CT. Paralysis of the larynx and pharynx. Surg Clin North Am 1980; 60:1079–91.

Schultz A, Niemtzow P, Jacobs S, Naso F. Dysphagia associated with cricopharyngeal dysfunction. Arch Phys Med Rehabil 1979; 60:381–6.

Smith AW, Mulder DW, Code CF. Esophageal motility in amyotrophic lateral sclerosis. Mayo Clin Proc 1957; 32:438–41.

Smith RA, Norris FH. Symptomatic care of patients with amyotrophic lateral sclerosis. JAMA 1975; 234:715–7.

Vantrappen G, Janssens J, Hellemans J, Coremans G. Achalasia, diffuse esophageal spasm, and related motility disorders. Gastroenterology 1979; 76:450–7.

Weider DJ, Tingwald FR. Dysphagia as initial and prime symptom of tetanus. Arch Otolaryngol 1970; 91:479–81.

Wolf S, Almy TP. Experimental observations on cardiospasm in man. Gastroenterology 1949; 13:401–21.

3

Mechanical Disorders of Swallowing

Michael E. Groher
Elizabeth Enderle Gonzalez

Patients with mechanical swallowing disorders evidence difficulty secondary to the loss of sensory guidance of the structures necessary to complete a normal swallow. The central and most of the peripheral neurologic controls for deglutition are intact. The structures needed to complete the act are not. Even though causes and mechanisms of the neurologic and mechanical groups are different, some of the deglutitory problems are shared. These include sialorrhea (excessive expectoration of fluid resembling saliva), difficulty with mastication, oral and pharyngeal pooling, lengthened swallowing transit times, difficulty channeling food into the esophagus, and aspiration. For the purposes of this and subsequent chapters, aspiration is defined as the residual, unswallowed pharyngeal content that is drawn into the larynx and trachea by inspiration following an attempt at a normal swallow. It is to be differentiated from spillage of oral contents into the pharynx and/or larynx without elicitation of swallow; this is penetration. Most patients with mechanical dysphagia have had oral, pharyngeal, or laryngeal structures removed or reconstructed during surgery for cancer. There are, however, other causes that must be considered in the differential diagnosis. The most common of these are considered here.

ACUTE INFLAMMATIONS

Acute inflammatory processes that produce or exacerbate dysphagia are nonspecific reactions to injury of the oropharyngeal tissue secondary to fungal, bacterial, or viral agents, chemical irritants, or traumatic insults.

Acute inflammations of the oropharyngeal tissues alone may not create significant, extended dysphagia. They are particularly significant, however, when superimposed on other more obvious swallowing disorders such as pseudobulbar dysphagia or the dysphagia seen in elderly debilitated patients. Early recognition and treatment of acute inflammatory reactions can make the difference between success and failure in attempts at oral feeding. They should be ruled out in patients whose mental state or competence interferes with the ability to communicate oral pain and those who evidence unexplainable dysphagia or sudden refusal to eat. Early identification is important because most inflammations

53

can be controlled within a short period of time, and oral nutritional intake can resume.

Herpes Simplex

Viral in origin, a herpetic infection is characterized by round vesicles that break to form shallow ulcers surrounded by a narrow zone of inflammation (DeWeese and Saunders 1973). Typically, they are found on the lips; however, the pharynx and buccal mucosa may be involved. Palatal and pharyngeal ulcers create significant pain and discomfort on swallowing.

Ludwig's Angina

The most typical type of infection to occur in the submandibular space that may compromise swallow is Ludwig's angina. Odontogenic infections such as abscesses, caries, and postextraction infection are implicated in 70 to 85 percent of cases of Ludwig's angina (Williams et al. 1943; Patterson et al. 1982). Clinical manifestations of Ludwig's angina include massive swelling and displacement of the tongue. The floor of the mouth also will appear red, swollen, hard, and tender. Posterior extension may result in epiglottitis, with further compromise of the airway. If the patient is able to speak, he or she may have a muffled, "hot potato" voice. The neck exhibits a woody, tender swelling, especially in the suprahyoid region. Patients generally present with complaints of mouth pain, stiff neck, drooling, and dysphagia. Complications of a supramandibular space infection include asphxia, aspiration pneumonia, lung abscess, and tongue necrosis. Treatment of Ludwig's angina includes airway control, intravenous antibiotics, or surgical exploration and drainage.

Lingual Tonsillitis

Patients with lingual tonsillitis have symptoms similar to those of other throat infections, except they complain of pain in the medial pharyngeal region. Often they describe a lump in the throat associated with complaints of dysphagia. The mechanism of lingual tonsillitis can be confirmed by indirect mirror examination of the base of the tongue and pharynx.

Epiglottitis

Epiglottitis is an inflammatory disease that affects the supraglottic region and often results in acute respiratory distress due to airway obstruction. It is most commonly seen in children but has more recently been recognized with increasing frequency in adults (Hawkins et al. 1973; Kander and Richards 1977; Sarant 1981; Mayosmith et al. 1986). Patients often complain of sore throat, dysphagia, respiratory difficulty, muffled voice, drooling, and stridor (Schabel et al. 1977; Cohen 1984; Mayosmith et al. 1986). An incorrect initial diagnosis of streptococcal or viral pharyngitis is often made (Cohen 1984). A modified barium swallowing study may reveal abnormal enlargement of supraglottic structures. An epiglottis that is 8 mm or greater in width and aryepiglottic folds greater than 7 mm seem to suggest epiglottitis in adults (Schumaker et al. 1984). Maintenance of a competent airway is the most important factor in the treatment of patients with epiglottitis.

Acute Pharyngitis

Acute pharyngitis may be viral or bacterial in origin. The reddened inflammation that it causes in the oropharyngeal region frequently precedes the common cold, leading patients to complain of swallowing difficulty. It often is accompanied by a mild fever without any other complications. The pain and dysphagia subside within four to six days.

The most common bacterial form of pharyngitis is streptococcal. The diagnosis is confirmed by laboratory analysis. The patient has an acutely inflamed oropharynx with characteristic white or yellow follicles. Most complain of headache and muscle joint pain and have fevers that reach 103 degrees. Streptococcal infections respond well to a full course of antibiotics.

Lateral Pharyngeal Space Infections

Infections in the lateral pharyngeal space are classified as anterior or posterior depending on the location of the infection. Infections of the lateral pharyngeal space may be secondary to primary infection in the tonsil or pharynx. Clinical presentation of symptoms differs between anterior and posterior compartments. When the patient has an anterior compartment infection, the patient may present with dysphagia, trismus, chills, high fever, hardening and swelling of the mandibular arch, systemic toxicity, medial buldging of the lateral pharyngeal wall, and pain (Blomquist and Bayer 1988). Dyspnea occurs infrequently. An infection involving the posterior compartment is characterized by marked sepsis in the absence of trismus or tonsillar prolapse. Edema and swelling of the epiglottis and larynx may result in dyspnea. Sudden death syndrome, fatal myocarditis, and further complications are associated when the infection spreads to the retropharyngeal space.

Treatment of lateral pharyngeal space infections are similar to that of Ludwig's angina. Therapeutic management includes antibiotic therapy, surgical drainage, and airway maintenance. Surgical intervention plays a primary role in patient management rather than a secondary role as in Ludwig's angina (Blomquist and Bayer 1988). In addition, airway control is not required as often and is associated with fewer complications than in Ludwig's angina.

Retropharyngeal and Prevertebral Space Infections

Retropharyngeal and prevertebral space infections lie between the common pharyngoesophageal wall and the spine. Retropharyngeal space infections arise acutely from an adjacent abscess, most commonly from the lateral pharyngeal space, or following cervical trauma. Prevertebral space infections most often are secondary to chronic disease, such as osteomyelitis, whereas inflammation following trauma is associated with infected hematomas following vertebral fractures. A patient with a retropharyngeal abscess may complain of fever, sore throat, dysphagia, stridor, regurgitation, dyspnea, and stiff neck. Consequences of retropharyngeal space infections include meningitis, mediastinitis, epiglottitis, pneumonia, empyema, spontaneous rupture of the larynx with aspiration and asphyxiation, bronchial erosion, pyopneumothorax, and purulent pericarditis. Treatment for retropharyngeal space infection involves antibiotic therapy and surgical drainage.

Fungal Inflammation

One of the common fungal inflammations is candidiasis (thrush). Most frequently seen on the tongue, the lesions appear as soft, white, slightly elevated plaques (Keyes 1980) (Figure 3.1). If left untreated, the lesions cause associated pain and difficulty swallowing. They are more common in debilitated and immunosuppressed patients, in those who are undergoing extensive antibiotic therapy, and in patients receiving irradiation treatments. *Candida* species is the most common cause of odynophagia and dysphagia in patients with AIDS (Raufman 1988). Odynophagia may also occur in AIDS patients due to Kaposi's sarcoma. Kaposi's sarcoma is most commonly found on the hard palate, but also may be found in any part of the oral mucosa (Greenspan and Greenspan 1988). They are differentiated from other white plaques such as leukoplakia because they can be scraped away, leaving a raw, bloody surface (Keyes 1980).

Chemical Agents

Mucosal inflammation may result from exposure to chemicals. The subsequent pain interferes most often with the oropharyngeal stage of swallowing.

Chemical inflammation can result from the prolonged use of phenol (toothache drops). Other drugs that precipitate mucosal burns include aspirin, which causes irritation to the cheek lining, some gargles, and anesthetic throat lozenges when used excessively (Kerr and Ash 1978). The latter reduce oral sensation and invite traumatic lesions from persons who unknowingly bite their oral mucosa. Mucosal burns can be red or white, but represent a change in the normal pinkish mucosal lining. More severe inflammations have a whitish slough covering an intensely reddened area. The most severe form of a chemical burn, lye ingestion, can cause severe blistering of the entire digestive tract. The clinician should be aware that patients who undergo chemotherapy can develop painful oral ulcer-

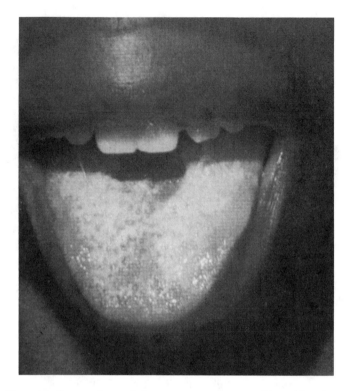

Figure 3.1 Fungal inflammations of the tongue appear as milky-white elevated lesions. (Reprinted by permission of the publisher, from Dreizen et al., *Postgrad Med,* 61 1977a.)

ations that interfere with swallowing. Drugs used in these regimens such as doxorubicin (Adriamycin), methotrexate, and cyclophosphamide (Cytoxan) can cause oral mucositis (Carl 1980).

TRAUMA

Other than major traumatic tissue losses such as those resulting from gunshot wounds, more frequently occurring injuries in the oral cavity are fairly benign and generally do not create significant swallowing complaints except when superimposed on other mechanisms of dysphagia. Examples include trauma from a toothbrush and mucosal irritation from ill-fitting dentures. Patients who complain of a poorly fitted denture can localize their pain. Clinical examination usually will reveal a reddened or whitish change in the mucosa at the point of contact where the patient has the sensation of most discomfort. Prolonged irritation can result in gingival hyperplasia (Figure 3.2) that results in soft, sometimes flexible masses of tissue that appear markedly inflamed.

Biting the sides of the lip, or more commonly, the cheek due to loss of

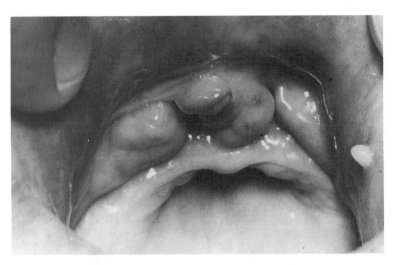

Figure 3.2 Gingival hyperplasia due to an ill-fitting denture. (Reprinted by permission of the publisher, from DeWeese and Saunders, *Textbook of otolaryngology,* 6th edition. St. Louis: The C. V. Mosby Co., 1982.)

sensation may create some swallowing discomfort. These lesions usually appear as small, irregularly shaped areas covered by a gray necrotic membrane surrounded by inflammation (LaVelle and Proctor 1978).

MACROGLOSSIA

An abnormally large tongue can interfere with the propulsive action of the bolus. The clinician should be aware of some of the conditions that may contribute to macroglossia that may be considered in the differential diagnosis. They include macroglossia secondary to lymphatic obstruction secondary to surgery or irradiation, hypothyroidism, mongolism, amyloid deposits, and lymphangiomatous or hemangiomatous processes. The speech and swallowing characteristics in a patient with primary amyloidosis affecting the tongue and cervical musculature have been described (Groher and Enderle, in press).

PHARYNGOESOPHAGEAL DIVERTICULUM

A pharyngoesophageal diverticulum, commonly referred to as Zenker's diverticulum in the cervical esophagus, is an abnormal muscular outpouching that forms either above the cricopharyngeus through Killian's dehiscence or from below through Laimer's triangle. The exact mechanism of pouch formation is unknown, although in small percentages it can be associated with esophageal disease, including traction diverticula, varices, achalasia, carcinoma, and hiatal hernia. Speculation that abnormal relaxation of the cricopharyngeus is the source of pouch formation is not substantiated by manometric evaluation (Knuff et al. 1982). Zenker's diverticula are more common in men in the sixth and seventh decades of life. They must become very large to produce dysphagic symptoms. Patients complain of regurgitation of undigested food, foul breath, fullness in the neck, weight loss, and nocturnal cough with aspiration.

MECHANICAL DYSPHAGIA SECONDARY TO CARCINOMA

The largest group of patients with mechanical swallowing disorders have had oral, pharyngeal, laryngeal, and esophageal structures removed, rearranged, or reconstructed secondary to surgery for carcinoma. Most often, combinations of these structures are involved.

Most clinicians are aware of the general rule for predicting significant dysphagic episodes following surgical excision: if less than 50 percent of an area or organ concerned with deglutition is removed, this will not interfere seriously or permanently with swallowing function (Conley 1960). A review of the pertinent literature suggests that we must use care when applying this rule.

First, the word "seriously" is nonspecific and can be defined in many different and subjective ways. Second, permanent dysphagia could mean that the patient has persistent dysphagia and cannot tolerate oral feedings, or it could mean that there will be difficulty initiating or completing a normal swallow, but oral feedings will be tolerated with limited success if supplemented by alternative methods. Differences in the permanence of the disorders suggest different treatment approaches and final outcomes. In short, the 50 percent rule is only a guide, and individual differences should not be overlooked. In fact, individual differences among patients who have had cancerous lesions and subsequent resections may not be related to the amount of the structure removed, but to factors such as preoperative and postoperative health, psychological reaction to the disability, and ability to learn adaptive swallowing techniques.

The 50 percent rule also applies if the structure in question is rearranged, or if adjacent structures are rearranged (Summers 1974; Weaver and Fleming 1978). Procedures on adjacent structures appear to carry a more negative prognosis for deglutitory recovery than does loss of mobility of those structures (Doberneck and Antoine 1974).

Sessions and co-workers (1979) implied that the 50 percent rule not be applied randomly to any swallowing structure. They pointed out that the original size of the lesion was not as important a prognosticator of dysphagia as was the area excised, and that resultant dysphagia could be predicted if surgical excision involved either the arytenoid cartilages or the base of the tongue. Logemann and Bytell (1979) analyzed swallowing transit times and motility in three separate groups of patients with head and neck resections. They concluded, "We cannot assume that the patient facing less ablative surgery will have only minimal functional problems in swallowing." Although this conclusion appears to stand alone, the differences in data interpretation once again come from how we define a minimal as opposed to a significant swallowing disorder. In fact, the overall success at oral feeding during and after the study period was not reported in the Logemann and Bytell (1979) data. Therefore, it is difficult to interpret the ultimate significance of dysphagia in those patients who have abnormal video-fluoroscopic findings with little ablative surgery.

An additional complication to the loss of structural function is the total or partial loss of sensation, or interruption of the neurologic afferent controls in the oropharynx that surgical procedures can precipitate. The use of tissue flaps to close surgical defects interferes with the normal sensation that provides adequate sensory guidance of the bolus needed to effect a normal swallow.

In addition to receiving surgical treatment for lesions, patients also may be candidates for irradiation in an effort to control the malignancy. There is agreement among clinicians that preoperative or postoperative irradiation predisposes the patient to dysphagic complications more than if this treatment were not undertaken (Summers 1974; Weaver and Fleming 1978; Sessions et al. 1979).

EXPECTED IMPAIRMENT FROM SURGICAL RESECTIONS

Following this introduction to mechanical deglutition disorders secondary to carcinoma, the impairment that can be expected from the most common types of resections is reviewed.

Oral Lesions

Cancers in the oral cavity may involve the anterior tongue, floor of the mouth and submental structures, mandible, and maxilla. Many times, more than one of these structures is involved. It is not unusual to have parts of the tongue, mandible, and floor of the mouth resected.

In general, patients with resected oral structures have difficulty with mastication, formation and retention of a bolus, and anteroposterior transport. Major resections of parts of the mandible and submental region can significantly alter the relationships among oral, pharyngeal, and laryngeal structures, resulting in disturbance of the sequential movements involved in swallowing. For instance, loss of the occlusal jaw relationships after mandibulectomy can interfere with mastication in such a way as to lengthen the oral phase of feeding. This can result not only in delayed and therefore poorly timed propulsion, but in premature attempts at swallowing because the delay is not well tolerated by most patients.

Patients with resections that involve the tongue (glossectomy) experience difficulty with bolus transport to the oropharynx. The question of how much this delay in schedule permanently interferes with the oral route of feeding remains somewhat controversial; most evidence supports the fact that even patients who lose all of their tongue can swallow.

After reviewing over 700 patients with resected tongue lesions (some had had preoperative irradiation), Frazell and Lucas (1962) reported that 40 of the 168 patients experienced transitory dysphagic complications, and only 13 of the 168 required permanent tube feedings. Other investigators have reported similar success, although most describe periods of transitory postoperative dysphagia that is dependent partially on the amount of tongue that is resected. Frazell and Lucas (1962) implied that the prognosis for recovery of swallow was better for those who did not have structures other than the tongue resected, such as part of the mandible or the submental region. They concluded that postoperative complications were correlated more positively with preoperative factors such as age and general health, size and position of the primary tumor, invasion of neighboring structures, and status of the regional lymph nodes.

Conley (1960) and Summers (1974) agreed that patients who lose up to one-third of the tongue have only transitory swallowing disorders. These resolve in two to four weeks without specific remediation of dysphagia.

Logemann and Bytell (1979) provided a more detailed analysis of the deglutition problems glossectomy patients might encounter one week after attempts at oral feeding. They studied by videofluoroscopy ten patients who had excision of lesions of the floor of the mouth and tongue (10 to 70 percent of those structures) with accompanying dissections of the anterior mandible and neck. All had difficulty forming and maintaining a bolus. Oral transit times were delayed, except in the two patients who had longitudinally divided tongue flaps. Eight of the patients were unable to chew because they could not orient material to the molar table. All experienced difficulty with anterior drooling. The swallowing stimuli (thin barium, cookie coated with barium paste, cookie with thin barium) often collected in the anterior and lateral sulci. Oral content of thick consistency was accumulated on the oral palate. Anteroposterior propulsion was disturbed and the bolus frequently spilled into the oropharynx before the patient was ready to initiate a swallow. This was true for all food consistencies used, except for the thin paste that required less oral effort and was associated with better transport times. Once the bolus was moved posteriorly, all patients could initiate a swallow.

Kothary and DeSouza (1973) used cineradiography in their analysis of 25 patients undergoing glossectomy. They found that these patients compensated well for poor lingual propulsion by increasing the use of the buccal musculature, inclining the floor of the mouth, and more prominent forward movement of the pharyngeal musculature.

Even though these problems exist in the early postoperative stages, reports in the literature suggest that patients with tongue resections uncomplicated by surgical involvement of related structures are able to take nutrition orally after no longer than a 1-month period of adjustment to their disability. Unfortunately, a significant number of patients must undergo resection of structures of more than the tongue to achieve adequate control of the cancer.

Patients with resections of the tongue, neck, floor of the mouth, and man-

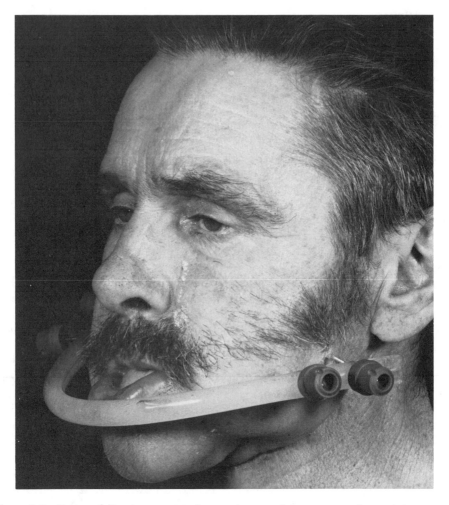

Figure 3.3 Patient following surgery for carcinoma of the anterior floor of the mouth and mandible with a right radical and left suprahyoid resection including the tongue. A right trapezius myocutaneous flap was used to reconstruct the oral cavity and a biphase appliance was used to temporarily fixate the mandible.

dible (Figure 3.3) have different degrees of dysphagia impairment: of the masticatory process, bolus control, and anteroposterior propulsion. Reconstruction of the structures in the mandibular region can create scar tissue contractures and temporomandibular joint pain interfering with normal mastication (Figure 3.4). Not only is it difficult to place food due to limited excursion, but subsequent swallows may be poorly timed because of abnormal occlusal relationships. These poor mandibular/maxillary contacts make biting and chewing more of an effort and tend to interfere with bolus formation.

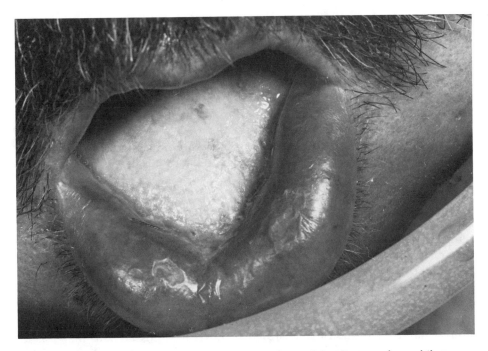

Figure 3.4 Floor of the mouth of the patient in Figure 3.3. Absence of a mobile tongue and a lower immobile lip made anterior/posterior propulsion difficult.

Oropharyngeal Lesions

Oropharyngeal lesions may include anterior tongue resections, as well as resections of the soft palate, retromolar trigone, tonsils, base of tongue, and superior and lateral pharynx. In general, patients with oropharyngeal resections may experience nasal regurgitation, decreased bolus transit, aspiration, and pharyngoesophageal segment dysfunction.

Patients who undergo glossectomy that includes the base of the tongue are susceptible to persistent dysphagia, although the majority can successfully eat orally. Donaldson et al. (1968) reported that 8 of 14 patients with total glossectomy had no dysphagia, while the remaining six had to rely on tube feedings. One of the six eventually had to undergo elective total laryngectomy to control the dysphagia. Myers (1972) reported a higher swallowing success rate in a series of 14 patients following glossectomy, all but one of whom were able to take nutrition orally. Summers (1974) noted that the majority of patients with glossectomy do well following surgery because they are able to protect their airway with an intact laryngeal sphincter.

Summers (1974) found that patients with composite resections required weeks or months to relearn swallowing, and that there usually is a much more pronounced degree of frustration with eating than for those who had only glossectomy. Conley (1960) supported this observation by noting that patients who had a hemiglossectomy with dissection of the floor of the mouth, adjacent mandible, and ipsilateral neck did recover the ability to swallow, but with some aspiration, coughing, and anxiety associated with swallowing attempts.

Patients who undergo glossectomy and bony palate resections lose the ability to generate the adequate force necessary to propel a bolus into the pharynx. Aspiration can occur due to loss of bolus control as well as nasal regurgitation. Lack of tongue strength and mobility results in an inability to generate the pressure required to move the bolus from the mouth to the pharynx (McConnell et al. 1987). This may result in premature leakage of contents into the pharynx, with subsequent aspiration or nasal regurgitation. For those with bony palate deficits a palatal stent may be placed at the time of surgery. However, it may not allow for complete occlusion between the oral and nasal cavity as air pressure may be lost along the lateral sulcus. For this reason, patients may complain of dysphagia, although it is transitory and they learn to compensate. Dietary modifications such as pureed food textures with thin liquids and head posturing techniques generally facilitate swallow.

Ablative surgery on the oropharynx usually includes combined resection of the soft palate and tonsillar pillars. This type of resection may interfere with transportation of bolus material through the pharynx because normal sensory input is interrupted due to reconstructive efforts using tissue flaps that contain no sensory innervation. These tissue flaps also interfere with swallow since they act passively rather than actively, resulting in the loss of the normal propulsive action supplied by the pharyngeal constrictor musculature. If the flaps are bulky, they also may interfere mechanically with the passage of a bolus.

Patients who must undergo glossectomy and submental resections not only may lose tongue propulsion and lip sensation, but the protective tilting action of the larynx provided by the hypomandibular constrictors is sacrificed. This can result in significant aspiration. Conley (1960) reported that patients who had undergone total glossectomy with bilateral dissections of cervical lymph nodes swallowed poorly, but if both superior laryngeal nerves, the hyoid, and the epiglottis were intact, they could swallow a liquid diet without aspiration.

Partial Laryngectomy

Partial laryngectomy is a general category of surgical resection of the pharyngeal and laryngeal region that seeks to control a malignancy while preserving vocal function and deglutition. These procedures are principally hemilaryngectomy and supraglottic laryngectomy.

Hemilaryngectomy

Definitions vary on what constitutes a hemilaryngectomy because some are complete and others are partial. Leonard et al. (1972) defined it as unilateral excision of the vocal fold plus extension to the anterior commissure or the vocal processes, or both. Weaver and Fleming's (1978) definition includes unilateral resection of the vocal fold, vestibular fold, ventricle, and superior laryngeal nerve with preservation of the epiglottis. The present discussion uses the latter definition. The typical resection that comprises a hemilaryngectomy is illustrated in Figure 3.5.

Weaver and Fleming (1978) studied a group of 11 patients undergoing hemilaryngectomy at periods of 6 weeks and 6 months postresection. The results showed that 7 of 11 had no swallowing difficulty with solids or liquids at either evaluation. Two patients had initial problems that resolved at 6 months, one failed to swallow adequately after 6 months, and one had recurrence of disease. The only patient who did not recover swallow had preoperative irradiation, neck dissection, and a postoperative fistula.

Leonard et al. (1972) found similarly encouraging results. Of the 75 patients with excised unilateral lesions that had not extended significantly, aspiration was not a problem except in those who already were debilitated and also had poor

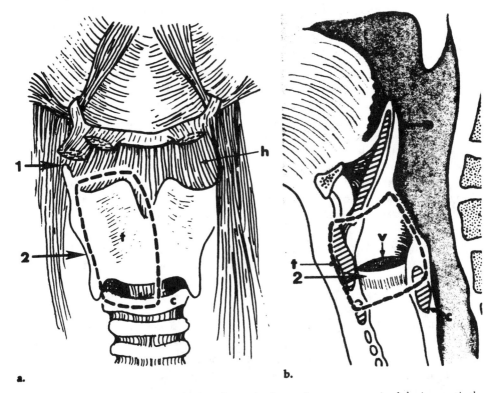

a.   **b.**

Figure 3.5 Frontal (a) and lateral (b) schematic views of structures excised during vertical hemilaryngectomy (enclosed within dashed lines). 1, level of the superior cornua of the thyroid cartilage; 2, level of the glottis; t, thyroid cartilage; c, cricoid cartilage; h, thyrohyoid membrane; e, epiglottis; v, laryngeal ventricle. (Reprinted with permission from Disantis DJ, Balfe DM, Hayden R, et al. The neck after vertical hemilaryngectomy: computed tomography. *Radiology* 1984: 151:683-7.)

pulmonary function. None of the 75 had an immobile vocal fold prior to surgery. The authors implied that this may have contributed significantly to their good results.

The results reported by Schoenrock and associates (1972) were less encouraging. After unilaterally severing and elevating the infrahyoid muscles to form a perichondrial muscle pedicle flap, the thyroid ala, arytenoid, and vestibular and vocal folds were removed. In addition, the ipsilateral superior laryngeal nerve was sectioned and the piriform sinus obliterated. Seven of the 11 patients who were studied 2 months postoperatively aspirated thin barium; one aspirated thick barium. Of the seven patients, only three subjectively complained of aspiration. Schoenrock's group (1972) attributed their findings to the fact that the larynx did not rise evenly on the excised side. This created a tilting of the larynx that directed the barium to the resected side, eventually spilling into the trachea. Cineradiography showed seven patients' larynges failed to meet the base of the tongue on the excised side during the swallow, thus offering limited protection against penetration into the trachea. In addition, normal sequential pharyngeal constriction was absent on the involved side, further contributing to aspiration. These authors noted that all seven patients had incompetent glottal chinks. Four of the seven could not achieve enough movement to get closure and three had good movement, but the functioning true vocal fold met the excised mucosal surface at a different level. It is interesting to note that even though aspiration in some of these patients was not subjectively apparent, it was demonstrated by chest radiography. This finding seemed to suggest that patients may be asymptomatic for a long period of time and then develop pulmonary complications, including minimal basilar pneumonia, pulmonary fibrosis, multiple lobe aspiration, aspiration pneumonia, and lung abscess.

Because there are alternatives to a complete hemilaryngectomy, such as laryngofissure and frontal lateral partial laryngectomy, fewer total hemilaryngectomies are being performed.

Supraglottic Laryngectomy

Supraglottic laryngectomy has several definitions. Weaver and Fleming (1978) defined it as a resection that "typically includes both false cords, both aryepiglottic folds, and one or both superior laryngeal nerves." Summers (1974) defined the resection as a "block resection of the vallecula, epiglottis, hyoid bone, aryepiglottic folds, ventricular bands, upper third of the thyroid cartilage, and thyrohyoid membrane." Flores and co-workers (1982) agreed with Summers and included the pre-epiglottic space. They pointed out that some supraglottic resections extend to include the resection of one arytenoid, the pyriform sinus (partial laryngopharyngectomy), and/or the base of the tongue. The careful reader will note the potential differences in data interpretation relative to supraglottic resections as different criteria for patient selection may bias the results. For the purposes of this discussion, a supraglottic laryngectomy includes resection of both vestibular and aryepiglottic folds and one or both superior laryngeal nerves (Weaver and Fleming 1978) (Figure 3.6).

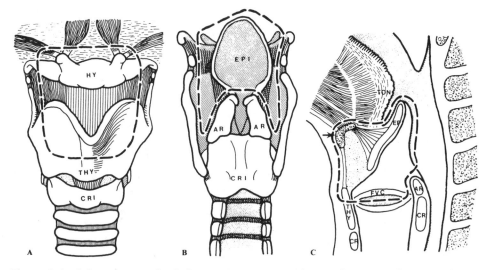

Figure 3.6 Subtotal supraglottic laryngectomy: surgical procedure. Line drawing of the larynx; dashed lines indicate the margin of resection. (A) View from the front; the surgeon resects portions of the hyoid bone (HY), thyrohyoid ligament, and thyroid cartilage (THY). (B) View from the rear; the resection includes the epiglottis (EPI), aryepiglottic folds, and portions of the piriform sinuses. The arytenoid cartilages (AR) are spared in routine operations; in extended procedures, a portion of one arytenoid may be shaved (CRI, cricoid cartilage). (C) View from the side; the resection extends into the vallecula and tongue base and removes the hyoid bone (arrow), pre-epiglottic fat, and false vocal cord (FVC). THY, thyroid cartilage; CR, cricoid cartilage; AR, arytenoid cartilage. (Reprinted with permission from Springer-Verlag, from Balfe DM. Dysphagia after laryngeal surgery. *Dysphagia* 1990; 5:20-34.)

Most investigators agree that supraglottic resections are not without dysphagic complications, especially in the immediate (2- to 4-week) postoperative period. The eventual severity and duration beyond this period appears to be highly variable, however, partly due to the fact that not all supraglottic resections remove identical structures, some patients develop postsurgical complications, and some receive either preoperative or postoperative irradiation. While a small majority eventually do swallow with minimal aspiration, resections that compromise the arytenoids and extend into piriform sinus and tongue base create significant and sometimes persisting dysphagia (Conley 1960; Staple and Ogura 1966; Litton and Leonard 1969; Summers 1974; Weaver and Fleming 1978; Flores et al. 1982). Loss of the tongue base apparently impairs glottic protection as the larynx is elevated. Loss of arytenoid mass also results in impairment of the glottis at the laryngeal level.

Sacrificing one superior laryngeal nerve (SLN) during supraglottic resection does not significantly interfere with swallowing, although bilateral excision carries a negative prognosis for pharyngeal deglutition (Shedd 1976; Weaver and Fleming 1978). Bocca et al. (1968) and Flores et al. (1982) did not find that bilateral excision of the superior laryngeal nerve influenced the severity or duration of dysphagia. In fact, the latter group reported that immediate success at deglutition (as a proportional percentage) was higher with bilateral SLN resections, although this was not statistically significant. They pointed out that this variable "probably should not be considered separately since preservation of one SLN is related to the preservation of the hyoid bone." Their patients with hyoid resections had a better prognosis for swallowing.

Weaver and Fleming (1978) measured swallowing competence of 23 patients following unilateral and bilateral supraglottic resections at 6 weeks and 6 months after surgery. All 23 had difficulty with both liquids and solids. After 6 months, 16 still had dysphagia that ranged from mild to persistent. The most severely affected patients also had had resections of the tongue base. Not one of the four who underwent bilateral supraglottic resections regained their normal swallow, although three were able to maintain their weight with acceptable levels of aspiration (e.g., no pulmonary complications). The one patient who had persistent aspiration had both superior laryngeal nerves severed and also had postoperative irradiation.

Staple and Ogura (1966) followed 36 patients with supraglottic laryngectomy who had excision of the epiglottis, both aryepiglottic folds and the pre-epiglottic space, vestibular folds, upper one-third of the thyroid cartilage on the affected side, and a smaller segment on the unaffected side. One-half of the 36 had initial periods of barium aspiration but regained their swallowing function so that oral nutrition could be maintained. Five patients evidenced persistent dysphagia but did well after 1 to 2 years. This led the authors to remark on the potential adaptability of the surgically interrupted swallowing mechanism. Because half of this group did experience some mild aspiration, a follow-up study (Staple et al. 1967) was done to assess the long-term effects on the lungs of mild aspiration. Chest films were taken at four months and an average of two and one-half years after surgery. At 4 months, 14 of the 27 patients reviewed had pneumonia. At 2 years, 13 of the 39 studied had pneumonia. The authors concluded that although patients who aspirated during these measurements had a poor prognosis for recovery of deglutition, the outcome was, in most cases, not fatal.

Flores and co-workers (1982) studied those particular factors that might correlate with success in oral deglutition in 46 patients following supraglottic laryngeal surgery. Most of the 46 received high-dose preoperative irradiation. All underwent a typical (Weaver and Fleming 1978) procedure. Some had additional resections, including the arytenoid, piriform sinus, and tongue base. Twenty-eight patients were able to rely solely on oral intake within five days after removal of the nasogastric tube. Nine experienced delayed recovery, but could rely solely on oral intake after 4 weeks to 5 months. Nine patients failed to swallow. The authors reported that age did not seem to be an important factor in predicting recovery, nor did preservation of the superior larynx or hyoid. Of the 15 patients in whom one arytenoid was sacrificed, a higher proportion (47 percent) failed to swallow than when both were preserved. Partial laryngopharyngectomy carried a negative prognosis for swallowing, although the most successful outcome in this group was in the only patient with preserved arytenoid function.

Logemann and Bytell (1979) studied eight patients with supraglottic laryngectomy with resections ranging from 10 to 50 percent of the tongue base. Fifty percent of the patients aspirated, with test materials falling diffusely into the pharynx in 75 to 92 percent. Laryngeal constriction was limited in one-half of the patients. This group also had some slowing of oral and pharyngeal transit times when compared with healthy persons.

Of 24 patients undergoing traditional and more extensive supraglottic resections, 16 aspirated thick barium paste, although in none was swallow incapacitated (Litton and Leonard 1969). Cineradiography revealed that 13 of the 16 had barium trapped over the laryngeal inlet and could not clear it on repeated attempts. All 16 who aspirated had pharyngeal involvement in addition to the supraglottic resection. Six also underwent tongue resections. The eight who did not aspirate all evidenced elevation of the laryngeal remnant and none had a resection that involved the pharyngeal wall.

Bocca's group (1968) reported on 223 cases of classic supraglottic resection. No patient received irradiation and only six experienced dysphagia incident to poor arytenoid movement. In the majority of cases, dysphagia subsided within 3 weeks. Of 192 patients who received irradiation only for treatment of supraglottic lesions, this therapy did not produce significant dysphagia in any (Fayos 1975).

Epiglottic reconstruction following supraglottic laryngectomy for the prevention of dysphagia has been successfully performed (Calcaterra 1985). Calcaterra demonstrated reconstruction of a neoglottis from an epiglottis microscopically free of tumor. The neoglottis functionally projects over one-half of the laryngeal inlet and diverts food to the piriform fossae. Calcaterra (1985) studied 14 patients over a 3-year period who underwent reconstruction of a neoglottis at the time of supraglottic laryngectomy. Of these 14 patients, most were able to swallow on their first attempt without significant aspiration, and none exceeded 3 days of intravenous or nasogastric tube feeds. Additionally, there were no instances of airway obstruction that required long-term tracheostomy.

There are numerous conclusions that become apparent when assessing the potential effects on deglutition following supraglottic laryngectomy. First, patients who undergo the classic resection without bilateral denervation of the superior laryngeal nerve experience mild and transitory dysphagia (Staple and Ogura 1966; Bocca et al. 1968; Weaver and Fleming 1978). If the resection extends into the piriform sinus, pharynx, or the tongue base, approximately one-half of patients have moderate to severe dysphagia, but may be able to tolerate limited oral feedings (Staple and Ogura 1966; Litton and Leonard 1969; Logemann and Bytell 1979).

Second, patients who do best after supraglottic resections have the following characteristics: a mobile tongue base (Staple and Ogura 1966; Shedd 1976; Weaver and Fleming 1978; Sessions et al. 1979), a larynx that rises far enough to meet the tongue base (Bocca et al. 1968; Litton and Leonard 1969), a resected hyoid bone (Flores et al. 1982), and a glottis that allows for bilateral approximation of the vocal folds (Staple and Ogura 1966; Summers 1974; Sessions et al. 1979; Flores et al. 1982). Support for myotomy (surgical relaxation of the cricopharyngeus muscle) at the time of surgery as a procedure to prevent aspiration is provided by Staple and Ogura (1976), rejected by Weaver and Fleming (1978), and is thought to be useful when the hyoid or arytenoid cartilage must be sacrificed (Bocca et al. 1967). Myotomy produces more immediate successful swallowing, but is not effective postoperatively in assisting patients who do not swallow well following supraglottic resection (Flores et al. 1982). Summers (1974) felt the myotomy should be considered in patients expected to have significant postoperative sialorrhea.

Laryngectomy

Even though the alimentary and respiratory tracts are separated surgically (see Figure 3.7), patients undergoing total laryngectomy still are at risk for dysphagic complications, especially in the acute stages of recovery. The reported incidence of dysphagia ranges from 10 to 58 percent (Balfe et al. 1982; Nayer et al. 1984). As might be expected, most of these focus on the physiologic changes the surgery might produce on the cricopharyngeus muscle. Early reports (Schobinger 1958) concluded that postoperative dysphagia was the result of the cricopharyngeus muscle in spasm. More recent investigations have shown that the cricopharyngeus fails to perform, but not necessarily in a spasmodic fashion.

Using manometrics, Hanks and colleagues (1981) concluded that following laryngectomy the cricopharyngeus was not spastic, but weaker. Summers (1974) pointed out that in the absence of stricture at this level, the cricopharyngeus performs in an incoordinated manner because of detached inferior constrictor muscles. Summers (1974) and Kirchner and colleagues (1963) are in agreement that the changes in cricopharyngeal function create a pharyngeal pseudodiverticulum that, in turn, may become the source of regurgitation. Such pseudodiverticula are found at the base of the tongue and in the posterior pharyngeal wall.

Following laryngectomy, the percentage of patients with postsurgical chronic dysphagia is poorly documented. In one study, five of ten patients developed dysphagia (Duranceau et al. 1976). Based on manometrics, all ten were found to have marked derangements in the upper esophageal sphincter.

Balfe et al. (1982) performed barium esophagrams on 45 total laryngectomy patients whose follow-up ranged from 6 months to 17 years. Forty of these patients had pharyngeal symptoms and 26 complained of dysphagia. Of the 40 patients with pharyngeal symptoms, the final diagnosis included recurrent neoplasm (15), benign stricture (14), fistula (13), cricopharyngeal muscle dysfunction (12), second primary in the esophagus (2), and abscess (1). Seventeen patients had more than one abnormality. The effect of irradiation on swallow is not described in this study, or to what extent dysphagia interfered with oral intake.

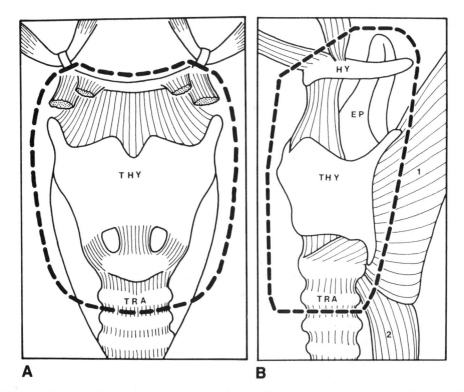

A **B**

Figure 3.7 Total laryngectomy: line drawings of the surgical procedure. (A) Frontal view; the surgeon removes the hyoid bone, thyroid cartilage (THY), cricoid cartilage, and often the first tracheal ring (TRA). (B) Lateral view; the posterior margin of the resection severs the connections of the inferior constrictor (1) and cricopharyngeus (2) muscles. HY, hyoid bone; EP, epiglottis; THY, thyroid cartilage; TRA, trachea. (Reprinted with permission from Springer-Verlag, from Balfe DM. Dysphagia after laryngeal surgery. *Dysphagia* 1990; 5:20-34.)

Kirchner and Scatliff (1962) used cineradiography to examine 43 laryngectomized patients for dysphagia at differing periods of time following surgery. Of the 26 examined immediately postoperatively, they found 12 had dysphagia. Eight of the 12 had fistulas and 4 did not. Even though the majority of the 43 eventually could take their nutrition orally, some had anterior pouch formation with regurgitation, constant accumulation of food and mucus, and complaints of a foreign body sensation.

In a follow-up study, Kirchner and co-workers (1963) examined 35 patients with laryngectomy. They found that dysphagia was caused by a pharyngeal pseudodiverticulum resulting from separation of the pharyngeal suture line at its junction with the tongue base or by uncoordinated contraction of the detached pharyngeal muscles in the absence of stricture.

McConnel et al. (1986) used manofluorography to study 14 total laryngectomy patients in order to analyze the pharyngeal phase of swallow with respect to tongue propulsion, laryngeal movement, and constrictor contraction. Subjects were divided into two groups: nine without tongue impairment and five with tongue impairment. They found that the major functional change in the pharynx following total laryngectomy was increased pharyngeal resistance. Those without tongue impairment compensated by using increased lingual propulsion to overcome increased pharyngeal resistance, whereas those with tongue impairment could not. This resulted in increased pharyngeal transit times for the latter group. Factors discussed that may account for pharyngeal resistance include tongue impairment, anterior pouches, pseudoepiglottis, and pharyngeal or sphincter dismotility. While all of the patients with tongue impairment complained of difficulty swallowing, its effect on weight, diet selection, and nutrition was not documented.

There is some evidence to suggest that a higher percentage of the laryngectomized patients who also receive irradiation experience dysphagia. Three of the five patients examined by Duranceau and colleagues (1976) had postoperative dysphagia. Hanks et al. (1981) studied ten patients who were dysphagic following laryngectomy, seven of whom had received irradiation. This led the authors to conclude that although this number was small, irradiation may adversely influence upper esophageal motility.

Our own experience and that of Weaver and Fleming (1978) suggest that the large majority of those undergoing laryngectomy who have no medical complications swallow a soft diet after 14 days and that irradiation retards this recovery in a small number of patients. Most complain that they are unable to easily swallow tough meats and larger-sized boluses. Forty-seven of 59 laryngectomized patients reported postoperative dysphagia, but all were taking their nutrition orally after discharge from the hospital (Volin 1980). Only one had persistent dysphagia. There was no significant correlation between preoperative and/or postoperative irradiation and dysphagia.

Jung and Adams (1980) did a retrospective review of 226 laryngectomized patients. Of this group 36 (16 percent) experienced dysphagia; 16 had benign pharyngeal stricture, 14 with stricture due to recurrence; 4 had malignant esophageal cancer; and 2 had benign lower esophageal stricture. The majority had preoperative irradiation. Most of those who experienced dysphagia had laryngopharyngectomy. The authors suggested that the complaint of persistent dysphagia may be a sign of early recurrence, especially if the postpharyngeal space is wider than normal, or if patients have benign strictures.

Tracheoesophageal Puncture

The creation of a tracheoesophageal fistula during or after primary laryngectomy has been described as an alternate method for achieving communication (Singer and Blom 1980; Hamaker et al. 1985; Juarbe et al. 1986; Stiernberg et al. 1987; Maniglia et al. 1989). A tracheoesophageal fistula allows the patient to shunt pulmonary air from the trachea into the pharyngoesophageal segment, which acts as a vibrating source for the production of voice. In the usual circumstance a prosthetic valve is placed into the puncture site to facilitate voice and prevent aspiration.

Numerous surgical interventions for the production of alaryngeal speech have been described. None are without complications. Conley et al. (1958), Asai (1972), Taub and Spiro (1972), Staffieri (1973), Singer and Blom (1980), Panje (1981), Wetmore et al. (1981), Li (1985), Andrews et al. (1987), and Saito et al. (1989) have reported complications that may impact on swallow, such as aspiration or leakage of saliva and food; aspiration of the voice prosthesis; stenosis of the hypopharynx, tracheostoma, or esophagus; stomal and fistula infection; development of a secondary fistula; pharyngoesophageal spasm; and migration or progressive fistula enlargement.

Following the creation of a tracheoesophageal fistula, a stent or voice prosthesis may be in place at the tracheoesophageal site when oral feedings are begun. During these initial trial feedings, one should suspect leakage around the prosthesis if the patient coughs during swallow. Aspiration or leakage also may occur through the voice prosthesis. Inspection for dislodgement, proper fitting, or faulty functioning of the voice prosthesis should follow. A modified barium swallowing study performed with the stent or voice prosthesis in place is often helpful to determine the site and amount of aspiration or leakage when clinical information is not available.

Irradiation and Deglutition

It is not infrequent for patients who undergo conservative surgical resections for carcinoma also to receive either preoperative or postoperative irradiation, which produces many potential side effects that may further compromise swallowing. They include oral and pharyngeal inflammation with subsequent pain in the soft tissues and bone, a drying effect on the mucosal tissues, diminished volume and thicker consistency of saliva, changes in taste sensation, and loss of appetite. Not all patients experience these symptoms, but when they do, the severity and duration of effects on deglutition are highly variable (Dreizen et al. 1977a).

Loss of Saliva Flow

If irradiation is directed toward the salivary glands in sufficient amounts, patients experience a marked reduction of salivary flow. These changes tend to be permanent and irreversible (Frank et al. 1953); Dreizen et al. 1977b). Of 42 patients with oral cancers who received 260 rads per day, 5 days a week, salivary flow rates after mastication dropped to 57 percent after the first week, 76 percent after six weeks, and to 95 percent 3 years after irradiation (Dreizen et al. 1977b).

Hansen et al. (1970) studied the subjective complaints of 80 patients receiving irradiation for oral lesions. Seventy-eight percent experienced xerostomia during the second week of treatment. This complaint ranked first in a list of six. After 6 weeks the same individuals were troubled by xerostomia, and after 3 months it continued to be their major complaint.

When the salivary glands can no longer produce a normal mixture of serous and mucous saliva, deglutition is affected in two ways besides xerostomia: increased dental caries due to loss of the natural defense against decay, and accumulation of stringy mucus that has lost its lubricating abilities (Carl 1980).

Dental caries create pain during mastication if left untreated (Dreizen et al. 1977b; Weaver and Fleming 1978). Decay can begin on any tooth and progresses rapidly toward destruction of the dental crown (Dreizen et al. 1977a) (Figure 3.8). Accumulation of thick mucus can in itself mechanically interfere with swallowing (Figure 3.9). Hansen and colleagues (1970) found that an accumulation of stringy mucus was the second most common complaint (59 percent) after 2 and 6 weeks of irradiation. Patients reported that they were most uncomfortable when the dryness and thick mucus were at their highest point on the

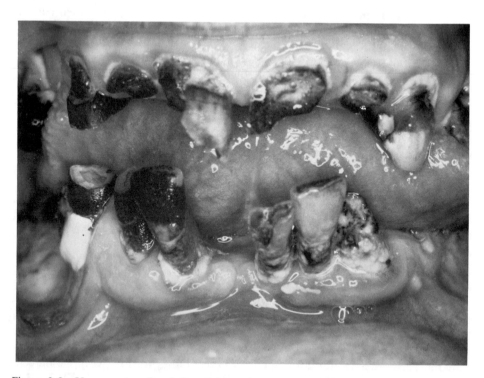

Figure 3.8 Xerostomia-related dental decay 2 years after radiotherapy in a patient with cancer of the tongue. (Reprinted by permission of the publisher, from Dreizen et al., *Postgrad Med* 61, 1977a.)

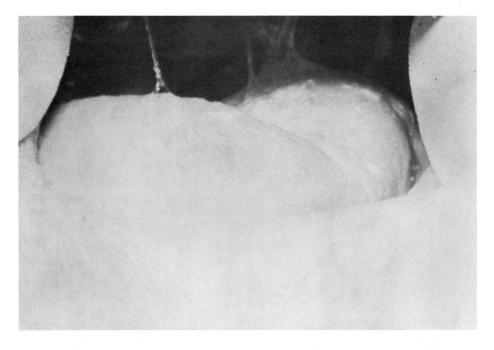

Figure 3.9 Patient with thick mucous secretions secondary to radiotherapy following resection of cancer of the tongue.

twelfth day of radiotherapy. These thick secretions also interfere with denture retention, tissue tolerance to the denture, and taste (Summers 1974).

Kuten and associates (1986) examined the effects of field arrangement, amount of salivary glands irradiated, clinical manifestations such as dryness of the mouth, taste impairment, dysphagia, salivary secretion, and composition, and oral yeast flora on 32 patients treated with external irradiation to the head and neck. The patients received either primary or postoperative radiation therapy and were divided into four groups based on the volume of area irradiated. After 1,000 to 2,000 cGy, 29 of the 30 patients developed a variety of oral symptoms, with each patient experiencing at least one symptom, including xerostomia (81 percent), taste impairment (62 percent), dysphagia (59 percent), soreness (37 percent), and increase in salivary viscosity (16 percent). Twenty-two percent of those patients who reported xerostomia were experiencing this symptom prior to radiotherapy. The examiners concluded that at least 50 percent of the parotid gland must be spared from the field of radiation in order to prevent severe dryness. The severity of oral symptoms was shown to increase as salivary gland involvement in the radiated field was extended. Decrease in salivary secretions was accompanied by an increase in salivary sodium concentration and oral yeast flora.

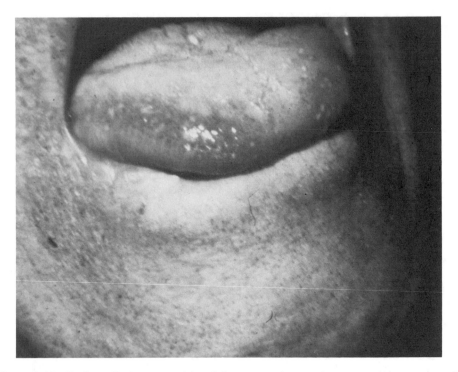

Figure 3.10 Early radiation mucositis of the tongue in a patient treated for cancer of the floor of the mouth. (Reprinted by permission of the publisher, from Dreizen et al., *Postgrad Med* 61, 1977a.)

Mucositis

Irradiation can produce significant inflammatory changes in the mucous lining, resulting in tenderness and burning not unlike a severe sore throat. A more marked form of these complaints may surface as mucositis (Figure 3.10). When the pain spreads to the pharyngeal mucosa, swallowing can be difficult. This discomfort is antagonized by coarse and highly seasoned foods. Hansen's group (1970) found that 33 percent of their patients complained that inflamed mucosa impeded swallowing. Three months following irradiation, patients no longer had this complaint. In their study of 32 patients, who received primary or postoperative head and neck irradiation, Kuten and associates (1986) found clinical manifestations of mucositis 3 weeks following the initiation of full-course radiation therapy. Patients were noted to have dry oral mucosa (53 percent), erythema of the mucosal surface (45 percent), and mucosal plaque formation (64 percent). They concluded that dysphagia was secondary not only to dryness caused by decreased salivary secretion, but more so to factors such as radiation damage to mucosal surfaces, edema, and infection. Dreizen et al. (1977a) reported that mucositis gradually improved spontaneously 3 weeks following termination of radiotherapy. Oral mucositis may also result from the use of chemotherapeutic agents such as adriamycin, methotrexate, and cyclophosphamide (Carl 1980).

Osteoradionecrosis

Osteoradionecrosis can result from oral mucosal destruction at the primary site of irradiation. Developing fibrosis and reduction of blood supply result in the formation of necrotic ulcers that if left untreated can invade bony structures through infectious processes. Ulcers can develop 2 to 3 months after radiotherapy or any time thereafter (Dreizen et al. 1977a). The resultant pain can impair oral feeding actions and swallowing to the point at which patients are not able to take nutrition orally. Patients are most vulnerable to osteoradionecrosis of the jaw during the 2 years following irradiation (Dreizen et al. 1977a). Spongy bones are more susceptible to osteoradionecrosis than flat bones. As a result, the mandible and zygomatic bones are more often affected than the mandible. A clinical example is presented in Figure 3.11.

Trismus

Patients who have difficulty with mastication in the form of tonic spasms during or following irradiation may be suffering from trismus. Trismus is believed to occur secondary to fibrosis of the muscles of mastication (Parsons 1984). Radiation-induced trismus occurs most often after irradiation of the nasophar-

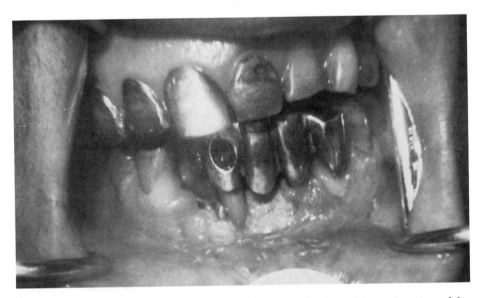

Figure 3.11 Osteoradionecrosis of the mandibular alveolar bone in a patient treated for cancer of the tongue. (Reprinted by permission of the publisher, from Dreizen et al., *Postgrad Med* 61, 1977a.)

ynx, tonsil, retromolar trigone, or paranasal sinuses. Patients who have received both surgery and irradiation are at greater risk of developing trismus than those patients who are treated with either modality alone (Parsons 1984). If severe trismus develops, dental extraction may become necessary for feeding. In addition, jaw excursions may be painful and limited. Temporomandibular joint exercises should begin following surgery and continue during and following radiotherapy to prevent the development of trismus. The success of therapeutic exercise methods depend on the severity of the fibrosis and patient compliance (Barrett et al. 1988).

Loss of Taste and Appetite

Patients often experience weight loss during radiation therapy due to a decreased ability to taste, chew, smell, and swallow. All of these factors contribute to a reduction in appetite. Hansen and associates (1970) reported that 53 percent of their patients experienced loss of appetite during and shortly after irradiation. Twenty-two percent said that this was due to a loss of taste, while the remaining 78 percent felt it was related to feelings of nausea and a general dissatisfaction with their diet. Acuity of taste is recovered rapidly at first and then more slowly. A tumor that is necrotic or infected also may predispose the patient to nausea and vomiting. Patients generally recover taste acuity 20 to 60 days following radiotherapy, and it fully returns after 120 days (Dreizen et al. 1977a). Others have reported specific losses of sweet, salt, and bitter tastes (Conger 1973; DeWys and Walters 1975). Sour and bitter tastes are suppressed more than sweet and salty; however, most patients complain that all food has lost its flavor (Jepson 1985). Aversions to meat and vegetable proteins have also been noted (Fleming et al. 1977). Such aversions can lead to loss of appetite, disinterest in food, and eventually, to poor nutrition. Severe loss of proteins, calories, vitamins, and minerals can lead to a nutritional deficiency type of stomatitis.

CERVICAL SPINE DISEASE

Osteophytic changes in the cervical spine that put undue mechanical pressure on the proximal pharynx or esophagus must be considered in the differential diagnosis of mechanical dysphagia.

Although pressure on the pharynx from the cervical spine is rare (Umerah et al. 1981), other investigators feel that it may just be overlooked as a potential cause and therefore is not as rare as once believed (Lambert et al. 1981). Radiographically, cervical osteophytes appear as bony projections from one or more of the cervical vertebrae, with displacement of the posterior pharyngeal or common esophageal wall. Typically, it is found in elderly patients with cervical spondylosis (Umerah et al. 1981) and usually is seen at the level of C4 to C7 (Lambert et al. 1981). Patients complain of pain at the cricopharyngeal level probably due to the pressure of food on the osteophytes (Umerah et al. 1981).

All patients complain that solids are harder to swallow than liquids (Lambert et al. 1981). In addition to dysphagia, other symptoms such as cough, stridor, hoarseness, and other laryngeal or pharyngeal disorders may be present (Girgis et al. 1982). A review of the history of spinal diseases and dysphagia is provided by Gamache and Voorhies (1980).

NASOENTERIC TUBES

Acutely ill patients may be placed on either enteral or parenteral nutrition as a primary means of nutritional support or as a supplement in patients with inadequate oral intake. Nasoenteric tubes may complicate oral feedings due to mechanical interference and by their association with an increased incidence of aspiration pneumonia.

We have clinically observed that large-bore nasogastric feeding tubes are more likely to interfere with the smooth passage of semisolid and solid bolus textures. Bolus residual may remain in the hypopharynx or be directed toward the airway. Consequently, in those patients who require supplemental nasoenteric feeding tubes it is preferable to have a small-bore feeding tube in place during dysphagia evaluations and when oral feedings are begun.

Enteral support using a nasogastric tube may lead to aspiration due to hypersalivation, depressed cough reflex, laryngopharyngeal injuries, gastroesophageal reflux, and dislodgement of the tube into the esophagus or trachea (Noone and Graham 1973; Alessi and Berci 1986). Risk factors predisposing a patient with nasoenteral feedings to aspiration pneumonia include reduced level of consciousness (less than alert and oriented), with consequent compromise in glottic closure and cough reflex, dysphagia from neurologic or esophageal mechanisms, vomiting, ilius or gastric dilation, and failure to maintain elevation of the head (Awe et al. 1966; Cameron and Zuidema 1972; Bartlett and Gorbach 1975; Torosean and Rombeau 1976; Metheny et al. 1986).

In a study conducted by Sitzmann (1990), 90 patients were reviewed who had been admitted to Johns Hopkins Hospital with a primary complaint of dysphagia. Patients were divided into two groups based on the etiology of dysphagia: neurogenic (43) and mechanical (47). All patients were placed on enteral (63 percent) or parenteral (37 percent) nutrition due to marked malnutrition. Patients with nasoenteric tubes had a 40 percent complication rate (aspiration or endotracheal placement of the tube), resulting in a 30 percent mortality. This mortality was significantly higher than seen with other treatment modalities, such as jejunostomy tube feedings and total parenteral nutrition. Both nasoenteric and gastrostomy tube feedings were associated with an increased risk of aspiration pneumonia. Sitzmann concluded that patients admitted to a hospital with the primary complaint of dysphagia that has led to severe malnutrition should not be placed on nasoenteric or gastrostomy feeding tubes until the dysphagia has resolved. It was also suggested that hospitalized dysphagic patients should be evaluated by cineradiography in order to rule out reflux or aspiration before oral or nasoenteric feedings are begun.

TRACHEOSTOMA TUBES

Tracheostoma tubes create a mechanical interference to swallowing by restricting normal laryngeal elevation. Loss of elevation compromises glottal protection and invites aspiration. Butcher (1982) reported that tracheostoma tubes increased the chances of aspiration by fixing the larynx anteriorly and preventing its axial rotation. Arms et al. (1974) demonstrated that one is at a greater risk for aspiration if a tracheostoma tube is in place.

Bonanno (1971) attempted to investigate the theory that tracheostoma tubes could contribute to dysphagia. He studied 43 patients who underwent elective or semi-elective tracheostomy for general surgery. All were considered to be poor pulmonary risks for general anesthesia. None had head or neck cancer. Previous medical health was not reported. Three of the 43 had postoperative dysphagia because, Bonanno felt, the tracheostoma tube appeared to be anchoring the trachea to the pretracheal strap muscles and the skin of the neck, thus limiting anterior elevation and rotation. Lack of this movement interfered with relaxation of the cricopharyngeus.

Stauffer et al. (1981) prospectively studied the complications and consequences of endotracheal intubation and tracheotomy in 150 critically ill patients. Of the 150 patients, 97 received only endotracheal intubation, 46 received tracheotomies following endotracheal intubation, and 7 received only tracheotomy. Of the 53 patients who received a tracheotomy, 51 were standard tracheotomies and two were cricothyroidotomies. The 8 percent incidence of aspiration was similar for those patients who received endotracheal intubation or tracheostomy. Two follow-up visits after extubation were conducted on the patients in this study in order to assess late complications. In the first follow-up visit, 47 patients were evaluated. The incidence of dysphagic complaints was not reported. During a second follow-up visit of 21 patients, dysphagia was reported by 38 percent of patients with tracheotomy and 8 percent of patients with endotracheal intubation.

It has been our experience that the incidence of dysphagia is greater in patients who have tracheostomy combined with surgical resection of the head and neck. In these cases, patients already have compromised deglutition, and the tracheostoma tube serves as an additional barrier to normal laryngeal elevation.

Patients who have cuffed tracheostoma tubes that are overinflated run the risk of esophageal obstruction from the pressure on the tracheoesophageal wall. The obstruction keeps nutrition from entering the esophagus easily, creating spillover and possible aspiration.

An additional complication is that the presence of the tube prevents expiratory air from being shunted superiorly, resulting in a decrease of expired air needed to clear the larynx after swallowing (Weaver and Fleming 1982). This reduction of the ability to clear the airway because of mechanical interference may impede rehabilitation (see Chapter 10).

SUMMARY

Mechanical swallowing dysfunction usually is the result of the oral and/or pharyngeal structures being surgically removed or altered. This impairs the displacement of food in the mouth and the bolus in the pharynx. Even though some patients have adequate sensory and motor components for oral and pharyngeal feeding postoperatively, most have significant dysphagia. Additionally, the majority have adequate cortical skills needed for the rehabilitation of feeding.

The dysphagia liability is increased by radiotherapy and/or chemotherapy. A careful evaluation of the pathology as discussed should assist the clinician in working out the diagnostic dilemmas that these patients often present. Treatment suggestions are provided in detail in Chapter 10.

REFERENCES

Alessi DM, Berci G. Aspiration and nasogastric intubation. Otolaryngol Head Neck Surg 1986; 94:486–9.

Andrews JC, Mickel RA, Hanson DG, et al. Major complications following tracheo-esophageal puncture for voice rehabilitation. Laryngoscope 1987; 97:562–6.

Arms RA, Dines DE, Tinstman TC. Aspiration pneumonia. Chest 1974; 65:136–9.

Asai R. Laryngoplasty after total laryngectomy. Arch Otolaryngol 1972; 95:114–9.

Awe W, Fletcher W, Jacobs S. The pathophysiology of aspiration pneumonia. Surgery 1966; 60:232–9.

Balfe DM, Koehler RE, Setzen M, et al. Barium examination of the esophagus after total laryngectomy. Radiology 1982; 143:501–8.

Barrett NVJ, Martin JW, Jacob RF, et al. Physical therapy techniques in the treatment of the head and neck patient. J Prosthet Dent 1988; 59:343–6.

Bartlett JG, Gorbach SL. The triple threat of aspiration pneumonia. Chest 1975; 68: 560–6.

Blomquist IK, Bayer AS. Life-threatening deep facial space infections of the head and neck. Infect Dis Clin North Am 1988; 2:237–64.

Bocca E, Pignataro O, Mosciaro O. Supraglottic surgery of the larynx. Ann Otol Rhinol Laryngol 1968; 77:1005–26.

Bonanno PC. Swallowing dysfunction after tracheostomy. Ann Surg 1971; 174:29–33.

Butcher BR. Treatment of chronic aspiration as a complication of cerebrovascular accident. Laryngoscope 1982; 92:681–5.

Calcaterra TC. Epiglottic reconstruction after supraglottic laryngectomy. Laryngoscope 1985; 95:786–9.

Cameron JL, Zuidema GD. Aspiration pneumonia: magnitude and frequency of the problem. JAMA 1972; 219:1194–6.

Carl W. Dental management of head and neck cancer patients. J Surg Oncol 1980; 15:265–81.

Cohen EL. Epiglottitis in the adult. Postgrad Med 1984; 75:309–11.

Conger AD. Loss and recovery of taste acuity in patients irradiated to the oral cavity. Radiat Res 1973; 53:338–47.

Conley JJ. Swallowing dysfunctions associated with radical surgery of the head and neck. Arch Surg 1960; 80:602–12.

Conley JJ, DeAmesti F, Pierce MK. A new surgical technique for the vocal rehabilitation of the laryngectomized patient. Ann Otol Rhinol Laryngol 1958; 67:655–64.

DeWeese DD, Saunders WH. Textbook of otolaryngology. St. Louis: CV Mosby, 1973.

DeWys WD, Walters K. Abnormalities of taste sensation in cancer patients. Cancer 1975; 36:1888–96.

Doberneck R, Antoine A. Deglutition after resection of oral, laryngeal and pharyngeal cancers. Surgery 1974; 75:87–90.

Donaldson RC, Skelly M, Paletta FX. Total glossectomy for cancer. Am J Surg 1986; 116:585–90.

Dreizen S, Daly TE, Drane JB, et al. Oral complications of cancer radiotherapy. Postgrad Med 1977a; 61:85–92.

Dreizen S, Brown LR, Daly TE, et al. Prevention of xerostomia-related dental caries in irradiated cancer patients. J Dent Res 1977b; 56:99–104.

Duranceau A, Jamieson G, Hurwitz A, et al. Alteration in esophageal motility after laryngectomy. Am J Surg 1976; 131:30–35.

Fayos JV. Carcinoma of the endolarynx: results of irradiation. Cancer 1975; 35:1525–32.

Fleming SM, Weaver AW. Clinical management of dysphagia in head and neck cancer patients. Dysarthria, Dysphonia, Dysphagia 1982; 1:80–84.

Flores TC, Wood BG, Koegel L Jr, et al: Factors in successful deglutition following supraglottic laryngeal surgery. Ann Otol Rhinol Laryngol 1982; 91:579–83.

Frazell EL, Lucas JC. Cancer of the tongue: report of the management of 1,554 patients. Cancer 1962; 15:1085–99.

Gamache FW, Voorhies RM. Hypertrophic cervical osteophytes causing dysphagia. J Neurosurg 1980; 53:338–44.

Girgis IH, Guirguis NN, Mourice M. Laryngeal and pharyngeal disorders in vertebral ankylosing hyperostosis. J Laryngol Otol 1982; 96:659–64.

Greenspan D, Greenspan JS. The oral features of HIV infection. Gastroenterol Clin North Am 1988; 17:535–43.

Groher ME, Enderle EE. Mechanical dysphagia secondary to macroglossia: a case report. Dysphagia, in press.

Hamaker RC, Singer MI, Blom ED, et al. Primary voice restoration at laryngectomy. Arch Otolaryngol 1985; 111:182–6.

Hanks JB, Fisher ST, Myers WC, et al: Effect of total laryngectomy on esophageal motility. Ann Otol Rhinol Laryngol 1981; 90:331–4.

Hansen D, Meyer E, Werner H. Function disorders of the oral cavity as a side effect of radiotherapy. Z Laryngol Rhinol Otol 1970; 49:534–41.

Hawkins DB, Miller AH, Sachs GB, et al. Acute epiglottitis in adults. Laryngoscope 1973; 83:1211–20.

Jepson J. Nutrition in patients irradiated for head and neck cancer. Nutritional Support Services 1985; 5:27–30.

Juarbe C, Shemen L, Eberle R, et al. Primary tracheoesophageal puncture for voice restoration. Am J Surg 1986; 152:464–6.

Jung TT, Adams GL. Dysphagia in laryngectomized patients. Otolaryngol Head Neck Surg 1980; 88:25–33.

Kander PL, Richards SH. Acute epiglottitis in adults. J Laryngol Otol 1977; 91:295–302.

Kerr DA, Ash MM. Oral pathology. Philadelphia: Lea & Febiger, 1978.

Keyes KS. Oral mucosal diseases. In: Paparella MM, Shumrick DA, eds. Otolaryngology: head and neck. Philadelphia: WB Saunders, 1980; 2136–47.

Kirchner JA, Scatliff JH. Disabilities resulting from healed salivary fistula. Arch Otolaryngol 1962; 75:46–54.

Kirchner JA, Scatliff JH, Dey FL, et al. The pharynx after laryngectomy. Laryngoscope 1963; 73:18–33.

Knuff TE, Benjamine SB, Castell DO. Pharyngoesophageal (Zenker's) diverticulum: a reappraisal. Gastroenterology 1982; 82:734–6.

Kothary PM, DeSouza LJ. Swallowing without tongue. Bombay Hosp J 1973; 15:58–62.

Kuten A, Ben-Aryeh H, Berdicevsky I, et al. Oral side effects of head and neck rotation: correlation between clinical manifestations and laboratory data. Int J Radiat Oncol Biol Phys 1986; 12:401–5.

Lambert JR, Tepperman PS, Jimenez J, et al. Cervical spine disease and dysphagia. Am J Gastroenterol 1981; 76:35–40.

LaVelle CLB, Proctor DB. Clinical pathology of the oral mucosa. Hagerstown, MD: Harper & Row, 1978.

Leonard JR, Holt GP, Maran AG. Treatment of vocal cord carcinoma by vertical hemi-laryngectomy. Ann Otol Rhinol Larngygol 1972; 81:469–78.

Li SL. Functional tracheoesophageal shunt for vocal rehabilitation after laryngectomy. Laryngoscope 1985; 95:1267–71.

Litton WB, Leonard JR. Aspiration after partial laryngectomy: cineradiographic studies. Laryngoscope 1969; 75:887–908.

Logemann JA, Bytell DE. Swallowing disorders in three types of head and neck surgical patients. Cancer 1979; 44:1095–1105.

Maniglia AJ, Lundy DS, Casiano RC, et al. Speech restoration and complications of primary versus secondary tracheoesophageal puncture following total laryngectomy. Laryngoscope 1989; 99:489–91.

Mayosmith MF, Hirsch PJ, Wodzinski SF, et al. Acute epiglottitis in adults. N Engl J Med 1986; 314:1133–39.

McConnell FMS, Mendelsohn MS. The effects of surgery on pharyngeal deglutition. Dysphagia 1987; 1:145–51.

McConnell FMS, Mendelsohn MS, Logemann JA. Examination of swallow after total laryngectomy using manofluorography. Head Neck Surg 1986; 9:3–12.

Metheny NA, Eisenberg P, Spies M. Aspiration pneumonia in patients fed through na-soenteral tubes. Heart Lung 1986; 15:256–61.

Myers EN. The role of total glossectomy in the management of cancer of the oral cavity. Otol Clin North Am 1972; 5:343–55.

Nayar RC, Sharma VP, Arora MML. A study of the pharynx after laryngectomy. J Laryngol Otol 1984; 98:807–10.

Noone RB, Graham WP. Nutritional care after head and neck surgery. Postgrad Med 1973; 53:80–4.

Panje WR. Prosthetic voice rehabilitation following laryngectomy. Ann Otol Rhinol Laryngol 1981; 90:116–20.

Parsons JT. The effect of radiation on normal tissues of the head and neck. In: Million RR, Cassisi NJ, eds. Management of head and neck cancer. Philadelphia: J B Lippincott, 1984; 173–207.

Patterson HC, Kelly LH, Strome RR. Ludwig's angina: an update. Laryngoscope 1982; 92:370–8.

Raufman JP. Odynophagia/dysphagia in AIDS. Gastroenterol Clin North Am 1988; 17:599–614.

Saito H, Yoshida S, Saito T, et al. Simple mucodermal tracheoesophageal shunt method for voice restoration. Arch Otolaryngol Head Neck Surg 1989; 115:494–6.

Sarant G. Acute epiglottitis in adults. Ann Emerg Med 1981; 10:58–61.

Schabel SI, Katzberg RW, Burgener FA. Acute inflammation of epiglottis and supraglottic structures in adults. Radiology 1977; 122:601–4.

Schobinger R. Spasm of cricopharyngeus muscle as a cause of dysphagia after total laryngectomy. Arch Otolaryngol 1958; 67:271–5.

Schoenrock LD, King AY, Everts EC, et al. Hemilaryngectomy: deglutition evaluation and rehabilitation. Trans Am Acad Ophthalmol Otolaryngol 1972; 76:752–7.

Schumaker HM, Doris PE, Birnbaum G. Radiographic parameters in adult epiglottitis. Ann Emerg Med 1984; 13:588–90.

Sessions DG, Zill R, Schwartz SL. Deglutition after conservation surgery for cancer of the larynx and hypopharynx. Otolaryngol Head Neck Surg 1979; 87:779–96.

Shedd DP. Rehabilitation problems of head and neck cancer patients. J Surg Oncol 1976; 8:11–21.

Singer MI, Blom ED. An endoscopic technique for restoration of voice after total laryngectomy. Ann Otol Rhinol Laryngol 1980; 89:529–33.

Sitzmann JV. Nutritional support of the dysphagic patient: methods, risks, and complications of therapy. Journal of Parenteral and Enteral Nutrition 1990; 14:60–63.

Staffieri M. Laringectomia totale con ricostruzione di "glottide fonataria." Nuovo Arch Ital Otol 1973; 1:181–98.

Staple TW, Ogura JH. Cineradiography of the swallowing mechanism following supraglottic subtotal laryngectomy. Radiology 1966; 87:226–30.

Staple TW, Ragsdale EF, Ogura JH. The chest roentgenogram following supra-glottic laryngectomy. Am J Roentgenol 1967; 100:583–7.

Stauffer JL, Olson DE, Petty TL. Complications and consequences of endotracheal intubation and tracheotomy. Am J Med 1981; 70:65–76.

Stiernberg CM, Bailey BJ, Calhoun KH, et al. Primary tracheoesophageal fistula procedure for voice restoration: the University of Texas Medical Branch experience. Laryngoscope 1987; 97:820–4.

Summers GW. Physiologic problems following ablative surgery of the head and neck. Otolaryngol Clin North Am 1974; 7:217–50.

Taub S, Spiro RH. Vocal rehabilitation of laryngectomees. Am J Surg 1972; 124:87–90.

Torosean M, Rombeau J. Feeding by tube enterostomy. Surg Gynecol Obstet 1976; 143:273–6.

Umerah BC, Mukherjee BK, Ibekur O. Cervical syopondylosis and dysphagia. J Laryngol Otol 1981; 95:1179–83.

Volin RA. Predicting failure to speak after laryngectomy. Laryngoscope 1980; 90: 1727–36.

Weaver AW, Fleming SM. Partial laryngectomy: analysis of associated swallowing disorders. Am J Surg 1978; 136:486–9.

Wetmore SJ, Johns ME, Baker SR. The Blom-Singer voice restoration procedure. Arch Otolaryngol 1981; 107:674–6.

Williams AC, Guralnick WC. The diagnosis and treatment of Ludwig's angina: report of twenty cases. N Engl J Med 1943; 228:443–50.

4

Esophageal Dysphagia

William J. Ravich

A large number of subspecialties are involved in the evaluation and care of patients with swallowing disorders. Most subspecialists have a limited understanding of the knowledge and technical expertise of other fields. The following chapter offers a gastroenterologist's perspective on dysphagia of presumed and documented esophageal origin, written for clinicians from other subspecialties who wish to acquire a working familiarity with esophageal causes of swallowing problems and their management.

MECHANISMS OF ESOPHAGEAL DYSPHAGIA

The esophagus is a distensible tube, about 20 cm long, connecting the pharynx and stomach. It is separated from the pharynx by the upper esophageal sphincter (UES) and from the stomach by the lower esophageal sphincter (LES). Under resting conditions, the esophageal lumen is collapsed, a potential space that can distend easily to accommodate swallowed air, liquids, or solids. The act of swallowing initiates pharyngeal peristalsis as well as relaxation of both the upper and lower esophageal sphincters. The pharyngeal peristaltic contractile wave is propagated through the UES and continues down the length of the esophagus, pushing the swallowed bolus into the stomach (Figure 4.1).

Esophageal dysphagia can be caused by motor or structural abnormalities (Table 4.1). Structural mechanisms include luminal stenosis and, less often, luminal deformity. Motor disorders include abnormalities of esophageal peristalsis and of LES function.

STRUCTURAL DISORDERS
Esophageal Stenosis

Esophageal stenosis (narrowing) is conceptually the easiest mechanism of dysphagia to understand. When the lumen narrows, solid food may be too large to pass. Esophageal stenosis typically causes dysphagia for solid food dysphagia. In addition, the nature of the solid material ingested is important for symptom production. Dysphagia is more likely to occur when solids are tough or fibrous. Softer, more easily chewed foods are much less likely to cause difficulty. An exception to this tough food/soft food dichotomy is that many patients also

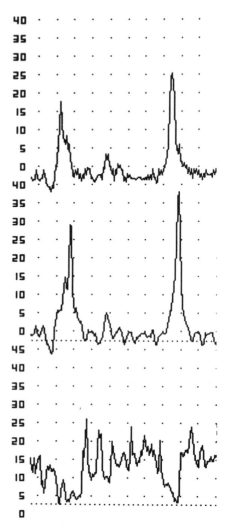

Figure 4.1 Normal esophageal peristalsis. In the manometric study shown here, the upper two pressure sensors are positioned in the body of the esophagus, 5 and 10 cm above the LES, while the bottom pressure sensor is within the LES segment. Swallowing initiates esophageal peristalsis, as well as LES relaxation. Peristalsis proceeds in an orderly fashion down the length of the esophagus. The LES remains open until the peristaltic wave passes through it, allowing the swallowed bolus to pass unimpeded into the stomach. Vertical scale, 1 increment = 5 mm Hg; horizontal scale, 1 increment = 2 seconds.

experience particular trouble with soft, absorbent foods such as bread or pasta, which swell when mixed with saliva during mastication.

There is a frequent overreliance on location of the sensation of food sticking. The common wisdom that patients "accurately localize symptoms to the site of obstruction" is often inaccurate. In fact, approximately one-third of patients with obstructing lesions of the distal esophagus point to the neck as the site of obstruction (Edwards 1974).

It is surprising how well some patients do despite dramatic degrees of stenosis. It is often stated, based on radiographic observations in patients with Schatzki's rings (Schatzki 1963), that patients with luminal diameters of greater than 18 to 20 mm are never symptomatic, whereas those with diameters

Table 4.1 Mechanisms of Dysphagia

Structural abnormalities
  Luminal stenosis
  Luminal deformity

Motor dysfunction
  Abnormalities of peristalsis
  Abnormalities of sphincter function

less than 10 to 12 mm are always symptomatic. Between these extremes, symptoms are variable both in frequency and severity, depending on the presence of associated motor dysfunction and the choice and preparation of food. The treatment of a stenosis is to open or remove the narrowed segment, depending on the specific cause.

Common intrinsic structural abnormalities that narrow the esophagus include mucosal rings, benign strictures, and malignant tumors.

Rings and Webs

The esophagus may be narrowed by a band of tissue composed of mucosa and submucosa. By tradition, this type of lesion is called a ring when located at the esophagogastric junction and a web when located elsewhere in the esophagus or hypopharynx.

Although classically described in patients with iron-deficiency anemia (sideropenic dysphagia), the vast majority of esophageal webs now seen are not associated with iron deficiency. Webs are frequently asymmetric, most often impinging on the esophageal lumen from the anterior wall (Figure 4.2A).

The most common band-like constriction of the esophagus is the Schatzki's ring. This lesion is typically symmetric and located at the esophagogastric junction (Figure 4.2B). Asymptomatic Schatzki's rings are detected in about 10 percent of the population (Goyal et al. 1971). The ring is always noted in the presence of a hiatal hernia. However, most hiatal hernias are not associated with Schatzki's ring. The etiology of a Schatzki's ring is unknown. They are rarely seen in childhood and generally present in middle age.

Webs and rings typically produce dysphagia for solids only. Patients often report that symptoms are intermittent and less likely to occur if they select their food wisely and chew carefully. Conversely, symptoms are more likely to occur if the patient eats out or carries on a conversation while eating, situations when the choice of food is more restricted and proper preparation of food before swallowing more difficult. The patient often must end the episode by inducing regurgitation. Once the episode is over, the patient is often able to return to the meal without further difficulty.

There is a limit to how far symptoms can be avoided by attention to the mechanics of cutting and chewing. When the lumen is severely compromised, the patient may find it impossible to maintain the level of attention required to remain symptom free without avoiding solids entirely. The patient may describe

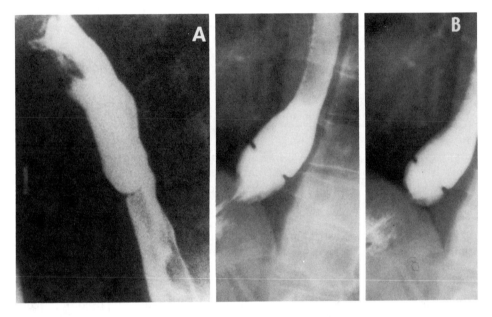

Figure 4.2 Webs and rings. Thin, band-like, stenotic lesions are generally referred to as rings when located at or near the esophagogastric junction, and webs when located elsewhere in the esophagus. (A) A web located at the pharyngoesophageal segment. (B) Schatzki's ring located at the esophagogastric junction. (Courtesy of Bronwyn Jones, MD.)

symptoms without any apparent progression in frequency or severity, going back for many years. Progression, when it does occur, usually is slow.

Radiographically, these lesions appear as thin (2 to 4 mm) bands that form shelf-like constrictions anywhere along the esophagus. Although radiologists occasionally refer to thicker lesions as webs or rings, these are probably short strictures or muscular contractions.

Treatment of webs or rings involves dilatation or rupture of the ring by any one of a variety of esophageal dilator systems. The ring is thin, nonfibrotic, and easy to dilate. Complete, or nearly complete, symptomatic relief can be anticipated. Dilatation may provide permanent relief, although a large proportion of patients will need periodic redilatation at variable intervals.

Benign Stricture

Strictures are rarely seen in children. The vast majority of benign esophageal strictures are acquired in adulthood as a consequence of esophagitis. In a circular structure like the esophagus, edema due to ongoing inflammation and fibrosis as part of the healing process occur at the expense of luminal diameter.

As with webs and rings, dysphagia is generally for solids only. However,

Table 4.2 Differential Diagnosis of Esophagitis

Gastroesophageal reflux
Infections (*Candida,* viral)
Trauma (prolonged nasogastric intubation)
Acute chemical ingestion (lye, industrial acids)
Drug-induced esophagitis (tetracycline, iron, potassium, quinidine, nonsteroidal, anti-inflammatory drugs)
Radiation
Skin conditions (pemphigus, cicatricial pemphigoid, epidermolysis bullosa dystrophica, lichen planus, toxic epidermal necrolysis, Stevens-Johnson syndrome)
Others (Crohn's disease, Behçet's syndrome)

dysphagia is progressive, with episodes becoming more frequent and severe over a period of months or years. As luminal narrowing increases, the patient reports trouble with food that previously caused no difficulty. Occasionally, stenosis can become so severe that even thick liquids cause dysphagia.

Because benign strictures are usually a sequelae of reflux-induced esophagitis, patients usually describe a previous history of heartburn or chest pain and may report the frequent use of antacids or other ulcer medications. However, in some patients the esophagus appears to be relatively insensitive to acid exposure. These individuals never experience significant reflux symptoms despite severe esophagitis and progression to stricture formation. While most benign esophageal strictures are a result of reflux esophagitis, any cause of esophagitis can cause stricture formation (Table 4.2).

Radiographically, a benign stricture is seen as a narrowed segment of esophageal lumen that may range from a centimeter to many centimeters long (Figure 4.3). The stricture usually is smooth and gradually tapering, with a symmetric lumen that follows the anticipated path of the normal esophagus. Ongoing inflammation may produce an eroded appearance along its course.

Proper management requires both treatment of the underlying inflammation and dilatation of the stricture. Treatment of the cause of esophagitis requires accurate diagnosis. While reflux is the most common cause of esophagitis, other possibilities must be considered, especially in the patient with atypical histories, an unusual distribution of inflammation, or failure to respond to reflux treatment.

Dilatation can often be performed using the same techniques available for a Schatzki's ring. However, the stricture may be relatively unyielding and require dilator systems that are stiffer. Effective dilatation is usually successful at improving symptoms, although edema from inflammation may result in less complete symptomatic relief than with a Schatzki's ring and in relatively rapid restenosis. Frequent dilatations are more often required in benign strictures than with Schatzki's rings. Even with complete cessation of ongoing inflammation, periodic dilatation may be necessary, especially during the first year after initial treatment, when maturation of the fibrotic reaction continues at the expense of luminal diameter.

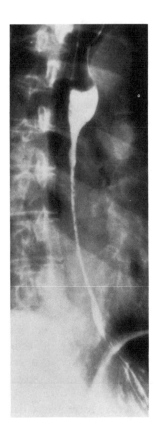

Figure 4.3 Benign stricture. This stricture is long and symmetric, with a lumen that tapers gradually. The lumen follows the anticipated line of the normal esophagus. The barium within the narrowed lumen has a somewhat irregular appearance due to the presence of erosions. (Courtesy of Bronwyn Jones, MD.)

Malignant Stricture

Although benign tumors may arise from the esophagus, the vast majority of clinically significant tumors of the esophagus are malignant. Most esophageal malignancies are squamous cell carcinomas, although cancers of the distal esophagus may be adenocarcinomas. Most esophageal adenocarcinomas appear to arise from Barrett's esophagus, a premalignant condition in which columnar cells replace the usual squamous epithelium covering the lower end of the esophagus as a result of severe gastroesophageal reflux.

As with other types of stenotic lesions, dysphagia is initially for solids only. However, it usually progresses rapidly, with dysphagia for soft foods and even liquids developing within a few months of the onset of symptoms.

Radiographically, esophageal malignancies appear as strictures of variable length. By the time of presentation, the cancer is usually many centimeters long and involves the entire circumference of the esophageal lumen, producing a stricture. The typical malignant stricture is characterized by its shelf-like proximal margins and irregular channel, which may diverge substantially from the anticipated course of the esophageal lumen (Figure 4.4). However, not all esophageal

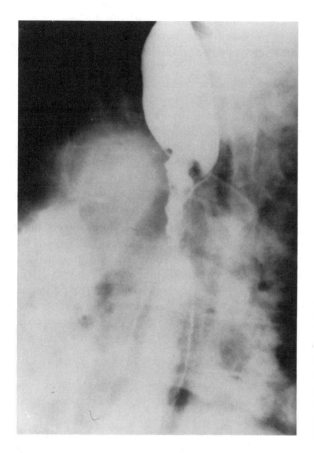

Figure 4.4 Malignant stricture. The stricture is circumferential. Characteristics distinguishing it from a benign stricture include the sharp, shelf-like proximal margin and the more irregular configuration of the stenotic segment. Unlike some malignant strictures, this stricture follows the anticipated path of the esophageal lumen. Compare the appearance to the benign stricture shown in Figure 4.3. (Courtesy of Bronwyn Jones, MD.)

cancers are obviously malignant on barium radiography, and occasional malignant-looking strictures may be benign (Ravich et al. 1986). For this reason, endoscopy with tissue sampling by biopsy and/or cytologic brushing is essential to distinguish between benign and malignant strictures.

Curative treatment is primarily surgical, although apparent cures by radiotherapy have been reported. Unfortunately by the time symptoms develop, the cancer is usually far advanced and incurable. The overall 5-year survival rate for esophageal cancer is only about 5 percent. Among those in whom resection for apparent cure is possible, the 5-year survival is only about 15 percent (Earlam and Cunha-Melo 1980).

For patients in whom curative resection is not possible, palliative resection is often still feasible and provides good symptomatic relief. In the past, a high perioperative mortality rate of about 29 percent, in combination with the infrequency of cure, made surgery unattractive (Parker and Moertel 1978). However with better nutrition provided by preoperative and perioperative hyperalimentation, the risk of palliative surgery has declined (Kinoshita et al. 1978).

Alternative approaches include dilatation, tumor ablation (thermal treatment to destroy tumor obstructing the esophagus) by means of laser or bipolar electrocautery, or stent placement. Each of these approaches is directed at opening the esophageal lumen to permit eating, in recognition that the major cause of early death in patients with esophageal cancer is malnutrition and aspiration pneumonia.

Dilatation generally provides limited and short-lived relief, but is useful in preparing for other forms of therapy. The choice between other modalities depends on specific features of the tumor and local technical expertise and resources. Endoscopic laser therapy and bipolar electrocautery can be used to destroy tumor tissue that blocks the esophageal lumen. This may provide a number of months of relief, allowing continuing oral intake. Should obstruction recur, treatment can be repeated.

An esophageal stent is a reinforced plastic or silastic tube with a large channel (about 11 mm inner diameter), which may be placed through the strictured segment to maintain luminal patency. The stent permits ingestion of a modified diet, concentrating on soft, easily chewed foods and purees. Since the development of thermal methods of treatment, the use of stents for palliation has decreased dramatically. However, they continue to be useful in certain situations, especially in the presence of a tracheoesophageal fistula that often complicates the natural history or treatment of esophageal cancer. In this situation, a properly placed stent can serve to maintain the esophageal lumen, while covering the opening to the airway.

Although endoscopic treatment with laser, bipolar electrocautery, or stent placement may be highly successful in reestablishing luminal patency, a substantial proportion of patients with esophageal cancer have poor appetites and are unable to gain weight. The early use of endoscopically placed gastrostomies should be considered in patients who fail to eat once the lumen is reestablished or who are scheduled to undergo chemotherapy or radiotherapy, treatments that may produce or exacerbate anorexia.

Luminal Deformity
Extrinsic Compression

Some degree of luminal deformity due to extrinsic compression by normal mediastinal structures (i.e., the aortic knob, the left mainstem bronchus, and the left atrium of the heart) is normally seen on barium studies and rarely, if ever, causes symptoms. More pronounced compression can occur with mediastinal pathology such as aortic aneurysm, cardiomegaly, congenital abnormalities of the large mediastinal arteries (e.g., aberrant subclavian artery), enlarged mediastinal lymph nodes, and lung cancer. The elasticity of the contralateral wall tends to minimize symptoms until compression is far advanced. By the same token, dilatation is usually ineffective because the force of dilatation is absorbed by the elastic, uninvolved wall. Effective treatment, when necessary, would require shrinking or removing the mass-producing compression. Unfortunately, this is often not practical in those patients in whom compression produces significant symptoms.

Esophageal Diverticulum

Compared with diverticula of the hypopharynx, esophageal diverticula are relatively rare and most often asymptomatic, even when they reach relatively large size. When symptoms do occur, they include dysphagia for liquids and solids and/or regurgitation of previously swallowed food back to the mouth.

Most often, esophageal diverticula are a consequence of downstream obstruction, either motor or structural in origin (pulsion diverticulum) (Figure 4.5). Presumably, increased pressure in the esophagus results in bulging at a point of relative weakness. Less commonly, diverticula can result from periesophageal inflammation, which causes traction on the esophageal wall (traction diverticulum). Although most traction diverticula occur in the midesophagus, most midesophageal diverticula, like their distal esophageal counterparts, are pulsion in origin.

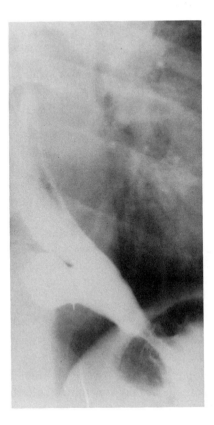

Figure 4.5 Esophageal diverticulum. A pulsion-type diverticulum located in the distal esophagus. Notice the narrowed appearance of the esophagogastric junction, suggesting the presence of a stricture. In most cases, esophageal diverticula are presumed to be caused by increased luminal pressure, secondary to motor or structural obstruction distally. (Courtesy of Bronwyn Jones, MD.)

Treatment of pulsion-type diverticula is only necessary if the diverticulum is symptomatic. Because of the frequent causative role of motor or structural disorders, it is important to look for these abnormalities. It may be difficult to distinguish between the underlying obstructive disorder and the diverticulum as a cause of symptoms. An attempt to treat the underlying cause of increased pressure, with dilatation in the case of structural obstruction or with drugs for dysmotility, is appropriate. In some patients, symptoms initially thought to be a consequence of the diverticulum improve significantly or resolve entirely with such conservative therapy.

Should medical management fail, surgical removal of the diverticulum is required. Surgery limited to diverticulectomy, however, is associated with a high incidence of early anastomotic leakage or late recurrence, probably because it fails to deal with the underlying cause of increased intraesophageal pressure and creates an area of relative wall weakness. Therefore, diverticulectomy should be combined with treatment of the underlying disorder, whether that be motor (with a surgical myotomy) or structural (with dilatation).

ESOPHAGEAL DYSMOTILITY
Classification of Esophageal Motility Disorders

An orderly, progressive peristaltic wave is not uniformly present after every swallow, even in individuals without dysphagia. The dividing line between normal and pathologic degrees of dysmotility is poorly defined.

In one study of 95 healthy adults (Richter et al. 1987), 5 mL wet swallow induced double-peaked contractions in 14.3 ± 22.4 percent of swallows, non-peristaltic contractions in 6.0 ± 10.3 percent of swallows, and nonpropagated contractions in 5.2 ± 1.5 percent of swallows. Interestingly, the frequency of simultaneous contractions was 0.8 ± 2.7 percent, substantially lower than previously reported. The incidence of abnormal contractions changes with bolus type, although not with age.

There have been a variety of schemes for the classification of esophageal dysmotility. In abnormalities of esophageal peristalsis, contraction amplitude may be too high or low, contraction duration prolonged, or the orderly progression of the contractile wave down the length of the esophagus uncoordinated. In abnormalities of LES function, the pressure may be too high or low, and relaxation may be incomplete. Finally, the esophageal body and the LES can misbehave separately or together. The individual characteristics of commonly described motility disorders are not necessarily unique. In many ways, the separation between entities is somewhat arbitrary.

Disorders of Esophageal Peristalsis

Motor dysfunction of the body of the esophagus may cause symptoms of dysphagia, chest pain, or regurgitation. Dysphagia is usually for liquids as well as solids, although not necessarily in equal measure. Chest pain may mimic that of cardiac disease and cause considerable concern on the part of both patient and physician. Although pain initiated or exacerbated by swallowing would strongly implicate the esophagus as the site of origin, a clear relationship to eating is often absent. Similarly, the presence of other symptoms implicating the swallowing mechanism would support the possibility that the esophagus is the cause of chest pain. However, cardiac disease is sufficiently common, especially in an older age group, that a cardiology evaluation may be justified.

Diffuse Esophageal Spasm

Esophageal spasm is a graphic term with imprecise meaning. The diagnosis of esophageal spasm is used quite freely among physicians, including gastroenterologists. All too often esophageal spasm is diagnosed on the basis of minor degrees of dysmotility seen radiographically or manometrically, or even on the basis of consistent symptoms in the absence of radiographic or manometric documentation. Esophageal spasm constitutes the end of a spectrum of nonspecific esophageal dysmotility, ranging from the abnormal contractions seen occasionally in normal individuals to the repeatedly high-amplitude, prolonged, simultaneous, and/or multiphasic contractions in the absence of any apparent peristaltic activity (Figure 4.6 and 4.7). While few would argue with calling the latter spasm, there is little agreement on where less severe abnormalities of esophageal peristalsis end and spasm begins.

An interesting feature of these criteria is the inclusion of high LES pressures and incomplete relaxations as an associated finding. LES dysfunction in diffuse esophageal spasm is well recognized, with failure of complete relaxation noted in one-third of patients (DiMarino and Cohen 1974). The presence of LES dysfunction in diffuse esophageal spasm and of spastic contractions in vigorous achalasia obscures the distinction between the two (see section in Achalasia).

Nutcracker Esophagus

In 1977, Brand et al. described a group of patients with chest pain or dysphagia, occurring in association with manometric findings of high amplitude, but normally progressive peristaltic waves (Brand et al. 1977). This syndrome, often called the nutcracker esophagus, is considered by some authorities the most commonly detected disorder of esophageal motility.

A number of questions surround the manometric pattern of the nutcracker esophagus. First, the criteria for diagnosis has changed over time. Originally described as a mean pressure of greater than 120 mm Hg, recent studies of normal individuals suggest that this value is too low, especially for the older population. Castell (1987) has suggested that, in order to avoid overdiagnosis, the term nutcracker esophagus should be restricted to patients with mean pressures greater than 180 mm Hg.

Second, the pressures measured during serial motility studies performed in the same individual may change substantially, resulting in the manometric inter-

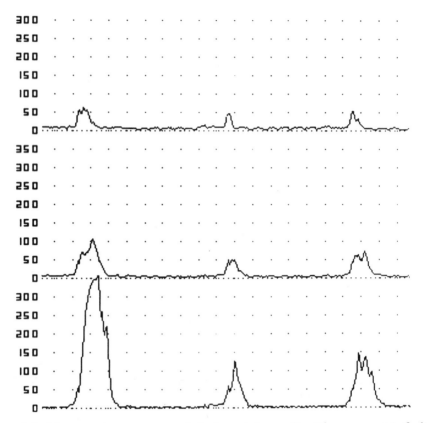

Figure 4.6 Manometric appearance of esophageal dysmotility. The manometric findings in esophageal dysmotility are characterized by simultaneous, multiphasic, high-amplitude, and prolonged contractions. These abnormalities may be present individually or in combination. As occasional abnormal contractions may be seen in normal individuals, the presence and nature of a disorder of esophageal motility requires evaluation of the frequency and characteristics of abnormal contractions. In the manometric study shown, all contractions are simultaneous and many are multiphasic. Although most contractions are of normal amplitude and normal duration, many are prolonged (greater than 6 seconds duration) and one pressure wave in the bottom pressure channel is greater than 350 mm Hg. Vertical scale, 1 increment = 50 mm Hg; horizontal scale, 1 bar = 5 seconds.

pretation changing from abnormal (i.e., nutcracker) to normal on different re-cordings in the same patient (Dalton et al. 1988). Interestingly, the pressures tend to be highest at the initial recording, suggesting that anxiety associated with the procedure may play a role in this manometric pattern.

Third, it is not clear why nutcracker esophagus produces symptoms. Barium esophagram studies demonstrate normal stripping function. While increased pres-

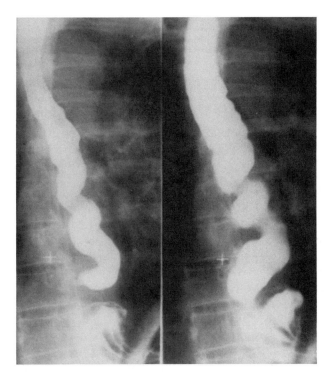

Figure 4.7 Radiographic appearance of esophageal dysmotility. A variety of patterns of abnormal peristalsis may be seen on barium radiography. In spot film, the silhouette of the barium column in the upper portion of the esophagus has a serrated appearance, whereas in the lower portion there is a "corkscrew" configuration. In addition, there is a hiatal hernia. (Courtesy of Bronwyn Jones, MD.)

sure could conceivably cause discomfort, most patients with high amplitude contractions during motility do not have pain at the time of the examination, and it is often difficult to appreciate differences between contraction amplitude and appearance during spontaneous episodes of pain that are witnessed manometrically. It is possible that the nutcracker esophagus represents a marker of patients with intermittent diffuse esophageal spasm.

Nonspecific Esophageal Motility Disorders

Disagreement about the criteria for esophageal spasm aside, a large number of patients referred to the esophageal function laboratory have abnormalities of esophageal motility in which the degree and type of motility abnormalities detected are not sufficient to be labeled esophageal spasm or nutcracker esophagus. Such lesser patterns of dysmotility are referred to as nonspecific esophageal motor disorders (NEMD). Their clinical significance remains unclear. On one hand, it is difficult to ignore the potential significance of disordered peristalsis in patients with dysphagia. On the other, similar degrees of abnormality are so frequently seen in normal volunteers, that their mere presence cannot be considered proof of causality.

Treatment of Disorders of Esophageal Motility

The medical therapy for esophageal dysmotility is often of limited benefit. A variety of smooth muscle relaxant drugs (nitrates, hydralazine, calcium channel blockers) have been used in an attempt to decrease esophageal contractile amplitude and repetitive contractions. Although some patients respond dramatically, many do not. Controlled clinical trials have thus far failed to demonstrate a convincing beneficial effect of these drugs on symptoms (Davis et al. 1987). Clinical experience suggests that symptomatic response is quite variable and often incomplete, that side effects related to the hypotensive effects of the drugs severely limit the use of these medications, and that patients who fail to respond to the first drug used, usually fail to respond to subsequently prescribed drugs.

The most common mistake in the treatment of esophageal dysmotility is to assume that the patient has a primary disorder of esophageal motility. Esophageal dysmotility is like anemia, a laboratory finding that requires further evaluation. Like anemia, there is a differential diagnosis of esophageal dysmotility. The most common cause of dysmotility is esophageal irritation, most commonly by gastroesophageal reflux. Disordered esophageal peristalsis also may result from esophageal obstruction, ganglion degeneration (i.e., vigorous achalasia), autonomic neuropathies (e.g., due to diabetes or alcohol abuse), or collagen vascular diseases (especially scleroderma and mixed connective tissue disease). Only those patients with esophageal dysmotility in the absence of an underlying etiology are considered to have a primary (or idiopathic) disorder of esophageal motility.

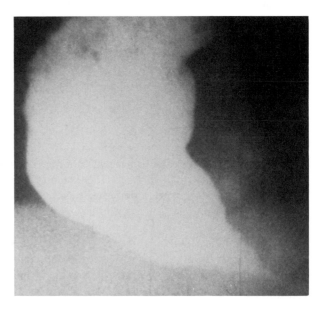

Figure 4.8 Radiographic appearance of achalasia. A barium esophagram with the patient in an upright position demonstrates the typical features of achalasia: a dilated esophagus and a smooth, tapering narrowing at the esophagogastric junction (the "parrot-beaked deformity"), holding up a column of barium mixed with retained food. In more extreme cases, the esophagus may take on a tortuous appearance (the "sigmoid esophagus"). (Courtesy of Bronwyn Jones, MD.)

Reflux-induced dysmotility is probably the most common cause of esophageal dysmotility and is more easily treated than idiopathic dysmotility. As heartburn is not always present, reflux should be considered in any patient with symptoms of esophageal spasm. Ironically, the drugs used in the treatment of idiopathic dysmotility may make reflux worse by further impairing LES pressure. Esophageal stenosis, another cause of esophageal dysmotility, may be missed occasionally by barium studies and endoscopy. Dilatation should be considered if there is any question of a structural obstruction.

Primary esophageal dysmotility accounts for only a minority of these patients. Whether idiopathic esophageal dysmotility is a single disorder or a number of disorders awaiting differentiation remains to be seen. Recent studies suggest that esophageal distention may be a cause of symptoms commonly attributed to spasm (Barish et al. 1986). The possibility that the pain of esophageal spasm derives from acute esophageal dilatation proximal to an area of spasm, rather than from the muscular contraction per se, must be considered.

ABNORMALITIES OF LOWER ESOPHAGEAL SPHINCTER FUNCTION
Achalasia

Achalasia is a condition in which a nonrelaxing, or incompletely relaxing, LES prevents the passage of swallowed material into the stomach. Patients usually present with dysphagia for both liquids and solids. Regurgitation is common, characteristically resulting in regurgitation of recognizable food, often many hours after its ingestion. The description of late regurgitation of undigested food is a feature seen in only a few causes of dysphagia, primarily achalasia and Zenker's diverticulum. During barium swallow, with the patient in the upright position, the esophagus is generally dilated and a column of barium of variable height is maintained above a tight esophagogastric junction (Figure 4.8). The possibility that this appearance could represent a tight esophageal stricture is ruled out at endoscopy when the endoscope passes into the stomach with mild-to-moderate resistance.

Although the impairment of LES response to swallow is key to the functional obstruction to the flow of food into the stomach, the motor abnormalities of achalasia include the complete loss of progressive peristalsis (Figure 4.9). In the classical form of achalasia, low-amplitude, aperistaltic contractions in the body of the esophagus are combined with a high or high-normal, nonrelaxing sphincter. The simultaneous low-amplitude increases in pressure with swallow are often attributed to pharyngeal pressure, transmitted into the dilated esophagus, rather than true esophageal contractile activity.

In recent years, the presence of a variant of achalasia, called "vigorous achalasia," has been recognized. In this condition, the typical LES findings of achalasia are associated with higher amplitude, prolonged, multiphasic contrac-

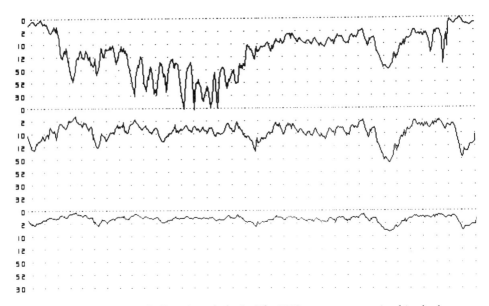

Figure 4.9 Manometric findings in achalasia. The LES pressure, examined in the bottom pressure channel during step-wise withdrawal of the manometric catheter from stomach (on the left) into the body of the esophagus (on the right), fails to relax with swallow. In addition, low-amplitude simultaneous pressure elevations in the body of the esophagus, examined in the upper two pressure channels, have replaced the normal higher amplitude progressive contractions. The pressure response that is observed is assumed to represent the effect of pharyngeal contraction on increasing pressure in a dilated esophagus. In the variant of vigorous achalasia, the typical LES findings of achalasia are combined with better defined simultaneous, often multiphasic, contractions, similar to those seen in esophageal spasm. Step-wise pull-through: vertical scale, 1 increment = 5 mm Hg; horizontal scale, 1 increment = 1 second.

tions, indicating that intrinsic esophageal motor response to swallowing, however deranged, is still present.

It also has been assumed that the complete absence of progressive peristalsis and the failure of LES relaxation represented the sine qua non of achalasia; a consequence of degeneration of the ganglion cells of the myenteric plexus. However, there have been reports of return of peristalsis after successful treatment. It has been suggested that the absence of progressive peristalsis is an artifact of the recording systems used, and that progressive peristalsis could be present, but unrecognized, until esophageal dilatation reverses after therapy (Vantrappen and Hellemans 1980). However cine or video recordings of barium esophagrams fail to support this suggestion. Peristalsis after treatment must be rare and may represent an early stage of disease.

More recently, complete relaxation of the LES has been described (Katz et al. 1986). Although conceptually earth-shaking from the esophagologist's perspective, the pattern of relaxation appears distinctly different from normal. It would appear to correspond to the limited degree of opening of the esophagogastric junction commonly noted on barium studies and does not require a complete reassessment of the manometric definition of achalasia.

The manometric features of achalasia are nearly, but not absolutely, pathognomonic. These include a lower esophageal sphincter with a high or high-normal resting pressure that fails to relax appropriately with swallow. In addition, there is a complete loss of progressive peristalsis. Occasional patients with identical manometric findings secondary to tumor infiltration of the esophagogastric junction have been described; a condition labeled "secondary achalasia" or "pseudoachalasia" (Kahrilas et al. 1987). This condition also has been described in a few nonmalignant conditions. Features that should raise suspicion of secondary achalasia include older age of onset, shorter duration of symptoms, modest dilatation of the esophagus, and rapid and profound weight loss.

Compared with other primary esophageal motor disorders, we usually are able to diagnose achalasia with confidence and treat it with success. Although achalasia involves motor abnormalities of both the esophageal body and LES, it is the LES dysfunction that is largely responsible for obstruction with resultant symptoms. Most patients are sufficiently symptomatic at presentation to warrant therapy. The major absolute indication for treatment is nighttime regurgitation, which puts the patient at risk for aspiration during sleep. Treatment also would be warranted if the obstruction is severe, nutrition is impaired, or the esophagus progressively dilates over time.

There are three treatment choices: smooth muscle relaxant drugs, pneumostatic dilatation, and surgery. All aim at decreasing LES pressure, thereby diminishing the resistance to the flow of food and liquid. None have a clinically significant effect on abnormal motor function in the esophageal body.

For many years it was said that there is no drug therapy for achalasia. However calcium channel blockers do lower LES pressure significantly and have been used for achalasia. Because esophageal transit, and therefore drug absorption, is problematic in achalasia, a sublingual route of administration is preferred. Although early reports suggested that most patients respond to calcium channel blockers, clinical experience has been less impressive. A recent double-blind, placebo-controlled trial (Traube et al. 1989), showed symptomatic improvement, but this improvement was rarely complete. Objective improvement in esophageal emptying could not be confirmed.

Sooner or later, most patients will require more definitive therapy. The choice between pneumostatic dilatation or surgery is most often dictated by local tradition. Few centers have extensive experience with both techniques as primary therapy. Either the initial therapy is pneumostatic dilatation, with the relatively few refractory patients proceeding to surgery, or myotomy, with the extremely poor risk patients sent for dilatation. Either way, the cards are stacked against the second choice. In a number of series, pneumostatic dilatation, using a number of different dilator types and techniques, provided good-to-excellent results in 60 to 94 percent of patients, whereas myotomy produced good-to-excellent long-term responses in 70 to 100 percent (Vantrappen and Janssens 1983).

Both pneumostatic dilatation and surgery have their advantages and limitations. Dilatation is less demanding technically, can be performed as an outpatient procedure, and costs less. The major risk is perforation, occurring in 0 to 4 percent of patients, depending on the series. Surgery requires greater skill, a prolonged recovery period, and greater cost. Mortality has been reported in 0 to 2 percent. A variable, but often high, incidence of clinically significant postoperative reflux-induced esophagitis and strictures has led to a lively argument in the surgical literature about technique, with a strong tendency among gastroenterologists to favor dilatation as an initial approach.

Isolated Abnormalities of Lower Esophageal Sphincter

LES dysfunction is not limited to patients with achalasia. As previously mentioned, incomplete relaxation of the LES occurs in perhaps one-third of patients with other evidence of severe esophageal dysmotility. In addition, occasional patients referred for esophageal manometry have isolated abnormalities of LES function, either a hypertensive LES pressure or incomplete relaxation in response to swallow. Few of these patients have any radiographically detectable impairment of function. They may represent a preclinical stage in the evolution of achalasia, abnormalities related to esophageal spasm during periods of otherwise normal peristaltic activity, or a secondary reaction to intragastric phenomenon in which the LES reaction is directed at preventing gastroesophageal reflux. In most patients, the explanation and clinical significance of isolated abnormalities of LES function cannot be determined.

MOTOR WEAKNESS

Intermittent impairment of contraction amplitude or peristalsis is relatively common. Radiologists frequently mislabel weakness as spasm when they see the escape of barium above the peristaltic wave. The distinction is important, as medication directed toward esophageal spasm, which generally decreases contractile amplitude, would be inappropriate if the problem actually is weakness. In practice, the esophagus can empty by gravity, and many patients with esophageal paresis are asymptomatic. Although some medications can increase esophageal contractility, their effect in patients with severe paresis usually is limited.

Severe esophageal weakness is relatively rare. It is most characteristically found in patients with collagen vascular disease, such as scleroderma and mixed connective tissue disease. The esophagus is the second most common organ involved in scleroderma (D'Angelo et al. 1969). Esophageal involvement varies from mild and nonspecific to the complete absence of a contractile response to swallow; a condition referred to as the sclerodermatous esophagus. Many of these patients have weak LESs. The resulting severe gastroesophageal reflux makes them particularly susceptible to esophageal inflammation and strictures.

GASTROESOPHAGEAL REFLUX DISEASE

Despite its name, heartburn (or the sensation of burning in the chest) is generally of esophageal origin. Heartburn is the archetypical symptom of gastroesophageal reflux, although it may occasionally represent a nonspecific response to other types of esophageal dysmotility. Patients with gastroesophageal reflux often complain of regurgitation of sour or bitter material with or without food.

Dysphagia associated with gastroesophageal reflux may be due to a variety of mechanisms. Gastroesophageal reflux, with or without esophagitis, is a common cause of esophageal dysmotility. It also can produce esophageal paresis. Finally, chronic inflammation of any type can cause strictures.

Our understanding of the pathophysiology of gastroesophageal reflux has progressed substantially over the past decade, but still remains incomplete. The major component of the "antireflux barrier" is the LES, probably acting in combination with the anatomic configuration of the esophagogastric junction. Reflux is most likely to occur when the pressure in the LES is low and when the esophagogastric junction is pulled up into the chest creating a hiatal hernia.

Other factors, however, play variable roles in different individuals. It now appears that the ability of the sphincter to prevent reflux is not simply a matter of the pressure of the sphincter measured during standard esophageal manometry. The sphincter pressure is dynamic, changing throughout the day under the influence of neural, hormonal, and mechanical influences. Additional factors that may either produce or exacerbate the severity of reflux include the neutralizing capacity of saliva, the ability of esophageal motility to clear refluxed material, and the efficiency of gastric emptying, which decreases pressure against the antireflux barrier.

Continuous pH monitoring permits the objective evaluation for reflux under near-physiologic conditions. The patient performs the activities of normal daily living, including eating, working, and sleeping. Continuous pH monitoring provides quantitative information on both the presence and severity of acid reflux. The incidence and duration of reflux events can be calculated and analyzed for the entire recording period and for segments of particular interest. The severity of reflux detected by pH monitoring correlates fairly well with the probability of esophageal inflammation and Barrett's esophagus (Iascone et al. 1983). Continuous pH monitoring is currently considered the best single test for the diagnosis of gastroesophageal reflux, with a sensitivity and specificity of approximately 90 percent (Richter and Castell 1983).

All reflux is not pathologic. Gastroesophageal reflux is a common physiologic event. Many apparently normal individuals describe heartburn on a regular basis. A study of apparently healthy hospital employees indicates that approximately 33, 14, and 7 percent complained of heartburn on a monthly, weekly, and daily basis, respectively (Nebel et al. 1976). It would appear that reflux is a feature of normal life and does not necessarily reflect a pathologic condition.

Continuous pH monitoring has demonstrated that the vast majority of normal individuals experience gastroesophageal reflux on a daily basis (De-Meester and Johnson 1976). Most reflux episodes in normal individuals are of short duration, occur during the day, and do not provoke any symptoms.

Although a variety of tests have been used to evaluate patients with presumed gastroesophageal reflux disease, continuous pH monitoring is the best test for the diagnosis of gastroesophageal reflux disease. Barium studies, although important in the evaluation of patients with dysphagia, confirm the presence of reflux in only the minority of patients with symptomatic reflux disease.

Esophagitis refers to inflammation of the lining of the esophagus. Esophagitis may vary in severity from microscopic inflammation, to mucosal edema, to frank erosions or ulcerations. Although the most common cause of esophagitis is gastroesophageal reflux disease, most patients with gastroesophageal reflux disease do not have esophagitis (Behar et al. 1976).

Treatment is directed at enhancing the strength of the antireflux barrier, improving esophageal clearance and gastric emptying, and decreasing the noxiousness of gastric contents. Antireflux therapy has three components: alteration in life-style, drugs, and surgery.

For many patients, reflux is provoked by dietary indiscretion and physical activity. Decreasing or eliminating foods that decrease LES pressure (e.g., fat, chocolate) or stimulate gastric acid production (e.g., coffee, tea) is important, especially in patients who ingest large amounts or note the association of symptoms with their ingestion. In some patients with reflux, dietary modification is enough to control symptoms. Smoking also impairs esophageal function and should be eliminated. In addition, patients are instructed to elevate the head of the bed on 6-inch blocks and avoid lying down within 2 hours of eating. These measures allow gravity to assist in reflux prevention and enhance esophageal clearance.

Self-medication with antacids is common in patients with heartburn. Unfortunately, antacids alone are rarely sufficient to control esophagitis. Antacids are primarily used for symptomatic relief in patients with intermittent, infrequent heartburn. Most patients with severe symptoms or esophagitis require more potent acid-lowering agents, most often one of the available histamine antagonists (the H_2-blockers), in combination with life-style changes.

Although prokinetic drugs (e.g., bethanechol, metoclopramide) have potentially beneficial effects on upper gastrointestinal motor function, they have generally been disappointing when used as single agents. The use of metoclopramide has been further limited by the frequent occurrence of neuropsychiatric side effects, including agitation, insomnia and lethargy. Prokinetic agents are occasionally used as adjunctive agents, in combination with H_2-blockers in patients with more severe disease.

The vast majority of patients can be controlled by the measures mentioned previously. Surgical intervention has generally been reserved for the occasional patient who has been refractory to medical management. A number of operations have been described, most involving reestablishing the intra-abdominal location of the esophagogastric junction (hiatal hernia repair) in combination with wrapping a portion of the stomach around part or the whole circumference of the lower esophagus (fundoplication). Surgery is effective in controlling reflux in approximately 80 to 90 percent of patients in whom it is used.

The introduction of a more potent class of acid-reducing drugs, the proton pump blockers, has demonstrated that acid plays a critical role in the production of symptoms even in the occasional patient who fails to respond clinically to H_2-blocker therapy. However, omeprazole, the only currently available agent within this class of drugs, is only approved for short-duration (2 months) treatment of gastroesophageal reflux because of concerns about the carcinogenic potential of long-term, profound acid suppression. It seems likely that omeprazole will be used as an alternative to surgery in patients with refractory reflux disease who are poor surgical risks.

REFERENCES

Barish CF, Castell DO, Richter JE. Graded esophageal balloon distention: a new provocative test for non-cardiac chest pain. Dig Dis Sci 1986; 31:1292–98.

Behar J, Biancani P, Sheahan DG. Evaluation of esophageal tests in the diagnosis of reflux esophagitis. Gastroenterology 1976; 71:9–15.

Brand DL, Martin D, Pope CE. Esophageal manometrics in patients with anginal type chest pain. Am J Dig Dis 1977; 23:300–4.

Castell DO. The nutcracker esophagus and other primary esophageal motility disorders. In: Castell DO, Richter JE, Dalton CB, eds. Esophageal motility testing. New York: Elsevier, 1987; 130–142.

D'Angelo WA, Fries JF, Masi AT, et al. Pathologic observations in systemic sclerosis (scleroderma): a study of 58 autopsy cases and 58 matched controls. Am J Med 1969; 46:428–40.

Dalton CB, Castell DO, Richter JE. The changing faces of the nutcracker esophagus. Am J Gastroenterol 1988; 83:623–8.

Davis HA, Lewis MJ, Rhodes J, et al. Trial of nifedipine for prevention of oesophageal spasm. Digestion 1987; 36:81–83.

DeMeester TR, Johnson LF. Patterns of gastroesophageal reflux in health and disease. Ann Surg 1976; 184:459–70.

DiMarino AT, Cohen S. Characteristics of lower esophageal sphincter function in symptomatic diffuse esophageal spasm. Gastroenterology 1974; 66:1–6.

Earlam R, Cunha-Melo JR. Oesophageal squamous cell carcinoma: a critical review of surgery. Br J Surg 1980; 67:381–90.

Edwards DAW. Diagnostic procedures: history and symptoms of esophageal disease. In: Vantrappen G, Hellemans J, eds. Diseases of the esophagus. New York: Springer-Verlag, 1974; 103–18.

Goyal RK, Bauer JL, Spiro HM. The nature and location of the lower esophageal ring. N Engl J Med 1971; 284:1175–80.

Iascone C, DeMeester TR, Little AG, et al. Barrett's esophagus: functional assessment, proposed pathogenesis, and surgical therapy. Arch Surg 1983; 118:543–9.

Kahrilas PJ, Kishk SM, Helm JF, et al. Comparison of pseudoachalasia and achalasia. Am J Med 1987; 82:439–46.

Katz PO, Richter JE, Cowan R, et al. Apparent complete lower esophageal sphincter relaxation in achalasia. Gastroenterology 1986; 90:978–83.

Kinoshita Y, Endo M, Nakayama K, et al. Evaluation of ten year survival after operation for upper- and midthoracic esophageal cancer. Intern Adv Surg Oncol 1978; 1: 173–200.

Nebel OT, Fornes MF, Castell DO. Symptomatic gastroesophageal reflux: incidence and precipitating factors. Am J Dig Dis 1976; 21:953–6.

Parker EF, Moertel CF. Is there a role for surgery in esophageal carcinoma? Am J Dig Dis 1978; 23:730–6.

Ravich WJ, Kashima H, Donner MW. Drug-induced esophagitis simulating esophageal cancer. Dysphagia 1986; 1:13–18.

Richter JE, Castell DO. Gastroesophageal reflux disease—pathogenesis, diagnosis, and therapy. In: Castell DO, Johnson LF, eds. Esophageal function in health and disease. New York: Elsevier, 1983; 151–175.

Richter JE, Wu WC, Johns DN, et al. Esophageal manometry in 95 healthy adult volunteers: variability of pressure with age and frequency of "abnormal" contractions. Dig Dis Sci 1987; 32:583–92.

Schatzki R. The lower esophageal ring: long term follow-up of symptomatic and asymptomatic rings. American J Roentgenol Rad Therapy Nuclear Med 1963; 90:805–10.

Traube M, Dubovik S, Lange RC, et al. The role of mifedipine therapy in achalasia: results of a randomized, double-blind, placebo-controlled study. Am J Gastroenterol 1989; 84:1259–62.

Vantrappen G, Janssens J. To dilate or to operate? That is the question. Gut 1983; 24:1013–19.

Vantrappen G, Hellemans J. Treatment of achalasia and related motility disorders. Gastroenterology 1980; 79:144–54.

5

Development and Impairments of Feeding in Infancy and Childhood

James F. Bosma

Feeding is central within the living experience of the young infant and it continues to be a major element of experience in the older infant and child. In the young infant, the manner of arousal toward feeding and competence in suckle feeding reflects the infant's general health and neurologic status. Conversely, many forms of neurologic impairment and some forms of systemic illness are associated with dysphagia. Failure to thrive is common, and frank malnutrition may occur rapidly in young infants. These may be associated with an increase in impairment, including dysphagia. In this reciprocating circumstance, the detection, evaluation, and therapy of dysphagia is strategic. This review is concerned particularly with evaluation of the performances of suckle feeding and of the later acquisition of voluntary oral manipulation and swallow of particulate foods in normal and the neurologically impaired individuals.

SUCKLE FEEDING

Our reference for description of suckle feeding is the normal young term born infant who has had several successful bottle feedings by a single care person; breast feeding is separately considered. Suckle feeding, in this circumstance, is a mature neurologic performance (Peiper 1963; Bosma 1986a; Blass and Teicher 1980; Selley et al. 1990a). It is consistent in its relation to arousal and in its initiating responses and sequences. It is consistent and efficient in actions of suckle, swallow, and adapted adjacent respirations. The efficiency of formula intake in relation to time varies between normal newborn infants, without relation to weight or incidental actions of the mother or care giver (Rybski and Gisel 1984; Rybski et al. 1984). This quality of performance is appropriate to stable coordination patterns, representing suckle and pharyngeal swallow, in the bulbar area neural networks. The infant is expected to rouse stably, with increasing readiness of rooting responses to oral area touching and prompt suckling on a nipple or equivalent object. The suckle action, perceived by the examiner's finger or imaged by videosonography or videoradiography, is a coordination of the tongue, the hyoid and mandibular muscles, and the lower lip. Videosonography in horizontal plane, with the ultrasound probe on the cheek (Figure 5.1),

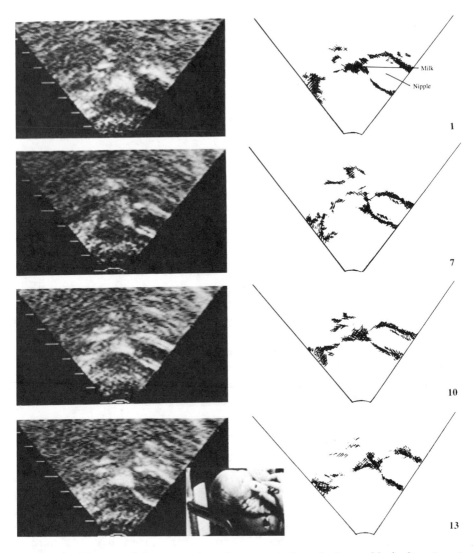

Figure 5.1 Ultrasound demonstration of tongue motions during suckle feeding. Imaging is in the transverse plane with probe held on the cheek; the video inset, expanded, shows the position of the probe. Selected video frames at 30 per second and derived tracings: frame 01, tip of the nipple is in reference contour; frame 07, tip of the nipple is compressed and the tongue dorsum is slightly separated from the tip of the nipple; frame 10, tip of the nipple is compressed and milk is expressed; frame 13, tip of the nipple is reopened nearly to reference contour.

demonstrates a posteriorward moving peristaltic wave. Each wave consists of a downward displacement followed by an upward displacement, effecting a succession of suction and nipple compression (Bosma et al. 1990). The peristaltic wave conveys the expressed bolus of formula toward the pharnyx. Sonography in transverse projection, with the probe under the chin (Figure 5.2), demonstrates that these vertical motions occur differentially in the medial portion of the tongue, into which the genioglossus muscle is inserted. By anatomic inference, the peristaltic motions of the medial portion of the tongue are accomplished by reciprocal coordination of the genioglossus and the transverse intrinsic lingual muscles, which relate the medial portion of the tongue and the adjacent lateral portion, into which the styloglossus and hyoglossus muscles are inserted. These intrinsic motions of the tongue, immediately effecting the milking actions of suction and nipple compression, are central within more general concerted motions of the tongue, lower lip, mandible, and hyoid. This composite of structures, the "suckle motor organ," is moved alternately upward and backward in relation to the palate and then downward and forward. These gross actions are coordinated with those of pharyngeal swallow.

Videoradiography in the lateral projection (Figure 5.3) demonstrates the conveyance of the suckled bolus from the nipple through the faucial isthmus, which is between the pharyngeal palate and tongue, through the pharynx, and into the esophagus. If suckle and swallow are in simple one-to-one sequence, milk filling of the oral accumulation area alternates rhythmically with pharyngeal swallow. If two or more suckles precede a swallow, bolus is accumulated adjacent to the junction of the oral, or bony, and pharyngeal, or muscular, palate and also in the valleculae, between the tongue, epiglottis, and pharyngeal palate and palatopharyngeal folds. These two accumulation sites are separate, as the faucial isthmus is closed after each conveyance of bolus.

The pharynx is moved extensively during swallow. Videoradiography in lateral and in posteroanterior projection demonstrates a peristaltic wave descending in the constrictor wall. The constriction begins at the level of cervical vertebra 1 and the oral, or bony, palate. At the beginning of swallow the palatopharyngeal isthmus is closed by combined action of the constrictor and palatine muscles. The descent of the peristaltic wave is demonstrated prominently in the constrictor wall. In some instances, a lucency is seen advancing ahead of the bolus through the lower portion of the pharynx and the pharyngoesophageal segment, indicating relaxation of the constrictor muscle. Simultaneously, the hyoid bone is moved upward and forward, and the tongue, having conveyed the bolus into the pharynx, is pressed posteriorward. The tongue is thus participating in the initiation of pharyngeal swallow. The larynx is raised, along with the hyoid, and also is undergoing closure. The pharyngoesophageal segment is stably closed except during swallow or retrograde transit by belching, regurgitation, or vomiting. It is opened during swallow by a combination of the inhibition that precedes the activation wave of peristalsis and of upward and forward displacement of the cricoid cartilage, on which the cricopharyngeus muscle and the suspensory ligament of the esophagus are attached.

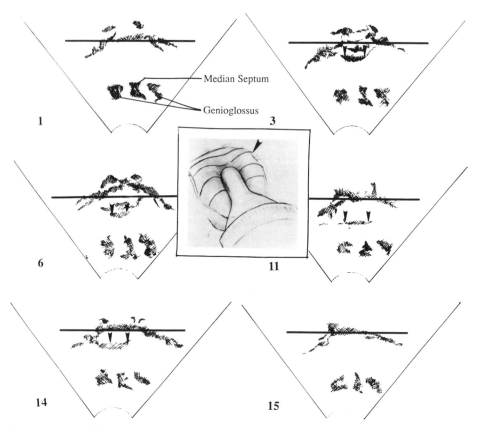

Figure 5.2(A) Ultrasound demonstration of tongue motions during suckle feeding. Imaging is in the coronal plane (arrow), with the probe in the submental area. The frames illustrate motions of the medial portion of the tongue, into which the genioglossus muscle is inserted, in relation to the lateral portions, into which the styloglossus and hyoglossus muscles are inserted. The arrows point to the superior margin of the medial portion. Frame 1: The superior margin of medial portion and of lateral portions are aligned. Frame 3: The margin of the medial portion is displaced inferiorly; milk is visible superior to the margin. Frames 6 and 11: The margin of the medial portion is displaced further inferiorly and milk is seen superior to the margin. Frames 14 and 15: Progressive return of the superior margin of the medial portion to alignment with the lateral portion.

During a rhythmic suckle feeding continuity, or run, the pharyngeal swallow coordination is accomplished in remarkable duplication. Exceptionally, during the initial swallow of a run, or during an isolated swallow, a small portion of the barium bolus may briefly penetrate into the laryngeal vestibule and be promptly and fully extruded again into the pharynx within 30 to 90 msec (one to three video frames).

The centers of respiration control and of feeding are developing simulta-

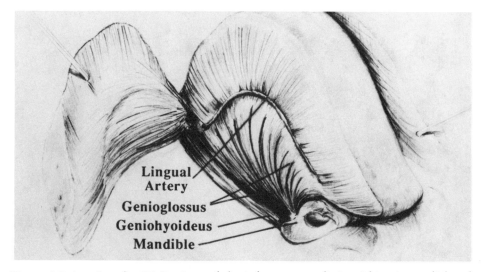

Lingual Artery
Genioglossus
Geniohyoideus
Mandible

Figure 5.2 *(continued)* (B) Sections of the infant tongue distinguishing its medial and lateral portions. The sections are approximately sagittal in the plane of the lingual artery. The right genioglossus is shown extending fan-like into the tongue from its attachment on the gonial process of the mandible. A portion of the genioglossus, which is extended toward the lingual artery, is in the pattern of gross bundles. Distally, the muscle is divided into small fascicles, similar in diameter to intrinsic lingual muscles.

neously in the brain stem. The coordination of individual pharyngeal swallows is consistently capable of superceding and displacing respiration (Doty 1968; Wilson et al. 1981; Miller 1982; Sessle and Henry 1989).

The alternation of pharyngeal actions in swallow and respiration are well shown in lateral-projection videoradiography, as the pharynx reopens after completion of swallow. During dyspnea, as in crying, the pharyngeal participation in inspiration is conspicuous, as it is enlarged transversely, with forward displacement of the tongue and hyoid, and is also enlarged vertically, with descent of the hyoid, larynx, and hypopharynx in relation to the basicranium and the midfacial skeleton. The inspiratory expansion of the pharynx is also well shown in the posteroanterior projection as a transverse expansion of the oropharynx and laryngopharynx. The expansion demonstrates the available mobility and also the resources of dilating muscles of the pharyngeal area. During expiration, the pharynx is constricted in each of these planes. The constriction is generalized and simultaneous, thus differing from the constriction of peristalsis and affording an additional criterion of pharyngeal area motor resources. Radiography in lateral projection during effortful expiratory constriction demonstrates near complete closure of the airway in the larynx and pharynx. The expiration may be valved at the glottis for phonation, grunt, or cough.

During rhythmic suckle feeding, respiration is incorporated into the rhythmic sequence, so that pairs of expiration and inspiration (less commonly the sequence of inspiration and expiration) are interposed between swallows (Wilson

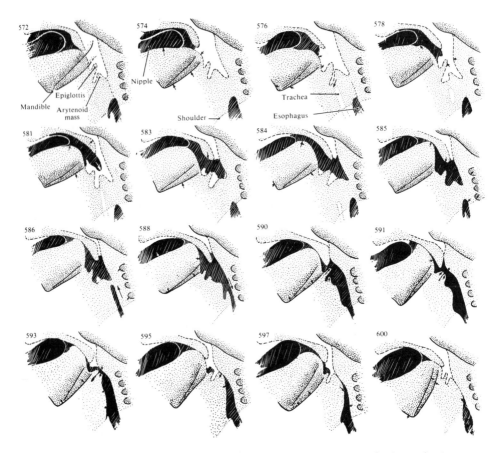

Figure 5.3 Cineradiographic frame tracings of established suckle feeding of a barium mixture at 50 frames per second. In frame 572, the undistorted nipple is within the mouth surrounded by barium. The barium bolus is retained in the primary oral accumulation area by apposition between the velum and tongue. The pharynx is open in respiration. In frames 574 to 584, the mandible and tongue are elevated and the nipple is compressed. Coincidentally, the increased mass of the free bolus penetrates the junction of the mouth and pharynx and fills the oropharynx. The reciprocal phase of the suckle performance is shown in frames 585 to 600, in which the mandible and tongue body are displaced inferiorward, allowing the nipple to resume its original contours; the velum and tongue are approximated, separating the oral and pharyngeal cavities. The pharyngeal stage of swallow occurs with elevation of the palate and anterior motion of the posterior pharyngeal wall, which is representative of general convergence of the posterior and lateral constrictor walls of the pharynx. The pharyngoesophageal segment is open in frames 588 to 593.

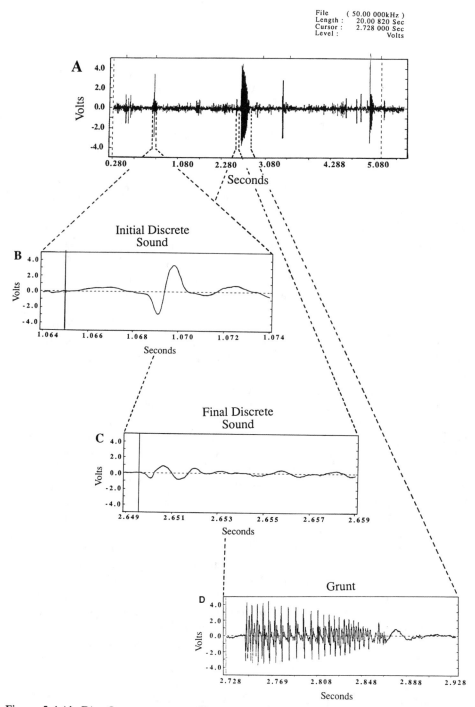

Figure 5.4 (A–D) Computer screen illustration of the cervical sounds of suckle feeding; normal newborn infant. Inset menu identifies file, sampling rate (50 kHz), total length (20+ sec), and cursor location (0 to 28 sec). (B D) Expanded items of compressed envelope display in A.

et al. 1981; Daniels et al. 1990; Bamford 1991). This incorporation may be delayed during a run, so that respiration is omitted between the first swallows. In some premature infants, and in occasional term or neurologically impaired infants, this feeding apnea may continue during the duration of the run, causing hypercapnia, hypoxia and secondary bradycardia.

Cervical auscultation, via stethoscope or a microphone over the larynx, is increasingly employed by clinicians in evaluation of feeding, particularly of the competence of pharyngeal swallow and the previously noted interactions of swallow and respiration (Logan and Bosma 1967). Cervical auscultation is employed in physiologic studies of swallow and respiration (Selley et al. 1990a). It demonstrates the bolus transit sounds and also abrupt, brief actions of the larynx and pharynx preceding and succeeding the bolus transit sounds (Vice et al. 1990). The initial discrete sounds and the final discrete sounds are each demarcated from the bolus transit sounds by a period, or zone, of diminished sounds. These acoustic correlates of swallow are demonstrated in Figures 5.4 and 5.5. These sounds demonstrate remarkable temporal stability of a suckle feeding run (Figure 5.6). In pharyngeally dysphagic infants and children, cervical auscultation may demonstrate the occasion or absence of pharyngeal swallow and also possible bubbling sounds, wheezes, or stridor, which may indicate the presence of unswallowed bolus or secretions in the airway.

The esophagus differs from the pharynx in structure, innervation, and pattern of performance in feeding. At the time of developmental acquisition of stable suckle feeding, esophageal peristalsis is also evident. Single boluses delivered from the pharynx are peristaltically conveyed, after a brief pause, down the length of the esophagus and through the esophagogastric junction (Gryboski et al. 1963; Gryboski 1965; Gryboski 1975; Boix-Ochoa and Canals 1976; Herbst 1989; Milla 1991). Each pharyngeal swallow briefly inhibits esophageal peristalsis so that, during a suckle feeding run, the boluses of successive swallows may accumulate in the esophagus. Transit of the accumulated milk into the stomach may be irregular, with little distinct peristalsis until the completion of the suckle feeding run. Neural control of the esophagus and the esophagogastric junction is incomplete in the infant and young child, permitting reflux of gastric contents into the esophagus (Gryboski 1975; Grand et al. 1976).

Neural control of the pharyngoesophageal segment is stable. Per manometry, the resting pressure in the pharyngoesophageal segment is increased by acidification within the esophagus, simulating reflux (Sondheimer 1983). The extent of increase in resting pressure is the same in infants known to reflux frequently and in normal infants.

CAUSES AND MECHANISMS OF SUCKLE FEEDING IMPAIRMENTS

The infant who transiently fails to initiate suckle feeding or who suckles or swallows poorly may be demonstrating current problems of feeding readiness or illness or injury. The clinician is more concerned about an infant who continues

Sounds of Swallow 12

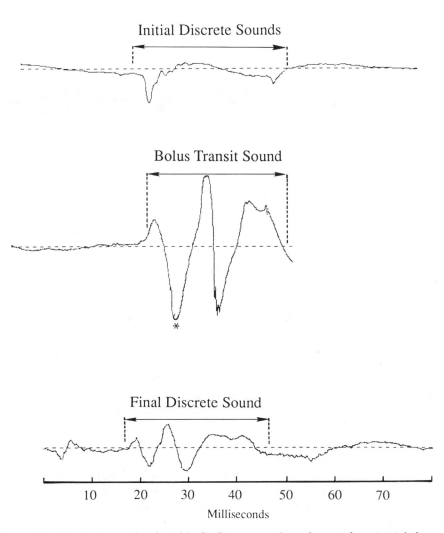

Figure 5.5 Cervical sounds of suckle feeding; normal newborn infant. Initial discrete, bolus transit, and final discrete sounds of swallow 12 in Figure 5.6, in which these sounds are shown in compressed form.

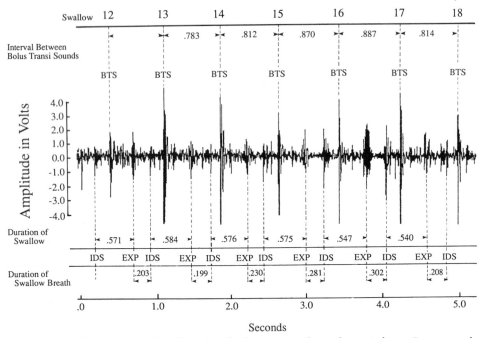

Figure 5.6 Cervical sounds of suckle feeding; normal newborn infant. Compressed display of first rhythmic suckle feeding run of infant 5, swallows 12 to 18 of a feeding run, indicating temporal intervals between events of swallow and swallow breath.

in feeding failure. The causes and mechanisms of continuing feeding failure probably lie in the developmental history of the mouth and pharynx and of the representations, or patterning, of feeding and of other oral and pharyngeal functions in the brain. Abnormalities of the mouth and pharynx or of the bulbar portion of the brain may have occurred during initial development in the embryo or small fetus. The resulting gross abnormalities of the mouth and pharynx or the brain are readily discerned. The greater challenge is to distinguish impairments of the development shared between the oral and pharyngeal area and the bulbar portion of the brain, which occurs later in development in the fetus and infant. This sharing is involved in the performance of suckle feeding. The sharing also is involved in participation of the pharynx and larynx in respiration and in the maintenance of the pharyngeal airway, which is the developmental prologue of postural control of the head and neck. The current concept of the development of this sharing is that it occurs by a reciprocating mechanism, i.e., sensory inputs from the mouth and pharynx during feeding stimulate the development of brain regions representing the various feeding movements, which then generate more refined movements. These, in turn, generate further performance-appropriate input. The system is thus reciprocating in both its peripheral and central aspects.

As clinicians gain experience with dysphagia in neurologically impaired infants and children, they are increasingly concerned with the development of the separate representations of these categorical functions in the medulla and at higher levels. It is necessary that abnormalities in the development of feeding be viewed from this perspective, because we then may understand the influence of abnormal early feeding performance on the pattern of feeding of the neurologically impaired child. Abnormalities of early respiratory and positional performances also are cumulative in their effects on performance in each of these categories. These categorical functions combine in their influences on the developing structure and form of the muscles and skeleton in the mouth, pharynx, and larynx. Thus, we may understand the mechanisms by which the peripheral effector structures grow and develop into shapes that further handicap the feeding performance.

For purposes of this review, the causes and mechanisms of suckle feeding impairments are classified into embryopathy of the oral and pharyngeal area, embryopathy of the brain and peripheral nerves, acquired neurologic impairments, acquired impairments of the mouth and pharynx, and iatrogenic mechanisms.

Embryopathy of the Oral and Pharyngeal Area

The embryogenesis of the pharyngeal and oral area is complex, because it is derived from convergence of the foregut with the branchial arches and with the cervical segmental muscles of the ventral median bar. The peripheral sensory and motor innervation is of corresponding diversity, as it includes the trigeminal, facial, glossopharyngeal, vagal, hypoglossal, and upper cervical nerves. The simplest impairments, in terms of detection and clinical management, are those of the tongue and palate. Infants who have hypoplasia of the tongue may achieve adequate suckle feeding by compensatory actions of the constrictor wall, pharyngeal palate, palatine folds, and hyoid suspensory muscles. The mandible and palate and other portions of the midfacial skeleton are adapted in shape so that they form functionally appropriate chambers about the hypoplastic tongue (Weinberg et al. 1969).

Analogously, an infant who has cleft palate, but who has normal feeding incentive and normal sensory inputs and central representations of suckle and swallow, may demonstrate remarkable motor compensations for this anatomic defect by muscles of the pharyngeal palate, adjacent constrictor wall, and tongue (Bosma et al. 1966).

A lesser degree of pharyngeal palate hypoplasia may be evidenced by cleft of the uvula or by a palate that is visibly short or lax under fingertip palpation. The lesser mass of the hypoplastic palate may be more clearly evidenced by radiography in lateral projection than by inspection or palpation. An infant who has palate hypoplasia may have greater problems of pharyngeal dysphagia, including nasal regurgitation, than does the infant with a cleft palate. The greater disability may be coincident with sensory impairment. The most extensive impairment associated with palatal hypoplasia or cleft is that described by Robin (1934), which includes retrusion and possible hypoplasia of the mandible and ptosis of the tongue, with secondary pharyngeal airway obstruction (Takagi et al. 1966; Bruston 1978; Rickham et al. 1978; Williams et al. 1981).

Embryopathy of the Medulla and Pons

The primary nuclei of the cranial nerves are distinguishable soon after the medullary portion of the brain stem achieves its basic form. The most common embryopathies are aplasia of motor nuclei and syringobulbia. Nuclear aplasia in the oral musculature is an infrequent but significant mechanism of suckle dysphagia, as part of the syndrome of aplasia. Aplasia in the hypoglossal or trigeminal motor innervation may cause impairment of the suckle actions. Aplasia in the facial innervation may cause general or discrete weakness in the orbicularis oris or in the fan-like arrangement of mimetic muscles, resulting in leak at the labial seal about the nipple. Aplasia of vagal striated motor innervations may cause weakness of the pharyngeal and/or laryngeal muscles. Since nuclear aplasia, or agenesis, may be disseminated throughout the striated motor system (Warkany et al. 1981), evidence of the syndrome of localized muscle weakness, hypoplasia, or contracture may be sought in other motor innervations, such as the extraocular muscles (Möbius' syndrome), or muscles in the trunk or limbs (Evans 1954; Goldblatt and Williams 1986; Cohen and Thompson 1987).

Expansion of the central canal in the bulbar area, or syringobulbia, may occur in isolation or as part of a more general myelodysplasia (Swaiman 1989). It may be associated with hypoplasia of primary nuclei (Sieben et al. 1971) or with impairment of performance coordination or regulation. Respiratory impairment may result from bilateral adductor vocal fold paralysis (Holinger et al. 1978) or from impairment of central regulation of respiration (Ward et al. 1986; Hays et al. 1989). We have seen failure of elicitation of pharyngeal swallow in two infants who had Arnold-Chiari malformation of the brain stem in association with lumbar myelomeningocele. In each, pharyngeal participation in respiration and cry and in airway maintenance was normal. In one comparably impaired infant, without radiographic evidence of malformation in the brain stem, an occasional swallow could be elicited in association with intensive suckling; these occasional swallows were seen by videoradiography to be normal in pattern. These selective impairments of swallow elicitation may imply a discrete lesion in the vicinity of nucleus tractus solitarius and adjacent internuncial cells of the swallowing center. This clinical topic awaits detailed comparison of bulbar impairments with the elegant demonstration of the brain stem that is now available by magnetic resonance imaging (Packer et al. 1985).

Acquired Neurologic Impairment

Dysphagia in infants is most commonly caused by neurologic impairment that is acquired in fetal or early postnatal life. The impairment may result from various respiratory or vascular problems that are shared by mother and fetus late in pregnancy or during delivery. The infant's respiration and neurocirculation may be impaired in the immediate newborn period. In spite of currently available therapy of Rh incompatibility, encephalopathy of hyperbilirubinemia may still occur. In many instances, no specific etiology of the impairment is identified.

Genetics has an increasing role in the diagnosis and evaluation of infants who have impairments of the oral and pharyngeal area, whether those impairments are of somatic structure or form or function. The postnatal period is the occasion for demonstration of certain metabolic problems that had been held in abeyance during pregnancy. The infant, as fetus, may have shared an endocrinopathy with the mother and then manifested it when the symbiosis was interrupted. For example, a diabetic mother's infant with hyperplasia of islet cells may be transiently hypoglycemic in the newborn period. A fetus may be defended by the maternal organism from its own metabolic anomaly, such as phenylketonuria. The first postnatal weeks or months may be a time of demonstration of progressive disorders, such as leukodystrophy or mitochondrial myopathy, which are not clearly related to the maternal–fetal symbiosis. The heritable problems, such as transient hypoglycemia in the infant of a diabetic mother or an infant with phenylketonuria, impair feeding by a mechanism of general depression or possible seizure. Progressive encephalopathy or neuropathy may specifically impair the oral or pharyngeal feeding actions.

Acquired Impairments of the Oral and Pharyngeal Feeding Apparatus

Acquired impairments of the oral and pharyngeal feeding apparatus are common but are usually benign and transient. Suckle feeding is usually diminished but not interrupted by acute upper respiratory infections; the infant has more feeding difficulties from nasal obstruction by secretions than by impairment of suckle or swallow. Similarly, oral mucositis of monilia (thrush) usually causes little impairment of suckle. Oral and/or pharyngeal lesions of herpes simplex cause feeding-related pain. In the infant with oral pain, from infectious, mechanical, or thermal inflammation of the mouth, suckle may be initiated and promptly discontinued, with indications of distress.

Iatrogenic Mechanisms

Some feeding impairments are incidental sequelae of pediatric care. The most common and increasing examples are those of infants who survive preterm birth and have been nourished parenterally and/or by enteric intubation for weeks or months. Thus, the infants have been deprived of oral feeding experience, and, perhaps, of spontaneous or pacifier-elicited suckling. Suckling deprivation is increased if the infant was ventilated via an orotracheal tube for a long time.

An analogous deprivation of oral feeding experience may occur during early postnatal surgery in or near the route of feeding, with the incidental effect of delaying the onset of oral feeding. The infant may have been adversely conditioned apropos of feeding, as by pain or distress associated with feeding, unskillful feeding, or interruption of the feeding schedule (Illingsworth and Lister 1964; Illingsworth 1969; Dowling 1977; Geertsma et al. 1985; Kaslon and Ruben 1978; Beraitis et al. 1981.)

In the circumstance of oral feeding impairment, the clinician is concerned with dual needs of nutrition and oral feeding experience. An infant who suckle feeds with variable competence, which possibly reflects the skill of different care givers, may graduate subtly into malnutrition. Conversely, an infant who is overtly malnourished, perhaps admitted to a hospital from a privation environment, may suckle avidly but may repair malnutrition only slowly. Intubation feeding, by nasogastric or gastrostoma tube, is indicated in either circumstance, in an effort to prevent possible neurodevelopmental failure associated with malnutrition (Cravioto and Arrieta 1979; Klein 1980; Prensky 1989).

PATTERNS OF SUCKLE FEEDING IMPAIRMENT

The evaluation of suckle feeding depends on an understanding of the actions and development of suckle and swallow and the relation of feeding to the infant's current state. Suckle feeding may be generally impaired, as in the infant who fails to arouse toward feeding, or impairment may be of feeding components, i.e., rooting and latching, suckle, pharyngeal swallow, or esophageal swallow. Clinicians are particularly concerned about an infant who fails to initiate rooting and latching during oral area stimulation, after the infant has been roused by gross movements of the limbs and trunk. The oral area stimulation should be in sequence of touching or stroking from the cheeks to the lips and thence to the tongue and lingual chamber (Morris and Klein 1987; Morris 1989). If the attempted elicitation of rooting by stroking the cheeks or the skin of the lips does not succeed in eliciting rooting, lip closure is evaluated by cross-wise stroking of mucosa of the inner lip (the pars villosa) (Bosma 1986a). Lip response may be a pattern of vertical closure, or pucker, or a pattern of eversion, or pout, appropriate to participation in suckle. The tongue and lingual cavity stimulation is usually by gloved finger, with the ball of the finger tip downward against the tongue. The stimulus motion is anteroposterior in direction. The response is enclosure by the tongue and lower lip graduating into anteroposterior tongue motions and then into the entire suckle motions, single and then rhythmic, of the tongue, lower lip, hyoid, and mandible. These gestures of evaluation of oral area responses are also the gestures employed in therapeutic stimulation, before feeding time, of the infant who demonstrates delay, deficiency, or variability of the oral stage of suckle feeding (Mueller 1972; Wilson 1977; Morris and Klein 1987, Morris 1989).

Failure of suckle elicitation in an infant who otherwise rouses well to stimulation outside of the oral area is found occasionally in infants who have had adverse conditioning experiences. The infant's aversion may be indicated at any stage of graduation toward suckle feeding, such as a disturbance during preparation for feeding or a negative response to rooting stimulation or nipple insertion. Suckling or suckle feeding may be initiated and then interrupted after a few swallows, possibly with the mouth then lax about the nipple. Restitution of feeding, in this circumstance, is a nursing or mothering skill. Often, it is necessary to continue nutrition by an indwelling soft nasogastric tube, which does not apparently impede suckle feeding.

The clinician is particularly concerned about an infant who suckles well but is impaired in pharyngeal swallow. This, again, may result from somatic embryopathy of form such as cleft or hypoplasia of the palate or cleft of the epiglottis or cricoid cartilage, or motor unit aplasia. The impairment may be of pharyngeal area sensory inputs, possibly combined with impairment in bulbar coordination of swallow, as in familial dysautonomia. Identification of the mechanism of selective pharyngeal dysphagia is aided by evaluation of other pharyngeal and laryngeal performances, including participation in tidal respiration, cry, and airway maintenance. For those with competence of nonfeeding performances of the pharynx and larynx, and incompetence in the suckle stage of feeding, selective pharyngeal dysphagia must be attributed to a localized lesion in the representation of swallow in the medulla. This selective impairment may be persistent. Cervical auscultation at the larynx, by stethoscope or by microphone and speaker, is useful in detection of pharyngeal swallow impairment, because the sounds indicate the event of swallow and also, if swallow of pharyngeal content fails to occur or is impaired, the sounds may demonstrate bubbles of respiration mixed with fluid, or choke, clearing, cough, or stridor. Further evaluation of pharyngeal dysphagia requires a videoradiographic study (Kramer 1989; Sivit 1991). Radiography may demonstrate that a marginally impaired swallow performs adequately if the formula is thickened, as by mixing with rice flour or with one of the recently available starch-based agents. If cervical auscultation is combined with videoradiography, with the acoustic recording on a channel of the video film, this combined recording affords a reference for the clinician who will subsequently guide the feeding care of the infant.

Suckle has been employed to facilitate swallow in an infant who has this selective impairment. Milk was delivered by syringe at the side of the pacifier. In this procedure, stethoscope auscultation was used to detect the effectiveness of this facilitation. Milk delivery was discontinued when swallows failed to empty the pharynx and retained swallow residua were evident, by audition, in the airway.

The normally feeding infant indicates satiation by attenuation of the suckle runs and increased frequency of feeding pauses. This attenuation can be distinguished from fatigue of the feeding effort, such as is found in myasthenia or myopathy or as in nonspecific fatigue of motor effort, as in some infants who have marginal cardiac or respiratory adequacy. The infant may actively grasp the nipple like a pacifier, with intermittent suckling, at the conclusion of feeding; this is noted particularly in breast feeding. At the conclusion of feeding, the young infant usually graduates into infant-pattern sleep.

Exceptionally, the infant may cry for a long time at the end of feeding. This postprandial crying, designated "fussiness" or "colic" has been attributed to inadequate burping, irritable bowel, or protein hypersensitivity (Illingsworth 1954; Wessel et al. 1954). Whether this prolonged crying is an individual difference in state regulation or a difference in parental tolerance may be difficult to discern (Taubman 1984). There is controversy whether an increase in carrying the infant during the day may have an effect on this problem (Barr et al. 1991).

ACQUISITION OF SUCKLE FEEDING IN THE PRETERM INFANT

The pharyngeal performances of swallowing of secretions, participation in respiration, and maintenance of an airway are adequate in small, viable, unimpaired preterm infants. The fetus has been swallowing since the twelfth week of gestation or earlier (Humphrey 1970). Fetuses near term are said to swallow 450 mL/d, a greater volume than in the first neonatal weeks (Golubeva et al. 1959). Prenatal ultrasound demonstrates frequent suckle actions.

Preterm infants have an oral and pharyngeal feeding experience that differs remarkably from that of a fetus in utero and of a term-born infant. Initial suckle, as early as 18 to 24 weeks gestation (Golubeva et al. 1959) is rapid, nonnutritive in pattern, and interspersed with nonspecific mouthing. Nonnutritive suckling concomitant with tube feeding is found to be associated with increased weight gain in preterm infants nourished by intubation (Measel and Anderson 1979; Field et al. 1982; Bernbaum et al. 1983). Field et al. (1982) showed that nonnutritive suckling also was associated with less restlessness and earlier achievement of bottle feeding. Nonnutritive suckling also increased polypeptide hormone release, with greater gastric secretion and earlier gastric emptying (Widstrom et al. 1988). In preterm infants without embryopathy of the oral and pharyngeal area or of the brain stem and without extensive acquired encephalopathy, this graduation toward mature suckle feeding progresses stably (Wolff 1968). The perioral elicitations of rooting are acquired later in development. Gryboski (1969) observed preterm infants sequentially from gestational week 32 and noted graduation of nonspecific mouthing into single or few nutrient suckles. At 35 to 36 weeks, suckling was in bursts or runs, interspersed with swallows. These observations are confirmed by Colley and Creamer (1958), Casear et al. (1982), Daniels et al. (1986), and Herbst (1989). Various sugars, particularly sucrose, elicit increase in suckling effort and duration of runs (Maller and Turner 1973; Steiner 1977; Ashmead et al. 1980). Tone in the esophagus and the esophagogastric junction is low in the early preterm infant, but tone in the pharyngoesophageal segment is comparable to that at term (Milla 1991). Esophageal peristalsis becomes more consistent and of higher amplitude as the preterm infant approaches term (Sondheimer 1983; Herbst 1989; Milla 1991).

Orogastric or nasogastric intubation feeding continues during these early feeding efforts, with supplementation of the oral feeding or replacement if the oral feeding attempt was unsuccessful. Of these methods, orogastric intubation is associated with fewer adverse effects on lung function than nasogastric intubation, in preterm infants smaller than 2,000 g. Awareness of the adverse effects of gavage feeding on compliance of the lung and chest wall and increase in diaphragmatic work requirement encourages the clinician toward oral feeding (Heldt 1988). The greatest risk to this progression toward oral feeding is that of interruption of feeding experience by reason of clinical exigencies, such as sepsis or other intercurrent illness. Illness of the preterm infant may occasion retrogression or actual loss of recently acquired advances in feeding. Orotracheal intubation for respiratory support particularly impedes feeding-equivalent experience, as the tube fills and immobilizes the mouth. Stabilizing flanges may cover the lips and cheeks. As increasing numbers of small preterm infants survive, the incidence and duration of respiratory assistance is increasing (Hack et al. 1991). The provision of oral feeding experience deserves and depends on the best available skills of the mother or other care person. If suckle feeding experience is not currently available, periods of passive suckle-equivalent oral stimulation should be provided (Morris 1989).

BREAST FEEDING OF THE PRETERM AND THE FEEDING-IMPAIRED INFANT

In the Western world, breast feeding of preterm and feeding-impaired infants has been largely replaced by formula feeding by nipple or by intubation (Jelliffe and Jelliffe 1978). Artificial milk-consistency feeding has been highly successful in nutrition and the nonmaternal care of infants, but these clinical advances have been detrimental to the mother–infant relationship. During gestation, the mother and infant are each prepared for suckle feeding. The mother has been furnished with a responsive lactation apparatus and with nipples that are well contoured for the infant's mouth and will be further adapted in form during each feeding (Erenberg et al. 1986). The mother is prepared in mind and spirit to provide the ambience that is so much a part of suckle feeding. The mother has olfactory cues to which the infant is responsive (Steiner 1977; Sarnat 1978; Schaal 1988; Sullivan et al. 1991). The mother also provides duplication of feeding circumstance. The milk is warm. Initially, postdelivery, it consists of colostrum. At each feeding, the infant's initial suckling usually obtains little milk, so that the dysphagia-liable infant's first swallows may be safer. Subsequently, the quantity of milk released varies with suckle effort and corresponding stimulation to lactation. Late in the feeding, and during the attenuation of effort at the end of feeding, the infant's swallows may be followed by phonation.

In Western hospitals, neonatal intensive care units customarily graduate a premature infant from nasogastric tube alimentation, of formula or expressed breast milk, to bottle feeding, using a premie nipple, and thence possibly to breast feeding, if the mother has been able to maintain milk production by breast pumping. However, recent studies have demonstrated that premature infants as young as 32 weeks gestational age or less than 1,500 g can be graduated directly to breast feeding, if the feeding coordination has been achieved (Meier and Anderson 1987; Meier and Pugh 1985; McCoy et al. 1988; Blackman 1991), and if the hospital routines can be adapted to permit flexibility in the time and duration of breast feeding. Breast feeding was found to be associated with greater stability of PO_2 levels than was bottle feeding (Meier and Anderson 1987). We anticipate that breast feeding of premature infants may become common practice in neonatal intensive care units in which this effort is well sponsored. Some intensive care units encourage mothers to express milk for intubation or bottle feeding of medically problematic postterm infants, with or without feeding impairment (Wilks and Meier 1988). No studies of breast feeding of dysphagic infants have been reported. The need for such studies in dysphagic infants is apparent, for these infants may be particularly in need of the resources and mechanisms of communication that breast feeding affords. In the face of these benefits of satisfaction and interpersonal exchange, it is important to recognize that the nutritional adequacy of breast feeding depends on the potential lactation efficiency of the mother and on the mother's lactation response state at the time of individual feeding. The preterm or dysphagic infant may fail to thrive with breast feeding, as a normal infant may occasionally fail to thrive (Evans and Davies 1977).

This experience of preterm infant feeding in modern contemporary nurseries is in striking contrast with the care of premature and small-for-dates infants born at high altitude in parts of the Andean mountains. As reported by Anderson et al. (1986) and Leeuw et al. (1991), these infants are swaddled and bound between the mothers' breast, with ad libitum access to nipple feeding.

TRANSITIONAL FEEDING

This is a time of graduation from exclusive suckle feeding of liquids to voluntary ingestion of physically varied foods. It is also a time of demonstration of various neurologic impairments of feeding actions. Recognition of these impairments depends on familiarity with the patterns of normal postsuckle feeding development.

The supplementation of suckle feeding by addition of discriminate oral awareness and voluntary oral feeding actions begins in the first postterm months. At term, the feeding-ready infant is fully preoccupied with the suckle feeding performance. During established suckle feeding, the infant may tolerate, and fail to respond to, other stimuli, including those of some painful clinical procedures. In some pharyngeally dysphagic infants, suckle feeding may continue in spite of nasal or laryngeal penetration of pharyngeal content.

Within a few weeks of term, volition and variation are added, usually near the completion of the suckle feeding session. The infant interrupts feeding to give visual attention or to phonate with the nipple still in place.

The graduation of oral responses and actions has been comprehensively described (Mueller 1972; Wilson 1977; Morris 1982; Morris and Klein 1987; Gisel 1988a; Morris 1989; Gisel 1991; Stolovitz and Gisel 1991). Spoon feeding of pablum or similar puree consistency foods at 4 to 6 months elicits mouth opening. The pablum is ingested by suckle actions. At this time, the infant's hand actions graduate from a finger or a fisted hand in the mouth to bringing manually manipulated objects into the mouth. This can include manual delivery of soft foods or of crisp but soluble crackers. Spoon feeding or independent hand feeding is graduated toward semiparticulate foods, such as small vegetal bits in a puree matrix.

Chewing

The acquisition of chewing and of biting skills are separate achievements. As noted previously above, the suckle feeding performance is oriented on the median portion of the mouth. Fluid consistency material usually does not penetrate into the lateral portion of the mouth adjacent to the molar alveolar ridges. The buccal recess of the infant (Figure 5.7) is minimal in area.

In young children, the oral manipulations of chewing differ qualitatively from the suckle-pattern manipulation of purees (Stolovitz and Gisel 1991). Chewing is a lateralized performance and is oriented about the molar area (Dubner et

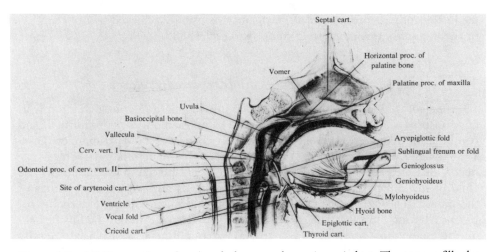

Figure 5.7 Midline section of oral and pharyngeal area in an infant. The tongue fills the lingual cavity, which is bounded in this demonstration by the oral palate, mandible, body of the hyoid bone, and mylohyoideus. The tongue is slightly separated from the oral and pharyngeal palate and is displaced anteriorly in this drawing. The pharynx is short in vertical dimension. The tip of the epiglottis approximates the uvula at the inferior end of the velum. The pharyngoesophageal segment is adjacent to the inferior margin of the cricoid cartilage; it is drawn in the open position. The infant's larynx differs notably from that of the adult. The arytenoid and corniculate cartilages are surrounded by a large mass of loose connective tissue, which diminishes the lumen of the laryngeal vestibule. The length of the vocal folds and of the ventricle is diminished in comparison with the internal diameters of the thyroid and cricoid cartilages.

al. 1978; Luschei and Goldberg 1981). The tongue has a major role in the chewing performance (Gisel 1988a) (see Figure 5.8). It shifts the oral content to the molar area and interacts with the buccal musculature to repeatedly place the food on the moving molar table. At the completion of mastication, the tongue transfers the food to the primary bolus accumulation area, adjacent to the junction of the bony and muscular portions of the palate. These various components of chewing are guided by subjective cues generated by voluntary manipulation of the food. Firm (solid) foods are more effective than viscous or pureed foods in elicitation of chewing (Gisel 1988b, 1991). The increasing chewing efficiency, to end-point of swallow, of normal children between 6 months and 2 years has been calibrated per videophotographic observation, using gelatin masses of differing sizes (Archambault et al. 1991). The initiation of swallow by conveyance of the bolus through the faucial isthmus is also voluntary. The young child may be seen to interrupt oral feeding and give attention to the swallow.

The mandibular motions of mastication are usually vertical in their early manifestation. The motions become principally transverse (grinding) and increase in efficiency. During transitional feeding, the sided incidence changes. At 2 years, 60 percent of chewing is on the right side; at 4 years, 60 percent is on left (Gisel 1988a). The achievement of chewing is not dependent on eruption of molar teeth; the entire coordination of mastication is usually achieved before eruption of the molars begins at 12 to 20 months (Gisel 1988b).

Evaluation of Chewing in Feeding-Impaired Children

Intraoral food manipulation is commonly impaired in young children who have disorders of oral area coordination. This manipulation in normal and coordination-impaired children has been described in a standard manner (Gisel 1988a; Gisel and Patrick 1988). Evaluation of this manipulation requires patience. Bits of cracker or readily softened candy are placed in the mouth by the child or the clinician and "followed" by inspections during passive openings of the mouth. The test material may remain on the tongue during externally apparent chewing motions. The material may be extruded through the lips or held on the tongue dorsum until swallowed. The material may be displaced laterally and not be retrieved (this is termed "squirreling"). In some children who have oral dyspraxia, chewing may be elicited by the care person placing particulate food on the molar table. At a lesser level of competence in such children, food placed on either molar table is moved by the tongue to its dorsum and there mashed by the tongue.

Infant-patterned suckle feeding is available in some orally dyskinetic children. They may retain rooting and latching responses. As part of their latching response, the head and neck are stabilized about a nipple equivalent. During videofluoroscopic study, barium-coated cracker bits deposited on the tongue of these children may be carried into the pharynx by suckle actions of the tongue and are swallowed.

Biting

Biting is separate from chewing in its coordination pattern and in the mechanism and schedule of its generation. Discrete voluntary biting can be readily distinguished from the sustained jaw closure that occurs in some forms of spastic dyskinesia. Biting on the nipple is first noted as a part of oral play at the end of suckle feeding. The infant of 6 to 12 months may bite objects that he or she brings to the mouth as a part of hand and mouth play. During transitional feeding the mouth may be voluntarily firmly closed by the jaw as well as by the lips during defensive resistance to feeding. During biting, the mandible is guided vertically in the midline toward such interincisor approximation as may be available in the child's arrangement of maxilla and mandible. The posteroanterior relation of the mandible and maxilla differ in biting and chewing. The mandible is commonly farther forward in biting than in chewing. The performance of biting is as liable to impairment as the performance of chewing in oral dyskinesia but its impairment is less well defined.

These graduations of oral skills indicate increasing awareness of food and other possible ingesta and increasing attention to oral actions. Selection or rejection of foods, and participation in feeding, is discriminate and is initially varied, possibly varying with the care person or the circumstance. Studies by Davis (1939) of young children offered trays of varied foods demonstrated nutritionally irregular selection during each meal but a nutritionally balanced diet over a period of days. Much of fluid intake during transitional feeding may continue to be by suckle feeding at breast or by bottle.

These developmental generations of the feeding performance are uniquely individual (Bosma 1976). They depend on the individual's accumulation of experience with foods, feeding circumstances, and culture. But this development also depends on variations in innate elements, including the array of oral mucosal sensory receptors. The resultant feeding patterns, which are carried into childhood, are a product of feeding satisfaction and failure. The feeding distortions, disruptions, and experiences of distress and failure to which the neurologically impaired infant and child are liable are mechanisms that subsequently influence the individual's feeding patterns. In some circumstances, noted in the following section, the dysphagic child's feeding pattern may be determined extensively by experiences of failure.

If semiparticulate food or small food bits are delivered into the mouth of a child who has impairment of chew and bite, the food may be partially prepared for swallowing by tongue mashing.

The motions of tongue mashing are similar, in external observation, to the early, vertical motions of chewing, but visualization of the oral cavity, by passive opening of the mouth or by videoradiography in posteroanterior projection, demonstrates that the food is not in the molar area. The tongue-mashed food, including particles, may be effectively swallowed. It is important to recognize, in this connection, that the feeding-related actions of the pharynx include more than swallow of accumulated secretions or of a food bolus delivered from the

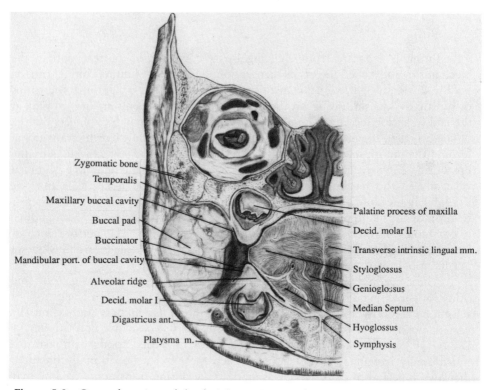

Zygomatic bone
Temporalis
Maxillary buccal cavity
Buccal pad
Buccinator
Mandibular port. of buccal cavity
Alveolar ridge
Decid. molar I
Digastricus ant.
Platysma m.

Palatine process of maxilla
Decid. molar II
Transverse intrinsic lingual mm.
Styloglossus
Genioglossus
Median Septum
Hyoglossus
Symphysis

Figure 5.8 Coronal section of the facial area in an infant. A section through the body of the tongue, symphysis of the mandible, oral palate, central portion of the nasal chamber, and buccal pad. The tongue fills the oral cavity, which in this plane is bounded inferiorly by the mandible and the mandibular ridge and laterally by the buccal wall.

mouth. The pharynx participates in more general performances of the upper portion of the alimentary tract, including gagging, vomiting, and rumination. The pharynx also participates with the larynx in the respiratory actions of coughing and choking and in the less effortful actions of clearing secretions or food residua in the trachea or the laryngeal vestibule.

Particularly during the first part of transitional feeding, the normal infant or young child gags or chokes mildly, with little distress or indication of alarm. A notable incidental videoradiographic observation in some neurologically impaired dysphagic children is that of regurgitation of pharyngeal content into the mouth by a simple constriction action of the pharynx; the content may then be expectorated or retained in the mouth until it is reswallowed. This pharyngo-oral regurgitation differs from choking or coughing, in that it is not associated with expiration. It differs also from vomiting in that the esophagus is not emptied upward and the child's pharynx and mouth are not in a vomiting or retching position.

MATURE FEEDING IN CHILDHOOD

The graduations from transitional into fully mature feeding reflect the increasing autonomy of person, the independent exploration of foods, leading to omnivorous diet, and independent use of feeding utensils. Drinking from cup or glass is increasingly skilled. The actions of food prehension and biting and the various actions of the tongue, buccal wall, and mandibular muscles in chewing and bolus selection are stabilized and become more automatic. Maturation of the coordination of the facial muscles about the mouth is an important element of graduation into mature feeding. The buccinator muscle controls the expanding sulcus lateral to the molars. This function becomes more important as the infantile sucking pad and the panniculus in the cheek are diminished and, with dental eruption and the change in form of the mandible, the mandible is increasingly separated from the maxilla. During chewing, the buccinator acts in a reciprocal manner with the transversely moving tongue to maneuver food on the molar table. The orbicularis oris and mimetic muscles are also changed in coordination pattern to achieve stable labial enclosure during intraoral food manipulation. This enclosure differs from that during suckle feeding, in which the lips are everted in pouting contour so that their inner aspect, adjacent to the pars villosa, approximates the nipple. During the suckle action, the lower lip, along with the tongue, mandible, and hyoid, is moved in relation to the nipple. During mature oral feeding in childhood, labial enclosure of oral content is in a vertical pattern. In the circumstance of incisor malocclusion, overbite, or prognathism, the upper or lower incisors may be included in the labial seal. Failure to achieve this labial seal, by any of its coordination mechanisms, results in spill or drooling (Sochaniwskyj et al. 1986; Harris and Purdy 1987). The sensory resources of the oral area pertinent to chewing and biting are substantially increased by eruption of the teeth. During childhood, the mouth is enlarged and, more significantly, is changed in form by enlargement and eruption of the teeth and by changes in dimension and form of the mandible and midfacial skeleton (Bosma 1975, 1985) (Figure 5.9). The anatomically related structures of the tongue, hyoid, and larynx descend in relation to the facial skeleton and the cervical vertebra. These changes in the facial and pharyngeal skeleton are related to changes in oral and pharyngeal feeding actions and also in the positional or postural actions of the head and neck and about the pharyngeal airway. These relations are reciprocal: the motor performances influence the form and position of the skeleton and related anatomy and, vice versa, these anatomic changes influence the displacements, but not the basic coordination pattern, of feeding and posture. The coordination pattern of pharyngeal swallow in the child who has achieved mature feeding is essentially similar to that in the adult, shown in Figure 5.10. The buccal space is enlarged by growth of the molars and their related alveolar structures and by diminution in the sucking pad and adjacent panniculus. Mastication and the lingual actions of selection and sizing of the bolus become more efficient. The entire suckle feeding sequence is retained throughout life although, in normal individuals, its corollary reflexes of rooting

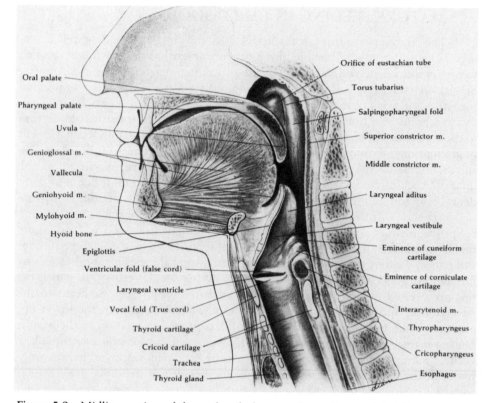

Figure 5.9 Midline section of the oral and pharyngeal area in an adult. This section, in comparison with that of Figure 5.7, demonstrates the result of postnatal growth of the oral and pharyngeal area. Note particularly the growth of the pharynx and larynx and the developmental descent of the larynx and adjacent pharynx in relation to the mandible and the cervical vertebrae.

and nipple latching are lost. Suckle feeding may continue to be a strategic mechanism of oral ingestion throughout life (Ramsey 1986).

FEEDING IMPAIRMENTS IN CHILDHOOD

The maturations of feeding actions and of the interaction of feeding and posture are of considerable significance in the feeding patterns and competencies of children whose feeding impairments originated in the fetus, the preterm infant, or the full-term infant. The impairments, which were manifested during transitional feeding, may simply be stabilized into lifetime patterns. This stabilization may be'at levels of feeding competence that are below their potential.

Alternatively, the child who demonstrates oral or pharyngeal dysphagia during the time of transitional feeding is liable to different, possibly increasing,

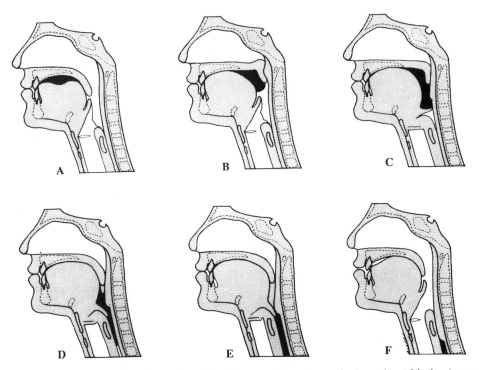

Figure 5.10 Summary schematic of the pharyngeal swallow of a large liquid bolus in an adult, as demonstrated by radiography in the lateral projection. (A) The bolus is retained in the oral cavity by approximation of the velum with the tongue; nasal portal respiration can be continued. (B) The bolus is conveyed through the faucial isthmus and into the oropharynx by the tongue. The velum is displaced upward and backward and is approximated by a protrusion on the posterior pharyngeal wall—the beginning of the pharyngeal peristaltic wave. (C) The bolus extends into the laryngopharynx. The epiglottis is tilted downward, and the hyoid and larynx are fully displaced upward and forward. The peristaltic wave is descending in the constrictor wall. (D) The bolus penetrates the opened pharyngoesophageal segment. The peristaltic wave has descended further. The upper portion of the palatopharyngeal isthmus has reopened. (E) The bolus has nearly traversed the pharynx. The peristaltic wave has reached the hypopharynx. The oropharynx is beginning to reopen. (F) The mouth, now empty, and the pharynx have returned to reference position. (Reprinted with permission from Springer-Verlag, from Donner MW, Bosma JF, Robertson D. Anatomy and physiology of the pharynx. Gastrointest Radiol 1985; 10:196–212.)

feeding problems at school age and puberty. These changes vary with the mechanisms of impairment. A malformation of the oral and pharyngeal area, the medulla and pons, or adjacent cranial skeleton may result in increasing impairment, or a pathologic process of the brain, musculature, or peripheral nerves may be progressive.

Increasing problems may result from social and environmental circumstances. Feeding efficiency may actually decline as the individual, along with his or her parents and care givers, attempts to achieve the mature feeding patterns of the family or other associates by use of feeding resources that are marginal or inadequate. The child and family may be unwilling to accept the available, and possibly more efficient, resources of suckle feeding or of pablum feeding by spoon or spout.

Embryopathy of the Oral and Pharyngeal Area

Most of the children who have embryopathy of the oral and pharyngeal area but who have intact or adequate neurologic mechanisms for postural, respiratory, and feeding performances are expected to continue in the linked development of performances and their effector anatomy.

In the child who has severe hypoplasia of the tongue, the physiologic compensations of the submental musculature, pharyngeal palate, and pharynx and the anatomic adaptations of the facial skeleton continue during childhood and puberal growth in the facial and pharyngeal area. The repaired cleft palate functions well, preventing nasal regurgitation, until the time of spontaneous normal diminution of the adenoid mass, when nasal regurgitation may occur, along with hypernasality.

Embryopathy of the Medulla and Pons

The oral and pharyngeal feeding actions of the children who have embryopathy of the medulla and pons depend on possible further anatomic changes in the area of the malformation and on possible late changes in an Arnold-Chiari malformation (Caviness 1976, Warkany et al. 1981). The adaptations and compensations noted previously may be available for the irregularly disseminated muscle deficiencies and contractures that may be a part of nuclear hypoplasia.

Dyscoordination in the Oral and Pharyngeal Area

The dysphagia problems of the school-age child who has dyscoordination in the oral and pharyngeal area vary with the pattern of the disorder. The feeding problems and adaptations of those who have athetosis or choreoathetosis are similar to adults who have these disorders (see Chapters 2 and 8.) The dysphagia problems of school-age and puberal children who have spastic disorder may increase. The hypertonus of the cervical extensors and the submental muscles and genioglossus, which become evident in some spastic quadriplegics in the time of transitional feeding, may be increasingly demonstrated in the child in the form of sustained hypertonus, with occasional surges during times of effort, as at meals. Increasing hypertonus, possibly associated with contracture of the craniocervical extensor and the mandible depressor muscles may handicap oral and pharyngeal feeding actions by a secondary mechanism of malposition of oral and pharyngeal structures. Chew and bite may be absent or minimal. Tongue mashing may still sufficiently prepare soft and semiparticulate foods for the child's pharyngeal swallow; this adequacy may be inferred from the child's freedom from coughing and choking at mealtime, and, more significantly, by history, which indicates no chronic lower respiratory disorder or frank pneumonia. Competence of pharyngeal swallow, by criteria of its promptness of occurrence, effectiveness of bolus transit, and absence of penetration into the larynx or the palatopharyngeal isthmus, can be evaluated by videoradiography (Kramer 1989; Sivit 1990). These children's liability to laryngeal penetration and dispersion of food during swallow or regurgitation from the esophagus and stomach can be evaluated by scintigraphic tracing of radionuclide-labeled foods (Ham et al. 1985; Espinola 1986).

The children who have dyscoordination of the oral and pharyngeal stages of feeding may also have impairments of respiration control in general and in respiration adjacent to feeding. These abnormalities of respiration coincident with dysphagia have been physiologically described by Kenny et al. (1989a). Kenny and associates (1989b) also have developed a Multidisciplinary Feeding Profile that provides a description of the anatomy of the oral and pharyngeal area in bulbar dyskinetic children and particulars of their feeding and respiratory performances. The Profile has been standardized (Judd et al. 1989) and can be employed as a reference for description of these children.

The increasing nutritional needs of the child must be considered. We are reminded of the need for frequent reassessment of feeding competence and routines. This reassessment must consistently include estimation of nutritional state, at least by weight progression and thickness of skin folds in areas that are least distorted by dyskinesia (Patrick and Gisel, 1990). In dysphagic children who are liable to malnutrition, there is a constant possibility of supplementation of oral intake by intubation feeding, via a nasogastric or gastrostoma route, on a schedule that interferes minimally with the incentives, actions, and satisfactions of oral feeding. Clinicians who care for dysphagic infants and children are now well aware of the liability of intubation feeding to increase gastroesophageal reflux and esophageal and esophagopharyngeal regurgitation (Raventos et al. 1982; Mollitt et al. 1985).

Progressive Encephalopathy

Feeding competence may be impaired in progressive encephalopathy. The mechanisms, neurologic form, and patterns of progression are reviewed in pediatric neurology textbooks (Swaiman 1989; Menkes 1990; Brett 1991). The impairment may be a nonspecific diminution in appetite and other aspects of feeding incentive or a more specific impairment of the oral and pharyngeal feeding actions. The pattern and severity of feeding impairment reflects the involvement of the bulbar area in the pathologic process. In the simplest and most easily managed pattern, the encephalopathy spares the bulbar area, so that nutrition can be maintained by infant-patterned suckle feeding.

A special concern is that of interaction of feeding with seizures in those progressive encephalopathies that are epileptogenic. The pattern of these inter-actions varies. Children who have seizure-free intervals may be fed at those times; the success of feeding depends on the perceptions of the care person. Occasionally, partial seizures with preserved consciousness may be associated with feeding in transitional or mature pattern. If these partial seizures are man-ifested only in the limbs, it may be possible to continue feeding. If, however, partial seizures are evidenced in the bulbar innervation, as by nystagmus, by twitches of the facial muscles, or by apnea, then oral feeding should be inter-rupted. In occasional examples, partial seizures appear to be diminished during stable suckle feeding. If the child is pharyngeally dysphagic, pharyngeal content entering the larynx may elicit laryngospasm, possibly graduating into grand mal seizures. Conversely, persons liable to laryngospasm can sometimes sense an impending episode and can avoid the episode, and possible further seizure activ-ity, by voluntary swallow. The subtlest correlation of feeding and seizure-like activity is that of syncope on swallowing, as reported in a 4-year-old child by Woody and Kiel (1986). Comparable episodes of syncope with bradycardia are described during esophageal swallow in adults (Levin and Posner 1972; Kalloor et al. 1977).

Static or Progressive Myopathy

The clinical pattern and sequence that results from progressive myopathy, such as that of nemaline or mitochondrial myopathy or muscular dystrophy (Swaiman 1989), in many respects, is similar to that of the child with acute anterior poliomyelitis. In either circumstance, impairment of feeding may be a sensitive indicator of bulbar impairment. Impairment of pharyngeal swallow may be critical to life. The progression of myopathic impairments may be irreg-ular in the muscles of the face, mandible, or tongue or in the intrinsic and the supporting muscles of the pharynx and larynx. Successive evaluations of feeding performance are essential. Optimally, these should include successive radio-graphic imaging at intervals determined by clinical changes in feeding competence or by calendar. On the basis of such evaluations, the clinician can modify the feeding routine, such as by exclusive use of suckle feeding by the use of a prosthesis by which to achieve a better match of the oral cavity to the atrophic or ptotic tongue, or by the use of intermittent sleep time or continual tube feeding.

Static or Progressive Peripheral Neuropathy

Familial dysautonomia (Riley 1974 Axelrod et al. 1974) is the type form of static or progressive peripheral neuropathy. It may be manifested by hypertonia and poor suckle in early infancy (Axelrod et al. 1987). Later in infancy and during transitional and mature feeding, feeding impairment results from defi-ciency of saliva and other secretions and from incoordination of pharyngeal and esophageal swallow (Silbiger et al. 1967). The syndrome is restricted to offspring of Eastern European Jewish ancestry and is identified by an absence of fungiform papillae on the tongue and by absence of local reaction to cutaneous injection of histamine. Other forms of congenital peripheral neuropathy (Axelrod and Pearson 1984) may be progressive and occasionally may be associated with self-mutilation of the lips, tongue, or hands, as well as with increasing oral and pharyngeal feeding impairment.

Diminution in oral sensory input also may result from loss of teeth, chronic periodontal inflammation, or extensive orthodontic work. Another possible mechanism of diminution of oral mucosal sensibility is that of dessication and chronic inflammation secondary to continuous, exclusive mouth breathing.

Acute Encephalopathy in Childhood

Acute encephalopathy with dysphagia may result from neurotrauma, tumor surgery, or encephalitis in a previously normal child. The circumstances and sequence of events in children is generally similar to that in adults. The acute occasion, in many instances, is associated with unconsciousness. If the initial impairment is severe and/or prolonged, the child may be fed by nasogastric intubation or gastrostoma and may be tracheotomized. Recovery of feeding and of other, related oral and pharyngeal functions depends on the nature and severity of the lesion of the bulbar sensory and motor nuclei and of the bulbar and suprabulbar representations of oral and pharyngeal performances.

The feeding impairments that may occur as effects of acute encephalopathy in school-age or pubertal children differ from those of comparable central lesions in the fetus or young infant. The differences are both in the brain and the oral and pharyngeal area. The mature or nearly mature brain has lesser plasticity and, therefore, has less potential for adaptation by surviving neural structures. The peripheral oral and pharyngeal structures presumably had been formed by normal development until the time of the injury. A newly acquired impairment, as by poliomyelitis, of the muscles of the face, mandible, tongue, or pharynx may actually be handicapped by an anatomically normal oral and pharyngeal skeleton. One must appreciate, however, that functional adaptation to the impairment on the part of the skeleton and other structures may begin promptly after function is resumed. In this circumstance of mismatch of performance with peripheral anatomy, use of an oral prosthesis may be helpful in regaining functional feeding. In experience with children recovering from acute bulbar poliomyelitic impairment of the mouth and pharynx (Bosma 1957a,b,c), we became aware of the varied succession of performance impairments and adaptive actions that reflect recovery of muscle strength, increase or release of muscle contracture, and increasing performance awareness and skill. In successive evaluations of children during recovery from feeding impairment due to acute suprabulbar central lesion, it is particularly important to evaluate infantile suckle and transitional puree feeding since these early functions may be differentially retained and available.

COMMUNITY AND PUBLIC RESOURCES FOR THE FEEDING-IMPAIRED INFANT AND CHILD

The special measures that are required to ensure adequate hydration and nutrition of infants and children who have neurologic feeding impairments are now commonly available in the Western world. These measures range from physical modifications of food and adaptations of food delivery implements and feeding procedures to direct alimentation by nasogastric or gastrostoma tube. In some instances, nutrition by these special means is not adequate, so that the children demonstrate growth retardation and malnutrition (Gisel and Patrick 1988; Patrick and Gisel, 1990). Nutritional failure demonstrated by successive observations of weight and skin fold thickness is an indication of need for changes in feeding routine and/or supplemental feeding by intubation.

The special feeding measures needed by these infants and children greatly increase the concerns and efforts of their parents or other care persons. The home environment commonly requires adaptation of personnel and space and, in many instances, special facilities, as for food preparation and storage and for custom feeding equipment. Increasingly, these handicapped infants and children are placed in day care centers or special schools. Selection of the care center is greatly influenced by the child's feeding requirements. Those who have similar needs for feeding assistance, or for intubation, are commonly further grouped at mealtimes. Such community-based centers have usually been generated by parent efforts. These aggregations and related clinical and daily care will be much increased by federal and state sponsorship and arrangement under US Public Law 99-457, An Act for Care for Handicapped Infants and Toddlers. We may anticipate that this further sponsorship and organization will result in more consistent reassessments and possible revisions and adaptations of feeding care, appropriate to changes in the child's feeding patterns and nutritional requirements. We reasonably anticipate that these aggregations of feeding-impaired infants and children, with attendant increase in expertise in their evaluation and care, will result in greater efficiency and use of oral feeding. An essential element of these special schools and centers is the successive evaluations of the competence of oral feeding, resulting in progressive changes in the choice of food texture, food delivery, or feeding mechanism in the center and in the home. Feeding competence can be sequentially evaluated by gross estimation of intake from notes of the care giver at test feeding, and this information can be converted by a dietitian into an intake estimation. In problematic situations or for investigative purposes a video-implemented, standardized, and quantified Gisel evaluation of feeding can be employed (Gisel 1988a, 1991). Competence of current and recent intake can be inferred from the child's nutritional state and increments of weight plotted on a weight-for-age chart. This information can be the basis for making decisions about intubation (Gisel and Patrick 1988; Patrick and Gisel, 1990), such as whether the intubation should be intermittent, as during night sleep, or continuous, and whether gastrostoma, with its attendant liabilities, is justified.

REFERENCES

Anderson GC, Marks EA, Wahlberg V. Kangaroo care for premature infants. Am J Nurs 1986; 86:807–9.

Archambault M, Millen K, Gisel EG. Effect of bite size on eating development in normal children 6 months to 2 years of age. Physical and Occupational Therapy in Pediatrics 1991; 10:29–47.

Ashmead DH, Reilly BM, Lipsitt LP. Neonates heart-rate, sucking rhythm, and sucking amplitude as a function of sweet taste. J Exp Child Psychol 1980; 29:264–81.

Axelrod FB, Nachtigal R, Dancis NR. Familial dysautonomia: diagnosis, pathogenesis and management. Adv Pediatr 1974; 21:75–96.

Axelrod FB, Pearson J. Congenital sensory neuropathies: diagnostic distinction from familial dysautonomia. Am J Dis Child 1984; 138:947–54.

Axelrod FB, Porges RF, Sein ME. Neonatal recognition of familial dysautonomia. J Pediatr 1987; 110:946–48.

Bamford O. Personal communication, 1991.

Barr RG, McMullan SJ, Spiess H, et al. Carrying as colic "therapy": a randomized controlled trial. Pediatrics 1991; 87:623–30.

Beraitis S, Kolb R, Sperling E, et al. Development of a child with long-lasting deprivation of oral feeding. Am Acad Child Psychiat 1981; 20:53–64.

Bernbaum JC, Peckham GJ, Pereira GR, et al. Nonnutritive sucking during gavage feeding enhances growth and maturation in premature infants. Pediatrics 1983; 1:41–45.

Blackman L. Personal communication, 1991.

Blass EM, Teicher MH. Suckling. Science 1980; 210:15–20.

Boix-Ochoa M, Canals J. Maturation of the lower esophagus. J Pediatr Surg 1976; 11:749–56.

Bosma JF. Studies of the pharynx. I. Poliomyelitic disabilities of the upper pharynx. Pediatrics 1957a; 19:881–907.

Bosma JF. Studies of the pharynx. II. Poliomyelitic disabilities of the lower pharynx. Pediatrics 1957b; 19:1053–79.

Bosma JF. Residual disability of pharyngeal area resulting from poliomyelitis. JAMA 1957c; 165:216–21.

Bosma JF, Truby HM, Lind J. Distortions of upper respiratory and swallow motions in infants having anomalies of the upper pharynx. Acta Paediatr Scand 1966; 163(suppl):111–28.

Bosma JF. Anatomic and physiologic development of the speech apparatus. In: Tower DB, ed. The Nervous System, vol. 3. Human communication and its disorders. New York: Raven, 1975; 469–81.

Bosma JF. Sensorimotor examination of the mouth and pharynx. In: Kawamura Y, ed. Frontiers of oral physiology. Basel: Karger, 1976; 2:78–107.

Bosma JF. Postnatal ontogney of performances of the pharynx, larynx and mouth. Am Rev Respir Dis 1985; 131(suppl):S10–S15.

Bosma JF. Anatomy of the infant head. Baltimore: Johns Hopkins University Press, 1986a.

Bosma JF. Development of feeding. J Clin Nutr 1986b; 5:210–8.

Bosma JF, Hepburn LG, Josell SD, et al. Ultrasound demonstration of tongue motions during suckle feeding. Dev Med Child Neurol 1990; 32:223–9.

Brett EM. Paediatric neurology. Edinburgh: Churchill Livingstone, 1991.

Bruston WR. Mandibular retrognathia. Neonatal Surg 1978; 137–42.

Casaer P, Daniels H, Devileger H, et al. Feeding behaviour in preterm neonates. Early Human Dev 1982; 7:331–46.

Caviness VS Jr. The Chiari malformations of the posterior fossa and their relation to hydrocephalus. Dev Med Child Neurol 1976; 18:103.

Cohen SR, Thompson JW. Variants of Mobius syndrome and central neurologic impairment. Lindeman procedure in children. Ann Otol Rhinol Laryngol 1987; 96:93–100.

Colley JRT, Creamer B. Suckling and swallowing in infants. Br Med J 1958; 12:422–23.

Cravioto J, Arrieta R. Stimulation and mental development of malnourished infants. Lancet 1979; 2:899.

Daniels H, Casaer P, Devileger H, et al. Mechanisms of feeding efficiency in preterm infants. J Pediatr Gastroenterol Nutr 1986; 5:593–6.

Daniels H, Devileger H, Minami T, et al. Infant feeding and cardiorespiratory maturation. Neuropediatrics 1990; 21:9–10.

Davis CM. Results of the self-selection of diets by young children. Can Med Assoc J 1939; 41:257–61.

Doty RW. Neural organization of deglutition. In: Code CF, ed. Handbook of Physiology, section 6, Alimentary canal. Washington, DC: American Physiological Society, 1968; 4:1861–902.

Dowling S. Seven infants with esophageal atresia: a developmental study. Psychoanal Study Child 1977; 32:215–57.

Dubner R, Sessle BJ, Storey AT. The neural basis of oral and facial function. New York: Plenum, 1978.

Erenberg A, Smith WL, Nowak AJ, et al. Evaluation of sucking in the breast-fed infant by ultrasonography. Pediatr Res 1986; 20, 409a (abstract).

Espinola D. Radionuclide evaluation of pulmonary aspiration: four birds with one stone—esophageal transit, gastroesophageal reflux, gastric emptying, and bronchopulmonary aspiration. Dysphagia 1986; 1:101–4.

Evans PR. Nuclear agenesis Mobius syndrome: the congenital facial diplegia syndrome. Am J Dis Child 1954; 30:247–254.

Evans TJ, Davies DP. Failure to thrive at the breast: an old problem revisited. Arch Dis Child 1977; 52:974–5.

Field T, Ignatoff E, Stringer S, et al. Nonnutritive sucking during tube feedings: effects on preterm neonates in an intensive care unit. Pediatrics 1982; 3:381–4.

Geertsma MA, Hyams JS, Pelletier JM, et al. Feeding resistance after parenteral hyperalimentation. Am J Dis Child 1985; 139:255–6.

Gisel EG. Chewing cycles in two to eight year old normal children: a developmental profile. Am J Occup Ther 1988a; 42:40–46.

Gisel EG. Development of oral side preference during chewing and its relation to hand preference in normal 2 to 8 year-old children. Am J Occup Ther 1988b; 42:378–83.

Gisel EG. Effect of food texture on development of chewing in children 6 months to 2 years of age. Dev Med Child Neurol 1991; 33:69–79.

Gisel EG, Patrick J. Identification of children with cerebral palsy unable to maintain a normal nutritional state. Lancet 1988; 1:283–5.

Gisel EG, Pollock NA. Eating skills: a review of current assessment practices. Occup Ther J Res 1988; 8:38–51.

Goldblatt D, Williams D. I an sniling! Moebius' syndrome inside and out. J Child Neurol 1986; 1:71–78.

Golf S. Swallowing syncope. Acta Med Scand 1977; 201:585–86.

Golubeva EL, Shuleikina KV, Vainstein II. The development of reflex and spontaneous activity of the human fetus during embryogenesis. Obstet Gynecol (USSR) 1959; 3: 59–62.

Grand RJ, Watkins JB, Torti FM. Development of the human gastrointestinal tract: a review. Gastroenterology 1976; 70:790–810.

Gryboski JD, Thayer WT, Spiro HM. Esophageal motility in infants and children. Pediatrics 1963; 31:382–95.

Gryboski JD. The swallowing mechanism of the neonate 1: esophageal and gastric motility. Pediatrics 1965; 35:445–52.

Gryboski JD. Suck and swallow in the premature infant. Pediatrics 1969; 43:96–101.

Gryboski JD. Gastrointestinal problems in the infant. Philadelphia: WB Saunders, 1975.

Hack M, Horbar JD, Malloy MH, et al. Very low birth weight outcomes of the National

Institute of Child Health and Human Development neonatal network. Pediatrics 1991; 87:587–97.

Ham HR, Piepsz A, Georges B, et al. Evaluation of esophageal transit in children and in infants by means of krypton-81m. Pediatr Radiol 1985; 15:161–4.

Harris SR, Purdy AH. Drooling and its management in cerebral palsy. Dev Med Child Neurol 1987; 29:805–14.

Hays MR, Jordan RA, McLaughlin FJ, et al. Central ventilatory dysfunction in myelo-dysplasia: an independent determinant of survival. Dev Med Child Neurol 1989; 31: 366–70.

Heldt GP. Effect of gavage feeding on the mechanics of the lung, chest wall and diaphragm of preterm infants. Pediatr Res 1988; 24:55–58.

Herbst JJ. Development of suck and swallow. In: Lebenthal E, ed. Human gastrointestinal development. New York: Raven, 1989.

Holinger PC, Holinger LD, Reichert TV. Respiratory obstruction and apnea in infants with bilateral abductor vocal cord paralysis, myelomeningocoele, hydrocephalus and Arnold-Chiari malformation. J Pediatr 1978; 92:368–73.

Humphrey T. Reflex activity in the oral and facial area of the human fetus. In: Bosma JF, ed. Second symposium on oral sensation and perception. Springfield, IL: Thomas 1970; 195–233.

Illingsworth RS. Three months colic. Arch Dis Child 1954; 29:165–74.

Illingsworth RS. Sucking and swallowing difficulties in infancy: diagnostic problem of dysphagia. Arch Dis Child 1969; 44:655.

Illingsworth RS, Lister J. The critical or sensitive period, with special reference to certain feeding problems in infants and children. J Pediatr 1964; 65:839–48.

Jelliffe D, Jelliffe E. Human milk in the modern world. New York: Oxford University Press, 1978.

Judd PL, Kenny DJ, Koheil R, et al. The multidisciplinary feeding profile: a statistically based protocol for assessment of dependent feeders. Dysphagia 1989; 4:29–34.

Kalloor GJ, Singh SP, Collis JL. Cardiac arrhythmias on swallowing. Am Heart J 1977; 93:235–8.

Kaslon K, Ruben RJ. Traumatically acquired conditioned dysphagia in children. Ann Oto Rhinol Laryngol 1978; 87:509–14.

Kenny DJ, Casas MD, McPherson KA. Correlation of ultrasound imaging of oral swallow with ventilatory alterations in cerebral palsied and normal children. Dysphagia 1989a; 4:112–7.

Kenny DJ, Koheil RM, Greenberg J, et al. Development of a multidisciplinary feeding profile for children who are dependent feeders. Dysphagia 1989b; 4:16–28.

Klein PS. Nutritional deprivation and retardation of cognitive functions. In: Mittler P, ed. Frontiers of knowledge of mental retardation, vol. 2. Biomedical aspects. Baltimore: University Park Press, 1980.

Kramer SS. Radiologic examination of the swallowing impaired child. Dysphagia 1989; 3:117–25.

Leeuw RD, Colin EM, Dunnebier EA, et al. Physiological effects of kangaroo care in very small preterm infants. Biol Neonate 1991; 59:149–55.

Levin B, Posner JB. Swallow syncope. Neurology 1972; 22:1086–93.

Logan WJ, Bosma JF. Oral and pharyngeal dysphagia in infants. Pediatr Clin North Am 1967; 14:47–61.

Luchei ES, Goldberg LJ. Neural mechanisms of mandibular control: mastication and voluntary biting. In: Brooks BV, ed. Handbook of physiology, vol. II. Washington, DC: American Physiological Society, 1981; 1237–72.

Maller O, Turner RE. Taste in acceptance of sugars in human infants. J Comp Physiol 1973; 84:496–501.

McCoy R, Kadowaki C, Wilks S, et al. Nursing management of breast feeding for preterm infants. Perinat Neonatal Nurs 1988; 2:42–55.

Measel CP, Anderson GC. Non-nutritive sucking during tube feeding: effect on clinical course in premature infants. J Obstet Gynecol Neonatal 1979; 8:265–72.

Meier P. A program to support breast-feeding in the special care nursery. Perinatology/Neonatology 1980; 4:43–48.

Meier P, Anderson GC. Responses of small preterm infants to bottle and breast feeding. Am J Matern Child Nurs 1987; 12:97–105.

Meier P, Pugh E. Breast feeding behavior in small preterm infants. MCN: Am J Matern Child Nurs 1985; 10:396–401.

Menkes JH. Textbook of child neurology, 4th ed. Philadelphia: Lea & Febiger, 1990.

Milla PJ. Feeding, tasting and sucking. In: Walker, et al., eds. Pediatric gastrointestinal disease. Philadelphia: Decker, 1991.

Miller AJ. Deglutition. Physiol Rev 1982; 63:129–84.

Mollitt DL, Golladay ES, Seibert JJ. Symptomatic gastroesophageal reflux following gastrostomy in neurologically impaired patients. Pediatrics 1985; 75:1124–26.

Morris SE. Development of oral-motor skills in the neurologically impaired child receiving non-oral feedings. Dysphagia 1989; 3:135–54.

Morris SE. Pre-Speech Assessment Scale: a rating scale for the measurement of pre-speech behaviors from birth through two years. Clifton, NJ: J.A. Preston Corp, 1982.

Morris SE, Klein MD. Pre-feeding skills. A comprehensive resource for feeding development. Tucson, AZ: Communication Skill Builders, 1987.

Mueller HA. Facilitating feeding and pre-speech. In: Pearson PH, Williams CE, eds. Physical therapy services in the developmental disabilities. Springfield, IL: Thomas, 1972; 283–310.

Packer RJ, Zimmerman RA, Bilanuik LT, et al. Magnetic resonance imaging of lesions of the posterior fossa and upper cervical cord in childhood. Pediatrics 1985; 76:84–90.

Patrick J, Gisel EG. Nutrition for the feeding-impaired child. J Neurol Rehab, 1990; 4:115–9.

Peiper A. Cerebral function in infancy and childhood. New York: Consultants Bureau, 1963.

Prensky AL. Malnutrition. In: Swaiman KJ, ed. Pediatric neurology: principles and practice. St. Louis: Mosby, 1989.

Ramsey WO. Suckle facilitation of feeding in selected adult dysphagic persons. Dysphagia 1986; 1:7–12.

Raventos JM, Kralemann H, Gray DB. Mortality risks of mentally retarded and mentally ill patients after a feeding gastrostomy. Am J Ment Defic 1982; 86:439–44.

Rickham PP, Ligter J, Irving IM. Neonatal surgery, 2nd ed. London: Butterworths, 1978.

Riley CM. Familial dysautonomia: clinical and pathophysiological aspects. Ann NY Acad Sci 1974; 228:283–7.

Robin P. Glossoptosis due to atresia and hypotrophy of the mandible. Am J Dis Child 1931; 48:541–7.

Rybski DA, Almli RC, Gisel EG. Sucking behaviours of normal 3-day-old female neonates during a 24 hour period. Dev Psychobiol 1984; 17:79–86.

Rybski DA, Gisel EG. Optimal and sub-optimal feeding behaviors of neonates. Phys Occup Ther Pediatr 1984; 4:37–48.

Sarnat HB. Olfactory reflexes in the newborn infant. J Pediatr 1978; 92:624–6.

Schaal B. Olfaction in infants and children in developmental and functional perspectives. Chem Senses 1988; 13:145–90.

Selley WG, Ellis RE, Flack FC, et al. Coordination of sucking, swallowing and breathing in the newborn: its relationship to infant feeding and normal development. Br J Disord Commun 1990a; 25:311–27.

Selley WG, Flack FC, Ellis RE, et al. The Exeter Dysphagia Assessment Technique. Dysphagia 1990b; 4:227–35.

Sessle BJ, Henry JL. Neural mechanisms of swallowing; neurophysiological and neurochemical studies on brain stem neurons in the solitary tract region. Dysphagia 1989; 4:61–75.

Sieben R, Hamida MB, Shulman K. Multiple cranial nerve deficits associated with Arnold-Chiari malformation. Neurology 1971; 21:673–81.

Silbiger ML, Pikielney R, Donner MW. Neuromuscular disorders affecting the pharynx (cineradiographic analysis). Invest Radiol 1967; 2:442–8.

Sivit C. The role of the pediatric radiologist in the evaluation therapy of oral and pharyngeal dysphagia. J Neurol Rehab 1990; 4:103–10.

Sochaniwskyj AE, Koheil RM, Bablich K, et al. Oral motor function, frequency of swallowing and drooling in normal children and in children with cerebral palsy. Arch Phys Med Rehabil 1986; 67:866–74.

Sondheimer JM. Upper esophageal sphincter and pharyngeal motor function in infants with and without gastroesophageal reflux. Gastroenterology 1983; 85:301–5.

Steiner JE. Facial expressions of the neonate infant indicating the hedonics of food-related stimuli. In: Weiffenbach JM, ed. Taste and development: the genesis of sweet preference. Bethesda, MD: National Institutes of Health, 1977; 173–88.

Stolovitz P, Gisel EG. Circumoral movements in response to three different food textures in children six months to two years of age. Dysphagia 1991; 6:17–25.

Sullivan RM, Taborsky-Barba S, Mendoza R, et al. Olfactory classical conditioning in neonates. Pediatrics 1991; 87:511–7.

Swaiman KF. Pediatric neurology: principles and practice. St. Louis: Mosby, 1989.

Takagi Y, Irwin JV, Bosma JF. Prone feeding of infants with Pierre Robin syndrome. Cleft Palate J 1966; 3:232–9.

Taubman B. Clinical trial of the treatment of colic by modification of parent-infant interaction. Pediatrics 1984; 74:998–1003.

Vice FL, Heinz JM, Giuriatti G, et al. Cervical auscultation of suckle feeding in newborn infants. Dev Med Child Neurol 1990; 32:766–8.

Ward SLD, Nickerson BG, Vander Hal, et al. Absent hypoxic and hypercapneic arousal responses in children with myelomeningocele and apnea. Pediatrics 1986; 78:44–50.

Warkany J, Lemire RJ, Cohen MM Jr. Mental retardation and congenital malformations of the central nervous system. Chicago: Year Book Medical, 1981.

Weinberg B, Christensen R, Logan W, et al. Severe hypoplasia of the tongue. J Speech Hear Dis 1969; 34:157–68.

Wessel MA, Cobb JC, Jackson EB, et al. Paroxysmal fussing in infancy, sometimes called colic. Pediatrics 1954; 14:421–34.

Widstrom AM, Marchini G, Matthiesen AS, et al. Non-nutritive sucking in tube fed preterm infants: effects on gastric motility and gastric contents of somatostatin. J Pediatr Gastroenterol Nutr 1988; 8:517–23.

Wilks S, Meier P. Helping mother express milk suitable for preterm and high-risk infant feeding. J Matern Child Nurs 1988; 13:121–3.

Williams AJ, Williams MA, Walker CA, et al. The Robin anomalad (the Pierre Robin syndrome): a follow-up study. Arch Dis Child 1981; 56:663–8.

Wilson JM. Oral-motor function and dysfunction in children. Chapel Hill, NC: Division of Physical Therapy, 1977.

Wilson SL, Thach BT, Brouillette RT, et al. Coordination of breathing and swallowing. J Appl Physiol 1981; 50:851–8.

Wolff PH. The serial organisation of sucking in the young infant. Pediatrics 1968; 42: 943–56.

Woody RC, Kiel EA. Swallowing syncope in a child. Pediatrics 1986; 78:507–9.

6

Clinical Examination for Dysphagia

Robert M. Miller

A comprehensive evaluation of a patient known to have or suspected of having dysphagia involves a number of medical and allied medical disciplines. The evaluation is intended to assess factors that relate to swallowing function, not to be diagnostic of the underlying disease, although it may either obviate or clarify the need for other studies. The word dysphagia, according to *Dorland's Illustrated Medical Dictionary,* is derived from the Greek *phagein,* meaning to eat. Conditions that could impair eating are numerous and diverse. Even considering the more limited definition of dysphagia such as "difficulty in swallowing," the complexity involved in comprehensive evaluations of patients with such complaints can be appreciated.

A comprehensive evaluation for dysphagia should be considered a team evaluation, as no one discipline can assess in detail all phases of swallowing. Without attempting to enumerate all of the disciplines that might contribute to a comprehensive dysphagia evaluation (see Chapter 14), and recognizing that responsibilities and expertise will vary from setting to setting, an outline of the relevant systems to be assessed and the methods available for evaluation is presented in Table 6.1.

One component of a comprehensive dysphagia evaluation is the clinical examination for dysphagia (CED). The CED is comprised of a detailed description of the subjective complaint or problem, the acquisition of a relevant health history, pertinent clinical observations, and a focused physical examination. Although it is ideal to record all of these components in detail, circumstances may require clinicians to modify the examination to fit the situation and the needs of a given patient. At a minimum, the CED should allow the clinician to (1) screen for the presence or absence of a swallowing impairment; (2) contribute information regarding the possible etiology of the dysphagia relative to its anatomic and physiologic basis; (3) ascertain the relative aspiration risk for certain patients; (4) determine the need for an alternative means of nutritional management; and (5) recommend additional tests and procedures necessary to diagnose and/or treat the dysphagia.

Disorders of swallowing may be found in diverse patient populations, e.g., following acute neurologic events and surgery of the head and neck. Dysphagia is also a manifestation of many subacute progressive neurologic diseases and

Table 6.1 Comprehensive Evaluation for Dysphagia

Factors Influencing Swallowing	*Methods of Assessment*
Oral phase	
Mental status, judgment	Screen orientation, language, visual-motor perception, and memory
Muscles of facial expression	Examine for symmetry at rest and during movement
Muscles of mastication	Palpate and gently resist movement
Mucous membranes	Inspect
Dentition	Inspect
Lingual muscles	Inspect at rest and on protrusion; resist movement
Orofacial sensation	Subjective; identify stimulus qualities
Pharyngeal phase	
Palatopharyngeal closure	Observe at rest and during phonation; stimulate gag reflex
Pharyngeal contraction	Stimulate gag; motion radiography
Extrinsic laryngeal muscles	Palpate larynx during swallow
Intrinsic laryngeal muscles	Indirect laryngeal inspection or fiberoptic examination
Cricopharyngeus muscle	Motion radiography
Esophageal phase	
Morphology of the esophagus	Motion radiography and endoscopy
Esophageal motility	Manometry and motion radiography
Gastroesophageal sphincter function, hiatal hernia, and reflux	Manometry, motion radiography, gastroesophageal scintiscanning, acid perfusion, pH monitoring, endoscopy, and biopsy

may be an isolated symptom found in otherwise stable elderly patients. The CED will need to be modified and adapted to fit the clinical setting and patient population. The procedures for performing the CED outlined within the chapter, therefore, should be viewed as general guidelines rather than a cookbook approach applied to every dysphagic patient.

WARNING SIGNS

Patients suspected of having swallowing dysfunction should undergo a CED as a minimum evaluation. There are several warning signs that should alert health professionals to the likelihood of dysphagia. The presence of a confused mental state or dysarthric speech in a patient with neurologic disease should be cause for special attention to the eating process. Since eating requires some degree of vigilance and planning, patients who exhibit poor judgment, perceptual impairments, or motor planning disorders following any form of brain damage are at risk for swallowing catastrophe. Similarly, dysarthric speech, characterized by slow, labored, or slurred articulation, nasal air emission, and hoarse or breathy voice, is a manifestation of the inherent weakness of muscles common to both speaking and swallowing. An additional symptom suggestive of dysphagia is excessive drooling (sialorrhea), which is often due to motor and/or sensory impairments of the swallowing mechanism. Frequent episodes of coughing and choking on food and sputum should be considered as warning signs for dysphagia. Prolongation of meals, unexplained weight loss, effortful chewing, or difficulty in the oral preparation of a bolus may all signify swallowing difficulty.

A patient's complaint of pain or obstruction during swallowing should be taken seriously as a warning for dysphagia. A clinical finding on indirect laryngeal examination of the pooling sign, or accumulation of food debris in the valleculae or piriform sinuses, suggests that the swallowing mechanism has failed to completely clear the bolus from the pharynx into the esophagus. Excessive pooling and the potential for tracheal aspiration may be appreciated on radiographic study of swallows.

THE EVALUATION

It is helpful when beginning an examination for dysphagia to have a procedural outline or worksheet available (Table 6.2). This will help to ensure that important data is not overlooked during the assessment.

Subjective Complaints

The history begins with information regarding the present complaint. Frequently, the subjective description of the problem will give the examiner significant clues regarding its cause. In many instances, however, history will not be attainable from the patient because swallowing problems are frequently associated with altered mental states and/or severely impaired speech. In these instances, information may come from a professional observer, health care attendant, family member, or medical records. Specific questions would address such issues as the duration of the problem, the frequency of swallowing difficulty, intermittent versus constant presence, and factors and circumstances that exacerbate or alleviate the problem.

It is particularly important to determine the relative influence of solid, semisolid, and liquid foods on swallowing. In general, patients who suffer from neurologic conditions that weaken or result in dyscoordination of the swallowing mechanism complain that liquids are more likely to cause choking than solids or semisolids (Linden and Siebens 1983). Since fluids will naturally spread as they move from the mouth through the pharynx into the esophagus, they require more precise channeling than solids, and therefore are more difficult for weak or uncoordinated motor mechanisms to control. Patients suffering from mechan-

Table 6.2 Clinical Examination for Dysphagia

I. Subjective Complaints
  A. Duration of the problem
  B. Frequency of swallowing difficulty
  C. Intermittent versus constant swallowing problem
  D. Factors exacerbating or relieving the problem
    1. Influence of solids, semisolids, and liquids
    2. Influence of hot and cold
  E. Associated symptoms
    1. Sensation of obstruction
    2. Mouth or throat pain
    3. Nasal regurgitation
    4. Mouth odor
    5. Choking or coughing while swallowing
    6. Pneumonia in the past
    7. Other respiratory symptoms (chronic cough, shortness of breath, asthmatic episodes)
    8. GE reflux (sensation of heartburn)
    9. Chest pain
  F. Ancillary symptoms
    1. Weight loss
    2. Eating habits
    3. Appetite changes/enjoyment
    4. Taste changes
    5. Dry mouth or saliva consistency changes
    6. Speech or voice changes
    7. Sleep disturbance
II. Medical History
  A. General health
  B. Family history
  C. Previous swallowing examinations
  D. Neurologic conditions
  E. Pulmonary disorders
  F. Surgeries
  G. Radiation
  H. Psychiatric/psychologic history
  I. Current treatments
  J. Medications
    1. Current and past
    2. Prescriptive
    3. Over-the-counter
III. Clinical Observations
  A. Feeding tube
  B. Tracheostomy (type of tube, cuff status)
  C. Nutrition/hydration status
  D. Drooling
  E. Mental status
    1. Attention

Table 6.2 Clinical Examination for Dysphagia *(continued)*

    2. Orientation
    3. Receptive/expressive language
    4. Visual perceptual-motor function
    5. Memory disturbance
IV. Clinical Examination
    A. Speech function (voice, resonance, articulation)
    B. Weight
    C. Peripheral swallowing musculature and structures
        1. Muscles of facial expression
        2. Muscles of mastication
        3. Pathologic reflexes
        4. Oral mucosa
        5. Dentition
        6. Pharyngeal palatine musculature
        7. Tongue
        8. Sensation
        9. Intrinsic laryngeal musculature
        10. Extrinsic laryngeal musculature
    D. Test swallows

ical obstructive conditions such as strictures, tumors, or webs generally report no difficulty swallowing liquids. They are likely to complain about solid food sticking or lodging in the throat or esophagus. Patients with esophageal motility problems or primary neuromuscular abnormalities of the esophagus may report dysphagia with both solids and liquids (Castell and Donner 1987). Although there is some correlation between the cause of the swallowing difficulty and consistency of the bolus, caution is recommended to avoid being misled.

The differential effect of hot and cold food boluses may have diagnostic significance. For example, cold liquids are known to reduce primary esophageal peristalsis and produce distension of the distal esophagus. Esophageal spasms may be produced by ingestion of cold liquids (Jones and Donner 1989). For patients with myotonic dystrophy, swallowing cold liquids often elicits a myotonic contraction in the pharynx and interferes with subsequent swallows. For most other patients with neuromuscular oropharyngeal dysphagia, cold liquids are recommended to facilitate swallowing.

In detailing the history, specific questions should be asked that address symptoms frequently associated with dysphagia.

Obstruction

Although many clinicians associate subjective descriptions of obstruction with tumors, strictures, webs, and diverticula, it is also a frequent complaint in patients with neurologic conditions that result in muscle weakness and/or incoordination and in those with esophageal motility disorders. The patient should be asked if food sticks and then directed to point to the level at which he or she senses the obstruction. Patients with cricopharyngeal dysfunction and those with a pharyngoesophageal (Zenker's) diverticulum usually describe the obstruction at the level of the thyroid cartilage (Jordan 1977). Those with pooling in the vallecula or piriform sinuses may also point to an area adjacent to the larynx as the site of obstruction. It should be noted, however, that the area in which the obstruction is sensed by the patient does not always correspond with the site of actual narrowing or blockage as this is demonstrated by radiography. Distal esophageal lesions, for example, may be referred to the lower neck (Edwards 1976).

A distinction should be made between the sensation of obstruction while swallowing and a "globus sensation" or foreign body feeling. Patients with either complaint should be examined because there is a high incidence of abnormality in both groups. The globus sensation may be an early symptom of hypopharyngeal cancer or organic esophageal disease, such as hypertensive upper esophageal sphincter (Castell and Donner 1987) or reflux.

Complaints of intermittent obstruction should not be dismissed as psychological. Patients with organic lesions, such as those with Schatzki's ring, may report intermittent difficulties that are exacerbated during periods of stress.

Mouth or Throat Pain

Odynophagia, or pain on swallowing, is rarely associated with dysphagia of central nervous system origin. Mouth or throat pain is more commonly related to infections, neoplasms, or mechanical obstructions in the oropharyngeal region.

Nasal Regurgitation

Patients should be asked about episodes of nasopharyngeal reflux, i.e., liquid or firm food moving up into the nasal cavity rather than down toward the esophagus. An occasional nasal penetration occurring in association with coughing is probably not significant. Frequent episodes of nasal regurgitation suggest some malfunction of the palatal and upper pharyngeal mechanism, or mechanical obstruction in the hypopharynx.

Mouth Odor

Foul mouth odors may be associated with a variety of conditions, including hygiene problems, oral retention of food, dental or periodontal disease, and oral-mucosal lesions that result in necrotic changes. An additional source for mouth odor is Zenker's pharyngoesophageal diverticulum. In these cases, food trapped in the sac can putrefy and emit a foul odor. These patients may also describe episodes in which food returns to the mouth, sometimes hours after a meal.

Choking or Coughing

The patient with complaints regarding swallowing should be questioned about episodes of aspiration in which food or liquid tends to go into the windpipe. Coughing or choking frequently while eating is another manifestation of aspiration. Although sensations of aspiration can occur with a variety of conditions, it is probably most common in neuromuscular disorders of swallowing.

History of Pneumonia

Evidence of recurrent aspiration pneumonia may be associated with either neuromuscular incoordination or weakness of the oropharyngeal swallowing mechanism or esophageal dysfunction. It can result from a patient's inability to protect the airway due to selective muscle paralysis. Paralysis of the vocal cords is particularly significant. Recurrent pneumonia also can be found in patients who have mechanical obstructions of the deglutitory tract, severe gastroesophageal and/or pharyngeal-tracheal reflux, and achalasia. The occurrence of aspiration pneumonia is grossly related to the severity of dysphagia.

Other Respiratory Symptoms

Conditions related to either oropharyngeal or esophageal dysphagia can cause a number of respiratory symptoms. Chronic coughing may be a manifestation of a failed oropharyngeal swallowing mechanism, causing pooled secretions to intermittently spill into the airway. Cricopharyngeal dysfunction, either as an isolated impairment or when associated with esophageal reflux, may also contribute to chronic coughing. Nocturnal coughing is classically associated with achalasia (Castell and Donner 1987).

Clinicians are developing a keener appreciation of the relationship between the deglutitory mechanism and pulmonary functions. In patients with either mechanical obstruction or neuromuscular esophageal disorders, respiratory symptoms including episodic coughing, wheezing, sputum production, and dyspnea may be found. Reflux and lower esophageal sphincter (LES) dysfunction are known to be etiologic factors in chronic obstructive pulmonary disease. There also is evidence to suggest that cricopharyngeal dysfunction may either precede or be secondary to chronic obstructive pulmonary disease in some patients (Stein et al. 1990).

Gastroesophageal Reflux

Gastroesophageal (GE) reflux is usually identified by patients as a sensation of heartburn or acid regurgitation. Additionally, patients may complain of a globus sensation, hiccups, halitosis, a sour taste, dry throat, or pain in the throat or tongue.

GE reflux results from failure of the LES to prevent stomach contents from reentering the esophagus. Reflux is a very common event. The potential for symptomatic GE reflux is probably great in patients with a hiatal hernia, a condition that is present in about 67 percent of persons over 60 years of age (Straus 1979). It is also found in patients with peptic strictures, esophageal cancer, neuromuscular esophageal motor disorders, and those with loss of tone in the LES due to scleroderma (see Chapter 4).

Severe or persistent cases of GE reflux may lead to esophageal mucosal irritation, esophageal muscle and sphincter dysfunction, laryngeal mucosal ulceration or granulomata, and/or aspiration of stomach contents, the latter particularly during sleep. Esophagitis, esophageal ulcer, and esophageal stricture are potential sequelae of reflux. Other less appreciated manifestations may be evident in the mouth and throat. Chronic pharyngitis, hoarseness, and loss of dental enamel may be evident. Among the pulmonary and cardiac symptoms related to reflux are exacerbation of asthma, chronic obstructive pulmonary disease, episodic apnea, bradycardia, and hypotension (Castell and Donner 1987).

Even when GE reflux cannot be appreciated on radiographic studies, the patient's report of symptoms associated with this condition should be taken seriously. When reflux is suspected, a trial of antireflux therapy can be effective in relieving pharyngeal symptoms of dysphagia (Jones et al. 1985).

Chest Pain

Chest pain may be a manifestation of an esophageal motor disorder. Pain that is not considered to be coronary in origin is one clue for diffuse esophageal spasm (Castell and Donner 1987). Intense esophageal pain is usually perceived substernally, with radiation into the back, jaw, neck, or down the left arm. It may be clinically indistinguishable from the pain of coronary artery disease (Pope 1977). Heartburn, and a similar retrosternal burning perceived by patients with dilated esophagus due to achalasia, are also important diagnostic clues.

Other Ancillary Symptoms

The previously mentioned symptoms are directly associated with an impairment at some level of deglutition, and the presence or absence of these symptoms lend diagnostic clues for the clinician. In addition to these major symptoms, questioning related to the following ancillary complaints allows one not only to discover additional diagnostic clues, but to assess the degree to which the swallowing dysfunction has affected the patient in important ways. Although most of the major symptoms often can be related to a level of impairment along the deglutitory tract, a thorough evaluation demands exploration of complaints that the patient may not relate to the swallowing disorder, e.g., speech or voice changes.

Weight loss is one of the best barometers for assessing the effects of a swallowing impairment. It is usually related directly to impaired nutritional intake, although it may reflect the effects of an underlying disease process. Reported changes in weight become the clinician's yardstick by which progressive dysphagia can be charted and the effectiveness of a feeding management plan is assessed.

A change in eating habits may suggest to the clinician impairments that can be related to a specific stage of swallowing. For example, foods or food types may be avoided due to specific muscle weakness, e.g., lettuce is avoided with early pharyngeal weakness. Eating time may increase or the patient may eat smaller meals to compensate when swallowing initiation is delayed or there is deglutitory muscle fatigue. Enjoyment of meals is frequently affected as swallowing difficulty increases, and questions related to appetite and the pleasure derived from eating should be asked. When possible, a description of the patient's previous day's meals and an estimate of the amount of fluid intake per day will be helpful.

Alterations of taste, mucosal dryness, and salivary consistency changes are known to affect appetite and may hinder the initiation of swallowing. Thickening of secretions may reflect a patient's chronically dehydrated state due to impaired swallowing of liquids or be related to mouth breathing, salivary gland function, or medications. Debilitated patients with extreme oral and pharyngeal mucosal dryness may not be able to swallow on this basis alone.

Since speech and swallowing are dependent on certain common neurologic, muscular, and anatomic factors, changes in speech or voice may parallel the development of swallowing difficulties. Patients should be asked if their speech has changed in any way, e.g., hoarseness or temporary loss of voice. A change in articulatory coordination or precision, interpreted by the patient as slurring or clumsy speech, usually reflects neurologic impairment. An isolated voice change may be either the consequence of neurologic, neoplastic, or inflammatory disorders, or related to GE reflux.

Dysphagia can cause sleep disturbance through a variety of mechanisms. Patients suffering from symptomatic GE reflux commonly suffer from sleep disturbance. In severe oropharyngeal dysphagia patients may be unable to keep their airway clear of secretions while reclining or sleeping. Presumably, this is one of the factors, along with food regurgitation, that contributes to disruption of sleep in patients with a Zenker's diverticulum.

Medical History

Information relevant to a patient's swallowing and nutritional status can often be obtained from the general health history. Family history is important because a number of conditions have a known genetic basis, e.g., muscular dystrophy, and others have a hereditary predisposition. The results and findings from any previous swallowing examinations should be noted. Special attention should be paid to neurologic history; cerebrovascular accident, head trauma, central nervous system infection, demyelinating disease, and motor neuron disease are particularly pertinent to dysphagia. Since dysphagia has been implicated as a major factor contributing to the genesis and exacerbation of some pulmonary disorders, particularly chronic obstructive pulmonary disease, attention should be given to any pulmonary conditions (Stein et al. 1990).

All prior surgery should be noted, particularly procedures involving the head and neck or gastrointestinal tract. When directed at the head and neck or mediastinum, radiation therapy can impair swallowing or exacerbate problems with deglutition.

Medications

Several medications influence swallowing. A list should be compiled of all medications currently prescribed and those that had been taken regularly in the past. Sedative drugs or those that cause disorientation and confusion can have a significant influence on swallow, particularly in brain-damaged patients. For example, slightly toxic doses of some anticonvulsants can add to the confusion of patients with brain trauma and cause decompensation of a previously marginal swallowing mechanism. Medications that potentially weaken muscles, such as some prescribed to reduce spasticity, may exacerbate existing swallowing problems. It is known that some moisture must be present in the mouth in order to elicit a swallow reflex; therefore, medications with an action or side effect of diminishing secretions and, thus, drying of the oral, nasal, and pharyngeal mucosae can adversely influence swallowing by delaying initiation of this reflex. Some medications, although they do not directly impair swallowing, may inhibit appetite or contribute to dehydration. Diuretics, often used to help in the control of hypertension, can exacerbate problems of dehydration in the patient with dysphagia for liquids.

Many antipsychotic drugs can lead to extrapyramidal symptoms such as dystonia, motor restlessness, pseudoparkinsonism, and tardive dyskinesia. Persistent tardive dyskinesia may present as hyperkinesis of the face, jaw, tongue, and upper esophagus, each of which may interfere with the initiation and control of chewing and swallowing. In some cases, neuroleptic drugs will cause dysphagia that is clinically indistinguishable from Parkinson's disease by blocking dopaminergic transmissions. For the psychiatric patient it may be difficult to determine the etiology for the swallowing impairment as it may be due to parkinsonism, tardive dyskinesia, anticholinergic drug, or other preexisting neurologic conditions (Weiden and Harrigan 1986).

Certain over-the-counter medications and prescribed topical anesthetics used to relieve a sore throat or tickling cough have the potential to impair swallowing. Some denture powders also contain topical anesthetics that could disturb oral and pharyngeal sensation.

In general, drugs appear to have very little effect on the function of the esophagus and are not known to cause motor disorders of the esophagus (Christensen 1976). However, β-adrenergic drugs, theophylline, alcohol, and tobacco have been reported to lower or overcome LES tone and promote reflux (Stein et al. 1990).

Clinical Observations

There are enumerable clinical signs that an experienced clinician will recognize in the interview and examination process. Some of these observations clearly will be related to the deglutitory process and may influence performance on subsequent examination. The presence of a feeding tube, its site of insertion, and size are significant. Attention should be given to any tracheostomy tube, its size, and the presence and status of a cuff. The patient's general nutritional state, whether appearing well nourished or cachectic, should be noted. A clinical impression should be formed regarding the patient's relative hydration status. A thorough nutritional assessment, including laboratory measures, should be included in a comprehensive evaluation of the patient with dysphagia. Additional observations might include the presence of drooling or the presence of towels and tissues for the purpose of controlling secretions. The patient's general behavior and emotional state should be clinically judged and may have significance in the final diagnostic impression.

Mental Status

Specific attention should be given to the assessment of the patient's mental status and ability to cooperate. This is especially true when dealing with patients with known or suspected central nervous system lesions contributing to dysphagia. Larsen (1981) described the problems experienced by patients with left- or right-sided brain damage. With right-sided hemiplegia and aphasia, for example, patients may become overwhelmed or confused while attempting to eat while engaging in conversation. Because of muscle spasticity in combination with the language disorder of aphasia, these patients are at risk for aspiration when trying to combine eating with speaking.

Conversely, Larsen describes right-sided brain-damaged patients as having problems with the praxis of eating; i.e., they are disturbed in organizing the motor sequence that would allow them to move food from plate to mouth. They are at risk of choking because of problems that relate to judgment, decisions of how much food to take in one bite, and how much to chew. These problems are discussed in more detail in Chapter 8.

A screening psychometric-type test can be used to assess perceptual and language functions to anticipate the type of eating problems that could occur and apply the appropriate rehabilitation procedures. Such screening tests should include (1) questions regarding the patient's orientation; (2) a series of simple verbal and written commands to assess language comprehension; (3) a task that requires the patient to name common objects or geometric forms to assess simple expressive language; (4) a written task to evaluate the patient's ability to spell several common words or write a phrase from dictation; (5) a verbal problem-solving task requiring the patient to interpret the meaning of a sentence or proverb; and (6) a visual perceptual-motor task in which the patient reproduces forms, such as a square, triangle, and cross.

Physical Examination

In most cases, the description of the problem and background data will dictate the appropriate course to follow in the physical examination. The detailed examination that follows may be used in part or in total, as the case requires. Since dysphagia is almost never purely psychogenic, all patients with swallowing complaints should be examined thoroughly.

The purpose of this examination for the clinical assessment of swallowing is to (1) establish a possible cause of dysphagia; (2) assess the patient's ability to protect the airway; (3) determine the practicality of oral feeding and/or recommend alternative methods for nutritional management; (4) determine the need for additional specific diagnostic tests, studies, or referrals; and (5) establish baseline clinical data that can be used to chart changes in feeding function of patients with progressively deteriorating diseases (Table 6.2).

Voice and Speech

The quality of a patient's speech should be assessed as a part of the swallowing evaluation. Speech is an extremely complex, overlearned behavior, and as such, serves as a barometer from which the examiner can assess the status of the neuromuscular system that also serves swallowing. Patients should be asked to sustain a vowel, with the examiner noting duration, quality (hoarseness, breathiness, and harshness), pitch, and intensity. Articulation should be assessed for precision and speed. The use of oral diadochokinetic tasks (forced rapid alternating movements) using consonant–vowel combinations is recommended. Both hypernasal and hyponasal resonance qualities should be noted. Hypernasality suggests impaired palatopharyngeal function. Hyponasality implies filling of the nasopharynx or occlusion of nasal passages.

For patients with unimpaired voice and speech, the clinician may reasonably conclude that the swallowing problem resides in either the late pharyngeal stage (cricopharyngeal function) or is related to esophageal and LES function. One would expect that the remaining physical examination would confirm the integrity of the peripheral sensory-motor swallowing mechanism. A final diagnosis in such cases would require additonal radiographic swallowing studies.

Weight

Weighing the patient is vital when examination data are to be used for charting changes in progressive disease, and when the clinician must assess the effectiveness of a nutritional management plan. These data also will be useful in leading to an understanding of the severity of a swallowing problem.

Muscles of Facial Expression

Facial muscles should be inspected both at rest and during active movement, comparing movement of the two sides for symmetry. The patient should be asked to make grimacing and puckering movements. When possible, the muscles should be palpated for any weakness. The examiner should look particularly at the patient's ability to seal the lips, having the patient puff out the cheeks and hold the air while manual pressure is applied to the cheeks. Lip closure is important in preventing loss of food anteriorly during the oral phase of swallowing.

Muscles of Mastication

The masseter is the most powerful muscle of mastication. It originates at the zygomatic arch and inserts into the angle of the mandible. The temporalis, which serves to adjust the jaw up, forward, or back, originates at the squamous portion of the temporal bone and inserts at the anterior border of the ramus. These two muscles of mastication should be palpated as the patient bites and chews. Gentle resistance can be placed on the mandible to assess the strength of these muscles. Excessive resistance could result in dislocation of the temporomandicular joint. Clinicians recognize that it is almost impossible to swallow with the mouth open.

The grinding action that occurs in chewing is produced by two sets of muscles, the external and internal pterygoids. Their action can be appreciated by instructing the patient to move the mandible from side to side in a rotary action. Again, gentle resistance can be applied to assess the relative strength of these muscles.

Pathologic Reflexes

There are a number of brain stem-level primitive reflexes associated with the chewing and swallowing mechanisms. Normally, these reflexes are inhibited in the adult by higher centers of the brain. Their presence in the adult patient suggests that these higher inhibitory centers are impaired. These pathologic reflexes are seen most commonly in patients with bilateral hemispheric or frontal lobe damage.

The suck reflex may be elicited either by tapping the upper lip with a reflex hammer or by stroking the vermillion border with a tongue blade. Movement of the lips in the direction of the stimulus is an abnormal response.

The bite reflex is often elicited in patients with severe neurologic lesions by touching the lips, teeth, or gums with a tongue blade and observing a strong closure of the jaw. This reflex can be particularly troublesome for the examiner, since it may prevent a good oral examination. Attempts to force a jaw open usually result in a stronger bite. The examiner should avoid strong resistance that could result in fracture or dislocation of the mandible. In some patients, spontaneous mouth opening will occur as a stimulus object, such as a spoon or food, is seen approaching the mouth. While the bite reflex can interfere with feeding management, this mouth-opening reflex can be used to aid in the feeding plan.

Oral Mucosa

The intraoral inspection should begin with an assessment of the mucosa. Dentures should be removed prior to this examination. Any pathologic lesions should be noted, and proper diagnostic procedures followed to determine its nature. In many cases this procedure involves consultation with an oral surgeon or otolaryngologist for examination and biopsy.

Particular attention should be paid to the moisture present in the oral cavity. Extreme dryness of the oral and pharyngeal mucosa can virtually prevent voluntary and reflexive swallowing. Thick, tenacious mucus can inhibit swallowing. Any residual oral debris should be noted.

Dentition

The condition of natural teeth should be noted. Painful teeth can inhibit eating and lead to impaired nutritional states. It should be recognized that dental plates block sensory receptors in the palate and gums that are contributory to the reflex stimulation of chewing. Dental consultation should be considered when dental or other oral disease or abnormality is suspected.

Pharyngeal Palate

The pharyngeal palatine musculature should be evaluated as a unit. In normal swallowing the palate should elevate and the pharynx constrict, allowing a properly masticated bolus to pass over the base of the tongue and enter the hypopharynx without regurgitation into the nasopharynx. Palatopharyngeal constriction should be assessed for symmetry during oral breathing, phonation, and tactual stimulation of the gag reflex. The gag reflex should be elicitable from either side, and the response should be compared on stimulation of each side. The gag is a highly variable reflex even among healthy persons. A diminished gag reflex is probably significant only when found in patients who have evidence of weakened or paralyzed pharyngeal palatine musculature, asymmetric gag reflexes, or other signs of cranial nerve dysfunction. Absence of a gag reflex does not automatically mean that the patient is unable to swallow or protect the airway (Linden and Siebens 1983).

Tongue

McConnel and associates (1988) compare the interaction of the tongue and pharyngeal muscles to that of a piston or plunger generating a propulsive bolus-driving force within a dynamic chamber. Lingual muscles should be examined for appearance and strength. In the edentulous or highly cooperative patient, palpation of the muscles can be revealing; atrophy, fasciculations, or abnormal movement should be noted. Recognizing that the tongue deviates toward the side of weakness, tongue strength can be grossly assessed by having the patient protrude the tongue. Tongue strength can also be evaluated by instructing the patient to push the tongue firmly against the inner cheek while the examiner resists the movement on each side.

Sensation

Chewing, salivary flow, and swallowing are all reflexes that are, in part, dependent on sensory stimulation. Sensations of hot, cold, pressure, and texture, carried by the trigeminal nerve, are known to stimulate chewing. Taste, which is carried by the facial and glossopharyngeal nerves, plays a role in stimulating salivary flow and, eventually, swallowing (see Chapter 1). If the gag reflex is absent, the patient drools, the mucosa is extremely dry, or food debris is retained in the mouth, some sensory loss involving oral structures may be suspected. Sensory loss alone is rarely the cause of dysphagia.

Many patients can detect and report sensory loss reliably, but in some instances clinicians may wish to test further. For purposes of evaluating functional swallowing, gross touch can be assessed on the face, lips, and buccal mucosa using a cotton swab. Taste can be evaluated by having the patient identify a small sip of juice or the flavors of salt, sour, bitter, and sweet applied to various areas of the tongue with a moistened cotton swab.

Indirect Laryngoscopy

Indirect laryngoscopy should be performed whenever possible as part of the swallowing examination. A complete examination, as visualized in Figure 6.1, should include inspection of the base of the tongue, vallecula, epiglottis, piriform sinuses, vocal and vestibular folds, and infraglottic area. Otolaryngology consultation should be initiated if suspicious mucosal lesions are observed. The vocal cords should be evaluated for function, with observation of symmetry of movement during quiet breathing, forced inhalation, and phonation. Vocal cord function is essential in airway protection during the pharyngeal stage of swallowing and for coughing.

Presence of the pooling sign, detection of food debris or secretions in the vallecula or piriform sinuses, is an indication that the swallow reflex has been incomplete in clearing the bolus from the pharynx into the esophagus. When pooling is observed adjacent to the aditus of the larynx, the probability of tracheal aspiration is high.

Test Swallows

In normal swallowing, a bolus is worked into the oropharynx by muscles of the lips, tongue, and cheek. As the swallow reflex begins, the muscles suspending the larynx contract and draw the larynx up to bury the epiglottis into the base of the tongue. The pharyngeal constrictors strip the bolus toward the cricopharyngeal sphincteric muscle, which opens ahead of the bolus and allows

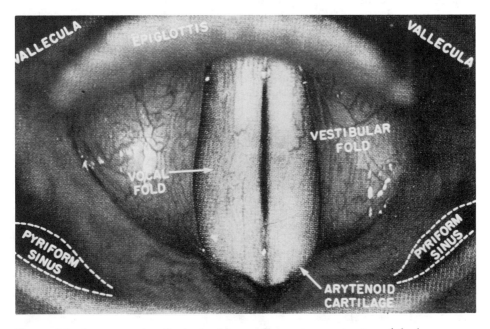

Figure 6.1 Structures visualized on mirror or fiberoptic examination of the larynx.

it to pass into the esophagus. An examiner can appreciate the moment of swallowing by placing a finger on the thyroid notch between the hyoid bone and the larynx and feeling the larynx move up and forward during the swallow reflex (Figure 6.2). If the muscles are weak or the reflexes inadequate, the examiner's finger may fail to be deflected by elevation of the larynx. In this case, the cricopharyngeus may fail to open properly and the epiglottis will not be adequately buried in the base of the tongue, thus leaving the airway unprotected.

On palpation of the laryngeal cartilages in some elderly patients, the larynx will be noted in an abnormally low position. This condition, laryngoptosis, may contribute to inadequate airway protection during swallowing.

Testing the adequacy of a swallow brings a certain degree of risk for aspiration. Coughing itself is not an indication that the patient is experiencing tracheal aspiration. In fact, the cough reflex is the final protective mechanism to prevent aspiration. The presence of an adequate cough reflex is necessary before an oral nutritional management program can be established. If the patient has lost or has an inadequate cough reflex, even test swallows with most foods and liquids are unsafe. Although a voluntary cough should be elicited and judged, the examiner should recognize that voluntary and reflexive coughs can be quite different in quality and effectiveness. Patients with cortical brain damage are frequently unable voluntarily to organize motor behaviors necessary to produce a good cough, but their reflexive cough is intact. Conversely, there are rare cases in which patients can voluntarily cough, but because of an impaired sensorimotor complex, the reflexive cough is lost. Measurement of vital capacity is sometimes a helpful adjunct in predicting the effectiveness of a cough reflex.

Initially, it is advisable to use a substance that is relatively safe if partially aspirated and to be absolutely certain that the patient is able to cough to protect the airway in case of aspiration. A spoonful of crushed ice is relatively safe and will provide a good medium for eliciting the chewing reflex because of its texture and cold stimulation to the receptors in the gums. The examiner should observe the chewing action and feel for laryngeal elevation to indicate that a swallow has occurred. Once it is determined that the patient adequately elevates the larynx and there is an adequate protective cough, the examination can proceed to using other substances with different textures and consistencies. During test swallows the examiner should take note of coughing, aspiration signs, or nasal regurgitation (see Chapter 8 for further discussion).

Some examiners attempt to demonstrate subtle weakness of the muscles and protective reflexes by testing swallowing under unfavorable circumstances. For example, it is known that the airway is more protected if a patient swallows with the head and neck flexed. Therefore, placing the patient in a posture with the neck extended and chin up may stress the swallowing musculature. Patients who can overcome this postural disadvantage are more likely to have an adequate swallow. Similarly, swallowing can be compromised by manually stabilizing the larynx and hyoid bone in order to bring out weakness of the muscles of laryngeal elevation (Figure 6.2).

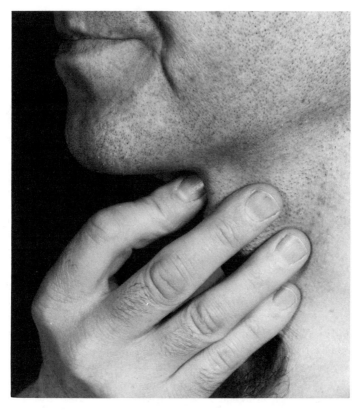

Figure 6.2 Manual stabilization technique of the larynx and hyoid bone.

Swallowing reflexes are subject to fatigue and warm up. Test swallows should be performed successively to evaluate for fatigability when the subjective complaint suggests this possibility. When the initial test swallow is judged to be inadequate due to coughing, additional tests may show improved function. This is particularly true when patients have pooled secretions in the valleculae and piriform sinuses. They may spill these secretions into the larynx when swallowing is stimulated initially, but improve with subsequent swallowing efforts.

Aspiration is difficult to evaluate. If a patient is observed to experience some choking or respiratory distress that is not immediately relieved by coughing, it is probable that some aspiration has taken place. Some examiners listen with a stethoscope placed against the larynx during the swallow and have learned to perceive a characteristic sound of air mixing with liquids that suggests aspiration. Change in a patient's color, gurgling breath sounds, and extreme breathiness or loss of voice may indicate acute aspiration. Objectively, aspiration can be documented by radiographic studies. During test swallows the examiner should also note nasal regurgitation. This is more common when testing with liquids. Following each swallow, the oral cavity should be inspected for retention of food. Patients with damage to the parietal lobe of the brain and unilateral neglect commonly pocket food on the neglected side.

Test swallows for patients with tracheostoma tubes present distinctive problems. Tracheostoma tubes have a tendency to tether the larynx and trachea, resulting in inefficient laryngeal elevation and tilting (Bonanno 1971). Sasaki and associates (1977) pointed out that the laryngeal closure reflex is weakened and dyscoordinated when the upper airway is bypassed by tracheostomy. The combination of the tethering effect and impaired protective laryngeal closure reflex leaves the larynx more susceptible to penetration, and the patient is less able to expel the material to prevent tracheal aspiration.

Testing patients who have cuffed tracheostoma tubes should be done with the cuff deflated. The trachea above the cuff should be suctioned before the cuff is deflated. Before testing swallow, the tracheostoma tube should be plugged for several seconds to assess the patient's ability to breathe through the larynx as well as the voluntary laryngeal cough. As in other patients, laryngeal elevation should be felt during a swallow.

Ice chips provide an adequate stimulus to elicit the initial swallows. Aspiration should be checked by using a stimulus that is dyed with a contrast color that can be detected in the trachea. As the patient drinks approximately 10 mL of colored solution, the examiner observes for evidence of aspiration. In a patient with inadequate swallowing and an unprotected airway, the solution may show up immediately in the trachea. The trachea should be suctioned and the contents examined for evidence of the colored solution. Color contrast solutions such as methylene blue tend to coat the entire oropharyngeal mucosa, and it is not unusual to find a very small amount of blue-tinged secretion in the tracheostoma several minutes after a test swallow. This is a very common finding and usually is not associated with inadequate swallowing (Cameron et al. 1973).

Greenbaum (1976) suggested a protocol for the decannulation of the patient who has a cuffed tracheostoma tube. The patient is required to drink 4 ounces of methylene blue-dyed water at intervals of 15 minutes for an hour. The trachea is then thoroughly suctioned, and secretions are inspected for evidence of blue coloration. If this test result is negative, the cuff is deflated for meals and at other times, with close supervision for 24 hours. Greenbaum added that even though a positive test result suggests aspiration, it is not automatically a contraindication to decannulation if the patient demonstrates adequate swallowing during meals with the cuff deflated.

Just as tracheostoma tubes can interfere with the swallow reflex and the protective reflexes in the larynx, nasogastric feeding tubes have the potential to interfere with normal swallowing by altering sensations in the pharynx and deflecting the bolus. A tube passing transnasally may force the patient to breathe from the mouth, thus drying mucosa and additionally impairing normal reflexes. Some patients may be further decompensated by even a mild degree of dehydration. The examiner must be cognizant of all mechanical and metabolic factors that impede swallowing and the protective reflexes. In some cases, before final decisions can be made to proceed with oral feeding plans, the patient's swallowing should be assessed with tracheostoma and nasogastric tubes removed, the mucosa moist, and the patient adequately nourished and hydrated.

Repeat Indirect Laryngoscopy

After testing a patient's swallow reflex, a repeat indirect examination of the larynx should be performed. Here again, evidence of excessive pooling of debris in the vallecula or piriform sinuses suggests that swallowing reflex has not completely cleared the bolus from the hypopharynx. Tracheal aspiration also might be appreciated by this repeat examination when the debris is visualized adjacent to the aditus of the larynx or subglottally. Langmore and associates (1988) have described a protocol for the fiberoptic endoscopic examination of swallowing safety that can be used to assess patients with oropharyngeal-stage dysphagia. Their procedure allows for laryngeal inspection before, during, and immediately following swallows of pureed food boluses.

ADDITIONAL STUDIES

The CED is not intended to be a definitive diagnostic evaluation for dysphagia, but rather, as was stated at the outset, it is one component of a comprehensive dysphagia evaluation. However, in some cases the findings of the CED will be consistent with a previously diagnosed condition, and this examination will be sufficient to establish an effective management and treatment plan. The CED should allow the clinician to determine the need for additional studies and specify those that are required to diagnose specific impairments of swallowing and related functions.

In order to make a proper judgment regarding the need for other studies of swallowing, clinicians must have considerable experience in conducting and interpreting a CED and in providing management for patients with dysphagia. A working knowledge of studies that may be appropriate for the evaluation of swallowing and related functions is essential. Dynamic radiographic swallows, ultrasound, manometry, manofluorography, electromyography, endoscopy, a variety of reflux tests, and nutritional assessment all have a place in the comprehensive evaluation of dysphagia.

Dynamic radiographic studies of swallowing, either cine radiography or videotaped modifications of barium swallows, are the best procedures available for visualizing the deglutitory muscles during function. Dynamic radiography is required for all cases of dysphagia in which the CED suggests that the problem is directly related to, or complicated by, a cricopharyngeal, esophageal, LES, or gastric impairment. Radiographic studies are necessary when the CED fails to determine the cause of dysphagia, the findings are not consistent with a previously diagnosed condition, and when the examination suggests multiple factors are contributing to the dysphagia. Radiography should be used in cases of unexplained aspiration pneumonia, and it may be useful to assist in determining the effectiveness of compensations in preventing aspiration.

Before automatically proceeding to radiography after the CED, one can reasonably ask whether or not the results are likely to alter the diagnosis or management in a given case. For patients with dysphagia that is caused by a well-documented etiologic event, e.g., stroke, or the symptoms and findings are consistent with a previously diagnosed disease, radiography may not be indicated unless the result is to be used as the determining factor in deciding on methods for nutritional management. For acute conditions necessitating intensive care unit observation, spinal cord injury cases, and many patients with limited mobility and/or access to appropriate radiographic equipment, the CED will be the only method available to assess swallowing, and the patient's management will be determined on the basis of this protocol.

REFERENCES

Bonanno PC. Swallowing dysfunction after tracheostomy. Ann Surg 1971; 174:29–33.

Cameron JL, Reynolds J, Zuidema GD. Aspiration in patients with tracheostomies. Surg Gynecol Obstet 1973; 136:68–70.

Castell DO, Donner MD. Evaluation of dysphagia: a careful history is crucial. Dysphagia 1987; 2:65–71.

Christensen J. Effects of drugs on esophageal motility. Arch Intern Med 1976; 136: 532–7.

Edwards DA. Discriminatory value of symptoms in the differential diagnosis of dysphagia. Clin Gastroenterol 1976; 5:49–57.

Greenbaum DM. Decannulation of the tracheostomized patient. Heart Lung 1976; 5: 119–23.

Jones B, Ravich WJ, Donner MW, et al. Pharyngoesophageal interrelationships: observations and working concepts. Gastrointest Radiol 1985; 10:225–33.

Jones B, Donner MW. How I do it: examination of the patient with dysphagia. Dysphagia 1989; 4:162–72.

Jordan PH. Dysphagia and esophageal diverticula. Postgrad Med 1977; 61:155–61.

Langmore SE, Schatz K, Olsen N. Fiberoptic endoscopic examination of swallowing safety: a new procedure. Dysphagia 1988; 2:216–9.

Larsen GL. Chewing and swallowing. In: Martin N, Holt N, Hicks DJ, eds. Comprehensive rehabilitation nursing. New York: McGraw-Hill, 1981; 174–85.

Linden P, Siebens AA. Dysphagia: predicting laryngeal penetration. Arch Phys Med Rehabil 1983; 64:281–4.

McConnel FMS, Cerenko D, Hersh T, et al. Evaluation of pharyngeal dysphagia with manofluorography. Dysphagia 1988; 2:187–95.

Pope CE. Motor disorders of the esophagus. Postgrad Med 1977; 61:118–25.

Sasaki CT, Suzuki M, Horiuchi M, et al. The effect of tracheostomy on the laryngeal closure reflex. Laryngoscope 1977; 87:1428–33.

Stein M, Williams AJ, Grossman F, et al. Cricopharyngeal dysfunction in chronic obstructive pulmonary disease. Chest 1990; 97:347–52.

Straus B. Disorders of the digestive system. In: Rossman I, ed. Clinical geriatrics, 2nd ed. Philadelphia: JB Lippincott 1979; 266–89.

Weiden P, Harrigan M. A clinical guide for diagnosing and managing patients with drug-induced dysphagia. Hosp Community Psych 1986; 37:396–8.

7

Radiologic Evaluation of Swallowing

Olle Ekberg

For the evaluation of swallowing, radiology is crucial. It allows evaluation of both function and structure of the organs involved. During swallowing of a radiopaque bolus (such as barium), movements of anatomic structures as well as bolus transportation can be studied in detail. On the dysphagia team the radiologist should act as a consultant to the other team members, selecting from different imaging modalities, i.e., videofluorography, cineradiography, computed tomography, magnetic resonance imaging, ultrasound, and nuclear medicine according to specific patient needs or disease entity. Choosing the correct imaging technique is dependent on the answers needed to solve clinical questions. Therefore, the radiologist's responsibility goes beyond the performance and interpretation of the barium swallow. The radiologist should contribute knowledge from other fields of radiology, such as neuroradiology, tying together information from different studies in addition to dynamic and/or static barium swallows. The radiologist also is responsible for technical aspects such as exposure technique and the identification and reduction of image artifacts. Even in the circumstance in which the modified barium swallow is directed by a speech/language pathologist, it is important that a radiologist is responsible for the quality of the imaging procedure. However, as a swallowing team member the radiologist must also be aware of the limitations of radiology for assessment of the course and treatment of function and structure.

Swallowing can be divided into four stages: oral, pharyngeal, pharyngoesophageal segment (PES), and esophageal. This subdivision is based primarily on anatomic considerations. However, there is overlapping function. The oral stage participates in ingestion as well as some events in the pharynx and in the voluntary initiation of pharyngeal swallow. The PES stage basically pertains to the inferior pharynx and the upper cervical esophagus. However, it should be understood that although physiologic dysfunction is the most frequent abnormality in the neurologically impaired patient, the coincidental presence of a morphologic abnormality is common (Goldstein and Zornoza 1978; Thompson et al. 1978). Therefore, a meticulous search for structural abnormalities is of strategic importance as these may add to swallowing problems.

Radiologically, swallowing can be described in terms of (1) displacement of a defined anatomic structure and (2) bolus movement. Moreover, there is a close relationship among the oral, pharyngeal, and PES components of swallow. The relation between these three components and the esophagus is less obvious (Ekberg and Lindgren, 1986). Therefore, all patients with dysphagic symptoms referred from the mouth, neck, or chest should undergo a complete radiologic evaluation (Halpert et al. 1985; Jones and Donner 1988; Levine and Rubesin 1990; Jones et al. 1985). However, swallowing dysfunction may be asymptomatic, especially in demented or mentally impaired individuals. The observation by a care giver that a patient has difficulty swallowing also should lead to a radiologic investigation. Other important indications for radiologic studies of swallowing are recurrent pneumonia, cough that may be due to chronic aspiration, and unintentional weight loss.

Radiologic evaluation is an extension of the physical examination and should be included as part of the sensory/motor examination of the oral cavity, pharynx, PES, and esophagus. The pharynx can be examined only partly during conventional neurologic evaluation (requiring radiologic evaluation to document its entire dimension). Most neurologically impaired patients with swallowing dysfunction do not undergo a radiologic swallowing study, even though there may be a reason to suspect dysphagia, as in voluntary restriction of diet choices, prolonged meal times, and postprandial heartburn. One of the explanations for this discrepancy is the fact that swallowing dysfunction is frequently not discovered at bedside evaluation (Linden and Siebens 1983; Splaingard et al. 1988). Further, some patients do not cough while aspirating and therefore are unlikely to be referred for a swallowing study. Another category of indication for radiologic swallowing studies is treatment planning. Even if there is a transition between diagnostic studies and treatment planning, these two studies have different focuses. All diagnostic procedures should be performed by the radiologist. In subsequent studies, the interaction with a speech/language pathologist is crucial in planning treatment. Therefore, swallowing studies fall into either of two categories: (1) diagnostic examination and (2) therapeutic examinations.

Patients referred for diagnostic evaluation of swallowing fall into either of two subcategories: (1) mild or moderate dysphagia and (2) severe dysphagia.

Mild or Moderate Dysphagia

Patients in this category usually have dysphagia of unknown etiology when referred for the radiologic study. They present with a feeling of "something getting stuck" while swallowing or of coughing during or after swallowing. In this category, the patient has no feeding problem and is not losing weight. Patients may complain of having to cut food finely, avoiding certain difficult-to-particulate foods, or having to eat slowly. The majority of these patients do not have a neurologic diagnosis when referred for the radiologic evaluation of deglutition. However, the majority will have swallowing dysfunction secondary to neurologic disease.

Severe Dysphagia

These patients have a severe feeding problem, and the presence of swallowing dysfunction is easily unrecognized. The purpose of the radiologic study is to assess the type and degree of feeding impairment, including airway protection and concomitant morphologic abnormalities. Treatment evaluation is usually needed. The videoradiographic study is inherently concerned with therapy, particularly if the study includes trials of adapted physical character of bolus and/or changes in posture as compensations for deficits.

RADIOLOGIC EXAMINATION TECHNIQUE

The radiologic examination takes advantage of the interaction between imaging radiation and materia. However, such interaction also has a potential harmful effect and may cause damage. Therefore, it is important to always perform the examination in such a way that radiation is kept to a minimum. Even more important is to avoid an unnecessary examination. However, if the indication for the radiologic examination is correct, the advantge of the study will always exceed the risk to the patient.

Feeding can be evaluated radiographically in most patients. Only patients who cannot be immobilized during deglutition need to be excluded. The effectiveness and contribution of the radiologic study in the circumstances of the patient who is resistant or has severe impairment depends on the patience and skill of the radiologist. The result of the study may determine whether the patient will be orally fed and, eventually, whether the patient can go home or to a long-term care facility. In patients who are difficult to examine, such as those with psychoses or mental retardation, sedation before the study is contraindicated as the results will be invalid.

The examination of the mild-to-moderate and the severely dysphagic patient is focused on two different goals. In patients with dysphagia of mild or moderate severity, one should look for the "worst swallow" (focusing on techniques to decompensate oral and pharyngeal deglutition). In patients with severe dysfunction, the primary concern is with treatment, focusing on techniques to elicit the "best swallow" as a method of compensation.

Cineradiography is optimal for monitoring minor dysfunction by reason of its excellent image delineation. For other patients, especially those who have severe impairment, videoradiography is preferable. Video allows a longer observation time because of lower radiation doses, is readily available, and is less expensive.

The examination should start with the patient in an upright position, either standing or sitting on the elevated foot plate of the x-ray stand (Figure 7.1). Patients who cannot be seated without support may be seated in a specially designed chair that fits on the footplate, or be seated in a wheelchair. Chairs may need to be narrow (17 to 19 inches) in order to fit between the table top

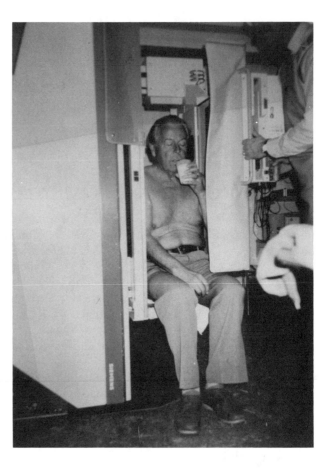

Figure 7.1 For radiologic evaluation of oral and pharyngeal swallow the patient can be seated on the footplate of the x-ray stand.

and the fluoroscopy unit. An erect position is ideal, but if the patient is unable to cooperate, any recumbent position can be used. However, such positioning will make assessment of function difficult because of the unfamiliar, oblique projection of the foodway.

Examinations of the Oral Cavity, Pharynx, and Pharyngoesophageal Segment

The examination begins in the lateral position with a brief assessment of phonation to view the velopharynx during phonation. The patient is instructed to say "candy" and "eeee." Evaluation of vocal cord mobility during phonation and breathing can be made after repositioning the patient to the frontal projection. Both observations are done without barium. Ideally, the swallowing study should start with boluses of high-density barium (250 percent weight/volume). It is important that the entire examination is video and audio recorded. Use of an audiotrack increases the information substantially. Ingestion should be from a cup, spoon, straw, or when applicable, any feeding device to which the patient is accustomed. In a patient with severe oral impairment, the pharyngeal phase may be elicited by injection of a small barium bolus (1 to 3 mL) directly into the pharynx through a soft tube. This may be placed into the pharynx either via the mouth or a nostril. Such techniques, however, are used only for examination and not for feeding. The patient should be allowed to self-feed, or be assisted as necessary. The patient should keep the ingested barium in the mouth until instructed to swallow. This interval should be 10 to 15 seconds and is intended to reveal failure of containment of the bolus. Three ingestions and swallows are observed. The patient is instructed to take a mouthful of barium. For the diagnostic examination, the size should be a normal bite size or slightly larger. The patient should be able to swallow it during one swallow attempt. It should be noted if the bolus swallowed is smaller than the volume ingested, i.e., considerable residue may be left in the mouth after swallow (Ekberg et al. 1988).

Severely impaired patients may reach the fluoroscopy suite without proper physical evaluation or medical histories. In a setting with a patient who is unable to self-feed and follow instructions, it is advisable for the radiologist to observe the patient swallowing water before positioning the patient on the x-ray table. Water is often accepted by the patient. Forced feeding should be avoided. If the patient or examiner is unable to get the water into the mouth, it is unnecessary to place the patient on the x-ray table. This water swallow test will serve as a screening device, saving much time and effort (Feinberg, in press). However, there are patients who report they are unable to swallow water, but can ingest enough barium for evaluation of function and structure. These patients may be found among those with a history of acute dysphagia and a suspicion of foreign bodies (Ekberg 1983a).

The first three bolus ingestions can be used to assess the oral stage and part of the pharynx. The field of view should include the area from the lips to the laryngeal vestibule in order to detect penetration of barium. An additional three swallows should be observed, centering the field over the pharynx and the PES. It is important to have the patient lower and move the shoulders posteriorly as they may obscure the PES. The patient is then moved into the frontal position, and two swallows including the oral cavity and two swallows including the pharyngoesophageal (PE) segment are observed. The previously mentioned schedule is a minimum of projections. If additional information is needed, more swallows should be recorded. After these swallows there usually is good coating of the mucosa of the oral cavity and pharynx, and double-contrast views should be obtained with the patient phonating ("eee"), or during slow expiration through almost closed lips, or during modified Valsalva. These double-contrast radiograms should allow detection of mucosal abnormalities as well as mass lesions (Ekberg and Nylander 1985; Rubesin and Glick, 1988; Rubesin et al. 1987). Films in lateral, frontal, and both oblique positions should be obtained (Figure 7.2).

Most patients tend to swallow with the head bent forward because it helps to close the laryngeal vestibule (allows for airway protection). However, patients

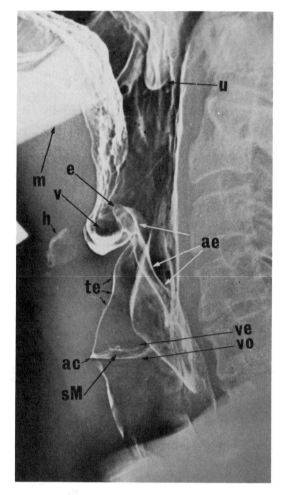

Figure 7.2 Lateral radiogram of the neck after barium swallow with coating of the mucosa. Contrast medium has reached the laryngeal vestibule and the proximal trachea. Anatomic landmarks are well visualized. Abbreviations: ac, anterior commisure; ae, aryepiglottic fold; e, epiglottis; h, hyoid bone; m, mandible; sM, sinus Morgagni; te, tubercle of the epiglottis; u, uvula; v, vallecula; ve, ventricular fold; vo, true vocal fold. (With permission from Ekberg O: Closure of the laryngeal vestibule during deglutition. Acta Otolaryngol 1982; 93:123–9.)

with poor tongue control often extend the neck in order to propel the bolus posteriorly into the pharynx. Some dysphagic patients, who do not have airway penetration with the head in the neutral position, penetrate when the head is extended. Few patients show the reverse phenomenon of being able to compensate for poor laryngeal closure when swallowing with the head extended (Jones and Donner 1988; Ekberg 1986b).

Therefore, the head should be in the neutral position. The easiest way of decompensating pharyngeal swallow is to tilt the head backward. Other methods may include increasing bolus size. In some circumstances the unfamiliarity and stress of the radiography room may create stress of sufficient degree to exacerbate pharyngeal dysfunction. This is best appreciated during the first swallow in the lateral projection for visualization of the laryngeal vestibule. Attempts to decompensate the swallow are not part of the normal routine, but may be made on patients who complain of swallowing in these positions, or in those who are symptomatic with studies in the neutral position.

Patients evaluated for severe dysfunction often have concomitant impairment such as hemiparesis and cognitive impairment that may interfere with positioning and/or cooperation. It is important to note that observations of anatomic details and structural displacement are the most crucial in mild or moderately severe dysphagia, while attention to bolus transport is the focus of attention in patients with severe dysphagia. Therefore, any projection for the severely compromised patient often is sufficient for obtaining needed information. A radiologic examination should determine whether severely duysphagic patients can achieve phryngeal swallow competence by any adaption of food or feeding. For treatment planning, the patient first should be examined in the same position as tht in which feeding occurs, followed by suggested changes in position, bolus size, or amount. Evaluation of pharyngeal function as well as closure of the laryngeal vestibule is difficult if the examination is performed in the oblique projection or in other nonstandard routines. Alteration in swallow during compensatory maneuvers by the patient or those suggested by the therapist, is notoriously difficult to evaluate. This often is due to low barium content of the bolus and obliteration of views. Therefore, it is important to standardize the examination as much as possible to validate observations of changes in function between studies on different occasions. Successive examinations should preferably be made by the same radiologist, employing familiar routines. The radiologist who completes the study is the one who should provide the written report. Consultations on radiographic studies obtained by other radiologists and from other hospitals may be meaningless if not accompanied by thorough details about technique.

Some examinations may start with the consistency of barium that is known to be more efficiently and safely swallowed. Usually in severe pharyngeal dysfunction this is barium of high density, with subsequent graduations of thick to thin fluid.

For evaluation of treatment strategies, the radiologist is assisted by the speech/language pathologist. The speech/language pathologist should be familiar with the patient's feeding problem and have performed a clinical evaluation. Both should be trained to implement a feeding care plan based on the diagnostic and treatment components of the examination. The precise description of the appropriate textures to be used is discussed in chapters on physical evaluation and treatment.

Esophagus

The examination should start with the patient in a standing position with double-contrast technique (Levine and Rubesin 1990; Ott 1988). The patient should swallow an effervescent agent, followed by 20 mL of water. The patient is instructed not to burp or belch and is then positioned in a left posterior oblique position and asked to gulp rapidly a cup (120 mL) of barium (250 percent weight/volume). This will open the lower esophageal sphincter, allowing the

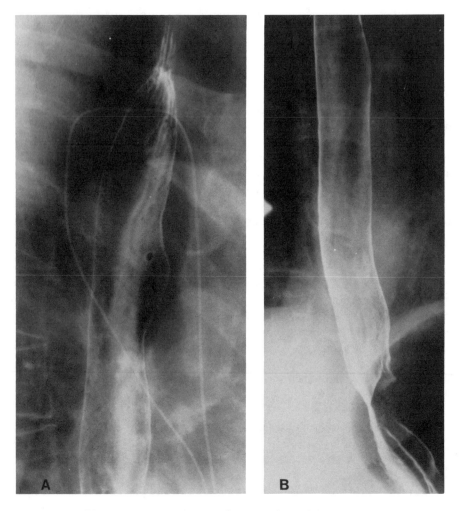

Figure 7.3 Double-contrast examination of a normal esophagus. (A) Proximal part. (B) Distal part.

carbon dioxide to rise and distend the esophagus (Figure 7.3). Rapid exposure of at least four spot films should be obtained covering the length of the esophagus. Because peristalsis causes the esophagus to collapse immediately after passage of the barium, timing of the exposure during the relatively brief period of distention is important. To fully document abnormalities, additional swallows may be necessary.

For functional evaluation of the esophagus the patient is then placed in a recumbent position, usually prone (Figure 7.4). The patient drinks from a cup through a straw. The patient is instructed to make one swallow at a time, as the examiner follows the tail of this bolus into the stomach. As new swallows abolish

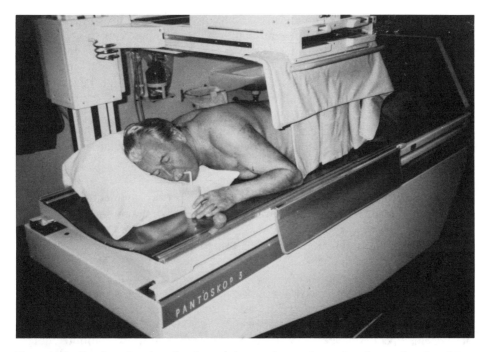

Figure 7.4 For functional evaluation of the esophagus the patient has to be placed in a recumbent position, usually prone.

ongoing esophageal peristalsis, it is important to instruct the patient to swallow just once. If necessary, the patient should be instructed to open the mouth and lower the mandible immediately after the first swallow because this makes an additional swallow difficult. Three to five single bolus swallows are observed. Following these swallows, the patient is instructed to gulp the remainder of the barium. This will distend the esophagus, and films should be obtained of the lower esophagus and gastroesophageal region. With air and barium in the stomach, the fundus and body of the stomach is screened in order to reveal structural lesions. Lesions in the gastric fundus may produce symptoms of obstruction (Jones and Donner 1988; Levine and Rubesin 1990). In one study, dysphagia was the predominant presenting symptom in five patients with carcinoma of the stomach (Halpert et al. 1985). Because patients are not fasting for this study, detailed evaluation of the stomach is not possible. The examination ends by testing for gastroesophageal reflux. This is done with the patient positioned first on the left side and then on the back so that barium pools in the gastric fundus. The gastroesophageal junction is then monitored as the patient turns to the right, coughs, and performs a straight-leg raising or Valsalva maneuver to increase the intra-abdominal pressure and elicit reflux. In patients with gross aspiration the esophageal component of the evaluation is limited. All diagnostic examinations also must include the esophagus, preferably at the same time as the oral and pharyngeal study. It is not enough to briefly observe the bolus dropping down into the stomach after the pharyngeal swallow. The esophagus must be examined carefully in every patient in order to detect the cause of dysphagia. In patients with pharyngeal abnormalities it is important to rule out accompanying lesions in the esophagus, which may add to, or be the source of, pharyngeal dysfunction. Patients with pharyngeal carcinoma have a significantly increased risk of coincident esophageal carcinoma (Goldstein and Zornoza 1978; Thompson et al. 1978). Boluses of varied texture and viscosity might be added to the study, but have a limited value in the diagnostic evaluation of the esophagus.

Additional Techniques

There are several circumstances in which the previously mentioned routine is changed. Most commonly this is accomplished by manipulating the bolus consistency. This may apply for the diagnostic portion of the examination, and always during the therapeutic part. As a test for how thin liquids are managed in the oral cavity and pharynx, a barium suspension of 140 percent weight/volume is used.

An extremely high viscosity is present in paste. This is used for studying pharyngeal and esophageal function. Paste is seldom seen to penetrate the laryngeal vestibule. In patients with poor primary peristalsis during liquid swallow, the extremely cohesive bolus of paste is regularly transported uninterrupted. Crackers soaked in high-density barium can be used for testing oral function to assess mastication and bolus formation.

Barium tablets 13 mm in diameter plus water or 140 percent weight/volume barium can be used for assessment of strictures. It is not necessary to use barium tablets if a stricture of less than 13 mm has been revealed with liquid barium. For the same purpose, a bagel bread sphere with a diameter of 10 mm can be used together with 5 mL of low-density barium (Curtis et al. 1987). If barium tablets are unavailable for assessment, a half standard marshmallow also can be used (Kelly 1961; Somers et al. 1986). An acid barium suspension with a pH of 1.7 has been advocated as a screening test for acid-induced esophageal pain (Jones and Donner 1988). The acid barium also can induce abnormal peristalsis. It is prepared by mixing 100 mL of barium suspension and 0.5 mL of concentrated hydrochloric acid (37 percent). The patient is studied first with a standard barium suspension in the prone position and then with the acid barium. A positive acid barium test result is present when normal peristalsis is replaced by segmental nonperistaltic contractions. After this test, 15 mL of antacid is given to neutralize remnants of acid barium left in the esophagus. The result is negative when esophageal function is unaffected.

When barium sulfate penetrates the lower airways, it is readily expectorated within a few days and produces few pulmonary complications. When massive, aspiration of barium may be fatal (Gray et al. 1989). Nonambulatory patients and those with known pulmonary disease can benefit from chest physical therapy to promote pulmonary drainage (Gray et al. 1989). If barium is retained in the lungs, it causes a benign short-term foreign body reaction within hours. Eventually, minimal fibrosis may follow after days or months (Ginai et al. 1984; McAlister and Askin 1983). Another variation in technique might include the use of water-soluble contrast medium such as Gastrografin (meglumine diatrizoate). Iodinated aqueous contrast media, however, produce a more intense acute inflammatory reaction with edema. Therefore, its use is contraindicated in patients with massive aspiration due to the risk for pulmonary edema if the contrast medium reaches the alveola. Barium sulfate, therefore, is the contrast medium of choice for the gastrointestinal tract, including the oral cavity, pharynx, and esophagus, except for those patients with a known or suspected perforation. The latter are often patients with postsurgical resections with a suspected anastomotic leak. Iodinated contrast media has low radiodensity, does not coat the mucosa, and gives suboptimal visualization of pathology. The only reason not to use barium to visualize a fistula is that barium trapped internally would cause difficulties in subsequent radiologic studies. With ample technique, however, including spot films before injection of new barium during the repeat study, these difficulties can be overcome.

SWALLOW INTERPRETATION

The oral, pharyngeal, PES, and esophageal stages of swallowing are precisely scheduled and symmetric and are readily appreciated radiographically (Curtis et al. 1985; Ekberg and Nylander 1982). Interpretation is done in slow motion by swallowing stage, following a precise scheme of sequenced observations.

Oral Stage

A normal individual is able to follow the instruction to drink from a cup and to take a bolus of appropriate size in a coordinated way. Liquid barium is not masticated or blended in the oral cavity. The bolus should be well contained in the oral cavity (Hamlet et al. 1988; Ekberg and Hillarp 1986). On instruction to swallow, the bolus should immediately be brought onto the posterior tongue. In the anteroposterior view the tongue dorsum is grooved to cradle the bolus in the swallow preparatory position (Hamlet et al. 1988). Delay in transfer and jerky tongue or jaw movements are abnormal.

Pharyngeal Stage

Pharyngeal swallow is then initiated. During eventual oral processing of the bolus, there is superior, inferior, and some anteroposterior movement of the hyoid bone. At the voluntary initiation of pharyngeal swallow, however, the hyoid bone moves distinctly superiorly and anteriorly. There is also a distinct apposition of the thyroid cartilage and the hyoid bone. The larynx and pharynx with the PES moves superiorly (Palmer et al. 1988). Peristaltic pharyngeal swallow is probably cued by bolus passage through the faucial isthmus, between the

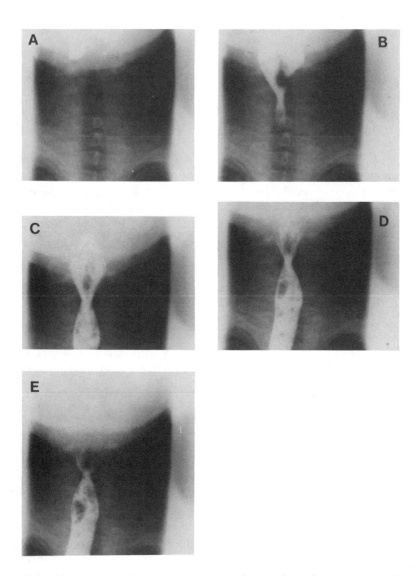

Figure 7.5 Cine sequence in (A–E) anterior and (F–J) lateral projections. The barium bolus is transported from the oral cavity into the cervical esophagus in a symmetric and synchronous way. The epiglottis is tilted down and the laryngeal vestibule is closed. The pharyngeal constrictor wave clears the pharynx from barium.

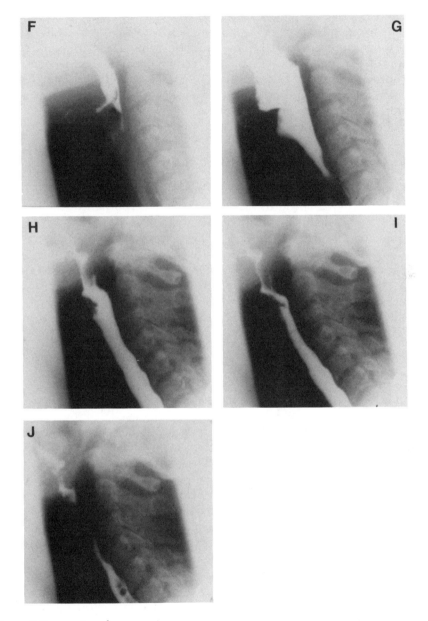

Figure 7.5 continued

tongue and the palate. Radiologically, it is convenient to use the beginning of the anterior hyoid movement as the starting point of pharyngeal swallow.

The tongue thrust propels the bolus posteriorly into the pharynx and further down into the PES and cervical esophagus, assuming the pharyngeal constrictor wall has normal compliance. The palatopharyngeal isthmus is closed by elevation of the muscular palate and constrictor convergence, which is mostly medialward of the lateral walls. No regurgitation of barium into the nasopharynx occurs in the normal patient (Figure 7.5).

Closure of the Airways

Closure of the airways occurs at four anatomically distinct and functionally separate levels: (1) the epiglottis, (2) the subepiglottic portion of the laryngeal vestibule, (3) the supraglottic portion of the laryngeal vestibule, and (4) the vocal folds (Ardran and Kemp 1952, 1956). The airways also are protected by an apposition of the thyroid cartilage toward the hyoid bone, leading to closure of the laryngeal vestibule. The vocal folds normally close before initiation of pharyngeal swallow and simultaneous with elevation of the larynx. The closure is best assessed in the anteroposterior view. Closure of the airways starts at the vocal folds and progresses in superior direction in a peristaltic-like manner (Figure 7.6).

Epiglottis

During resting conditions between swallows, the epiglottis is kept in an upright position (Ardran and Kemp 1967; Ekberg and Sigurjönsson 1982). During swallowing, the epiglottis first attains a horizontal position and then an inverted position (Figure 7.6). The first movement of the epiglottis (from an upright resting to a horizontal position) is passive and occurs synchronously with the elevation of the larynx. This movement is due to the anterior movement of the hyoid bone and the approximation of the thyroid cartilage to the hyoid bone. The epiglottis is bilaterally fixed by the pharyngoepiglottic plicae and, during laryngeal elevation and thyrohyoid approximation tilts to the transverse position, with these plicae as turning points (or fulcrum). During this movement the epiglottis maintains its hollow form, with its concavity in the cranial direction. The second movement of the epiglottis is from the transverse plane to the position where it is flipped into the esophageal inlet. During the latter movement, the epiglottis changes its shape to an inverted caudal, concave form. The inferior surface of the epiglottis is then pressed over the arytenoids. According to Fink and colleagues (1979), this movement can be explained by either a compression from side to side or by contraction of the thyroepiglottic muscles. The latter theory is compatible with the synchronous downward tilt of the epiglottis and compression of the subepiglottic portion of the laryngeal vestibule. The final contraction of the aryepiglottic musculature closes the superior laryngeal inlet more effectively, acting as the string in a tobacco pouch. The downward tilting

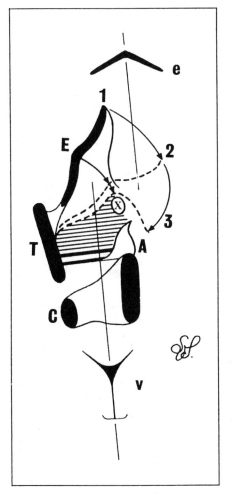

Figure 7.6 Schematic drawing of epiglottis and adjacent structures, seen from the left. The epiglottis is reproduced in its three different positions: 1, indicates resting upright position; 2, transverse position; 3, final down-tilted and inverted position. Hatched area represents closed supraglottic portion of the laryngeal vestibule. Abbreviations: A, arytenoid cartilage; C, cricoid cartilage; E, epiglottis; T, thyroid cartilage; e, horizontal position, free lip of epiglottis seen in coronal plane; v, closed vestibule seen in coronal plane; x, corniculate cartilage. (With permission from Ekberg O: Epiglottic dysfunction during deglutition in patients with dysphagia. Arch Otolaryngol 1983; 109:376–80.)

of the epiglottis occurs inconsistently in relation to peristalsis in the pharyngeal constrictors and in relation to the bolus location. It is also obvious that the epiglottis may or may not tilt down, regardless of bolus size. During dry swallows, the epiglottis tilts down to the horizontal position.

The Laryngeal Vestibule

The vestibule can be described as a bent tube, with an angle of about 45 degrees. This angulation divides the vestibule anatomically into a cranial (subepiglottic) and a caudal (supraglottic) segment. This subdivision also is valid from a functional point of view (see Figure 7.6). Simultaneous with the initiation of pharyngeal swallow (seen as the beginning of an anterior movement of the hyoid bone), there is an elevation of the pharynx and larynx, as well as an apposition of the thyroid cartilage to the hyoid bone by contraction of the thyrohyoid muscles. This apposition, together with contraction of the thyroarytenoid muscles (pars ventricularis), closes the supraglottic segment of the vestibule. At this time the arytenoids also are apposed by contraction of the interarytenoid muscles. Somewhat later and simultaneous with the final descent of the epiglottis, the subepiglottic segment of the vestibule is closed. This is affected by an apposition between the fixed portion of the epiglottis to the arytenoids and is due to contraction of the thyroepiglottic muscles as well as further elevation of the larynx. The two segments of the vestibule are thereby closed in two separate and distinct anatomic planes, which form a right angle to each other. The supraglottic segment is closed in a sagittal and vertical plane, while the subepiglottic segment is closed in a sagittal and horizontal plane.

Pharyngeal Constrictors

In the normal individual, the tongue sweep, including the posterior bulging of the tongue base, is followed by forward bulging of the posterior pharyngeal wall in a wave-like manner, starting superiorly and traversing inferiorly. The forward bulging wave normally is faint or absent in the superior constrictor area. A more conspicuous bulge, however, is regularly seen in the middle and inferior constrictors. This wave is much easier to observe in the frontal projection when the lateral pharyngeal walls are seen to oppose and form a wedge-crescent shape, with an acute angle superiorly. In the lateral projection the displacement of the anterior pharyngeal wall is more pronounced than the displacement of the posterior wall. The anterior wall displacement has three components. The most superior third is caused by the posterior bulge of the back of the tongue and is affected by the following muscles: constrictor superior, hyoglossus, styloglossus, and glossopalatinous. The middle third corresponds to the hypothyroid segment, including the inverted epiglottis and arytenoids brought posteriorly by the stylohyoid muscle and the middle pharyngeal constrictor. This posterior displacement occurs somewhat earlier than the activity in the constrictors posteriorly and laterally. The inferior component is at the level of the cricoid lamina. The posterior bulge of the cricoid is affected by the following muscles: the inferior constrictor, the stylopharyngeus, and the pharyngopalatinus. Abnormal pharyngeal clearance may be due to weakness in either of the previously described six components, three of which are anterior and three of which are posterior and lateral.

Normal pharyngeal constrictor activity is reflected in several ways during swallowing. Normal tone keeps the pharynx as a relatively straight tube without flaccidity and outpouchings. Therefore, the force created by the tongue's thrust can act on the bolus, propelling it down into the esophagus. Contraction of the constrictors is then seen as a peristaltic wave, stripping the barium from the pharynx and leaving only a thin coating on the mucosa. This peristaltic wave always is conspicuous in the frontal view and is regularly seen in the lateral view as a few millimeter deep, smooth indentation traversing inferiorly.

Monitoring the pressure gradients generated from the oral cavity, pharynx, and PES have revealed the importance of the tongue thrust and the compliance of the pharyngeal constrictors (Dodds 1989; McConnel et al. 1988a; Richter and Castell 1989). Moreover, the simultaneous recording of pressure and structural movement as well as bolus position have again emphasized the importance of laryngeal and pharyngeal elevation during swallowing.

Pharyngoesophageal Segment

The PE segment is composed of the most inferior portion of the inferior constrictor, the cricopharyngeus, and the most superior portion of the cervical esophagus. Between swallowing, the PES provides a barrier to air reaching the esophagus during inspiration and keeps refluxed or regurgitated material from the stomach and esophagus from entering the pharynx. During swallow the PES opens by a combined effect of cessation of muscle tone, elevation by the anterior movement of the hyoid bone and larynx, and by the intraluminal pressure of the bolus (Kahrilas et al. 1988; McConnel et al. 1988). During normal conditions there should be no indentation of the cricopharyngeal muscle posteriorly into the barium column when the PES is well distended. Some impingement may normally be seen early during the transport of the bolus through the PES. The PE segment also takes part in a peristaltic-like contraction with the constrictor muscles. The contracting wave continues uninterrupted from the oropharynx through the cricopharyngeus. In most persons there is a slight delay before the peristaltic contraction continues into the cervical esophagus.

Esophagus

Normal esophageal function is seen as a peristaltic wave traversing from the cervical esophagus that is elicited by pharyngeal peristalsis. During liquid barium swallows, normally only a thin coat of barium covers the mucosa. However, loss of peristaltic activity at the level of the aortic arch, where the transition between striated and smooth muscle occurs, is regularly seen and should not be considered abnormal.

The Influence of Bolus Type and Head Positioning

Compared with a low-density barium bolus, the high-density barium preparations have a slightly slower oral and pharyngeal bolus transit time not recognizable during fluoroscopy (Dantas et al. 1989). However, the effect on upper esophageal sphincter function is significant. The sphincter opening and closing is later. The duration of sphincter opening is longer, the flow rate is lower, and the maximal anterior hyoid movement is greater. The sagittal sphincter diameter is also greater (Dantas et al. 1989).

Solids (tablets) and semisolids (marshmallows) are supposed to reveal strictures in the esophagus. The bolus is halted above and then helps to distend the narrow segment. Especially with the tablet, the exact size of the narrowing can be assessed.

Evaluation of chewable food like crackers is difficult as it requires processing, chewing, and containment. With this stimulus, only a gross assessment of oral cavity and pharyngeal clearance, as well as penetration and aspiration can be made.

ABNORMAL SWALLOW

In terms of what abnormalities can be expected on the four different anatomic levels, a rule of thumb is that dysfunction is by far the principal abnormality in the oral cavity and pharynx. In those with motility dysfunction of the PES, structural abnormalities may coexist. In the esophagus, structural abnormalities predominate (Ekberg and Wahlgren 1985a,b).

Oral Stage

In patients with neurologic disease, oral dysfunction regularly predominates over pharyngeal dysfunction (Ardran and Kemp 1956; Ardran et al. 1957; Murray 1962; Donner and Siegel 1965; Donner and Silbiger 1966; Silbiger et al. 1967; Bosma and Brodie 1969a,b; Calne et al. 1970; Ekberg and Wahlgren 1985a,b; Veis and Logemann 1985; Robbins et al. 1986; Ekberg et al. 1986; Kim et al. 1987; McConnel et al. 1988; Horner et al. 1988; Robbins and Levine 1988; Dantas et al. 1989). Rapid ingestion or the inability to restrict size of oral content may produce severe abnormalities. In the same way, defective containment characterized by leakage of barium is abnormal. This may occur either anteriorly through the lips, laterally into the buccal pouches, or posteriorly into the pharynx where it potentially may reach the airways if the laryngeal vestibule is not closed (Figure 7.7). Incoordinated, jerky movements of the tongue and jaw or chewing gestures are abnormal when a liquid bolus is held in the oral cavity. Delayed transfer of the bolus within the oral cavity into a ready-to-swallow preparatory position is abnormal. An abnormal tongue thrust can be difficult to appreciate and is characterized by slow and weak posterior movement of the posterior tongue. Usually there is lack of effacement of the valleculae as well as retention in this region. Abnormalities in the oral phase of swallowing, including impaired lingual movement or soft tissue defects, generally lead to delayed oral transit and clearance of the oral bolus with retention of barium. Premature spill of barium into the pharynx may be accompanied by failed initiation of swallow, aspiration, or both. The pharyngeal phase may be delayed, but once initiated is normal.

Patients with incoordinated, weak, or jerky tongue movements commonly cannot correctly position the bolus on the tongue. Accordingly, the tongue cannot displace the bolus posteriorly. There is a strong correlation between an abnormal anterior movement of the hyoid bone and overall abnormal oral and pharyngeal functions as well as defective opening of the PE segment (Dodds 1989). Abnormal

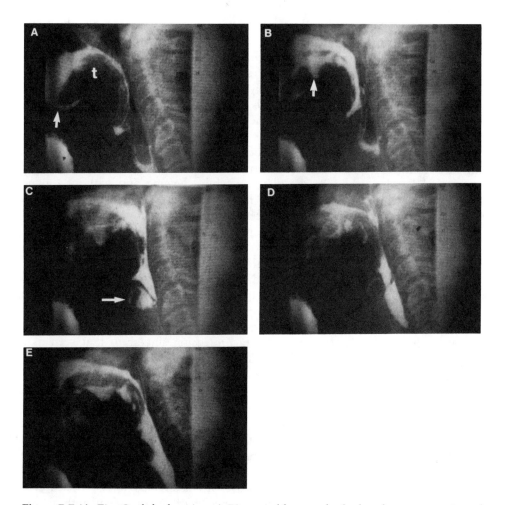

Figure 7.7 (A–E) Oral dysfunction. A 73-year-old man who had undergone resection of a part of the tongue and the floor of the mouth due to carcinoma. (A and B) After having ingested the barium, part of the liquid bolus flows anteriorly and laterally over the tongue (t). (C) The barium flows posteriorly into the pharynx without being gathered as a bolus. A large amount of barium reaches into the pharynx without any initiation of pharyngeal swallow. Barium also reaches into the open laryngeal vestibule (arrow). The epiglottis, however, is partly inverted. (D) Due to the defective elevation of the PE segment it does not open and barium is trapped in the pharynx. (E) When the patient elevates the mandible with his hand, the PE segment opens and there is elicitation of pharyngeal swallow.

initiation of the pharyngeal stage of swallow is easily appreciated when the bolus is conveyed into the pharynx without the pharynx being elevated and without occurrence of constrictor activity. Lack of anterior displacement of the hyoid bone is a conspicuous indicator of a serious abnormality. Demonstration of dissociation between the oral and pharyngeal stages depends on observation of structural displacement. Except for this failure of voluntary elicitation of pharyngeal swallow, the oral, as well as the pharyngeal stages of swallow basically appear radiologically normal.

The wide range of normalcy can be observed during chewing and swallowing of a mixture of solid and liquid, especially while talking, when the barium and/or solid is brought into the pharynx while chewing and without tongue propulsion. In this circumstance, what happens to the bolus is more important than observing pharyngeal wall displacement. It is commonly difficult to distinguish leak (whether due to defective sensory input or weak musculature) from compensatory delivery of the bolus into the pharynx.

Barium reaching superiorly into the nasopharynx is consistent with defective closure of the velopharynx secondary to either soft palate dysfunction or defective function of the superior pharyngeal constrictor. Medialward movement of the lateral pharyngeal walls is more pronounced and easy to appreciate than is the anterior movement of the posterior constrictor wall. Compensation may be in the form of a Passavant's ridge, a protrusion similar to that seen as a compensatory maneuver in speech or in patients with cleft palate.

Pharyngeal Stage

Abnormal hyoid movement is seen either as lack of anterior displacement, or a total absence of movement. The latter is rare. Motion also may be delayed in relation to bolus positioning, i.e., the bolus is in the pharynx before (more than 1 sec) hyoid elevation. This is an indicator of dissociation between oral and pharyngeal stages and is a frequent cause of misdirected bolus. Absence of thyrohyoid apposition is always abnormal and is often coincident with airway penetration.

Defective elevation of the larynx and pharynx is usually due to abnormal hyoid bone elevation, abnormal thyrohyoid apposition, defective contraction of palatopharyngeal muscles, or any combination of these factors.

Abnormal vocal fold apposition is seen in patients with involvement of the recurrent laryngeal nerve.

Epiglottis

Abnormal movement of the epiglottis is common and always indicative of pharyngeal dysfunction.

Defective secondary movement of the epiglottis from a horizontal to an inverted position is common (Figure 7.8). This is seen as the epiglottis remaining in the horizontal position (Curtis and Sepulveda 1983; Ekberg 1983b). However,

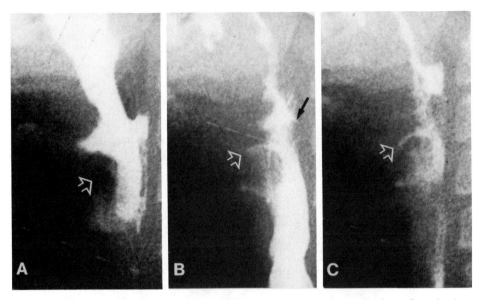

Figure 7.8 (A–C) Sequence from a cineradiographic examination in lateral projection during barium swallow. Defective tilting down of the epiglottis that is halted in a horizontal position (i.e., the second stage of tilting down is missing). (Arrow, tip of the epiglottis). There is delayed closure of the laryngeal vestibule and barium contrast medium reaches into the subepiglottic portion (open arrow). (With permission from Ekberg O, Nylander G: Cineradiography of the pharyngeal stage of deglutition in 150 individuals without dysphagia. Br J Radiol 1982; 55:253–7.)

there is a variety of abnormalities where the epiglottis tilts down incompletely. This might indicate a variable degree of incoordination of muscle function or a varying degree of paresis. Immobility of the epiglottis is seen as absence of the first movement. However, there is movement that is regularly transmitted from the back of the tongue. Therefore the epiglottis is never completely immobile.

Laryngeal Vestibule

Defective closure of the supraglottic portion of the laryngeal vestibule causes the bolus to reach the airways (Figure 7.8). In the majority of patients with abnormal closure of the supraglottic portion of the laryngeal vestibule, closure is accomplished too late. The barium will reach into the lumen of the vestibule and either will be expelled superiorly into the pharynx or inferiorly into the trachea beyond the vocal folds (Curtis and Sepulveda 1983; Ekberg 1982) (Figure 7.9). Complete absence of closure of the supraglottic vestibule is rare and is seen only in patients with a defective thyrohyoid apposition. The closure of the supraglottic portion of the laryngeal vestibule is crucial to protection of the airways. When the bolus extends beyond this point, it is a

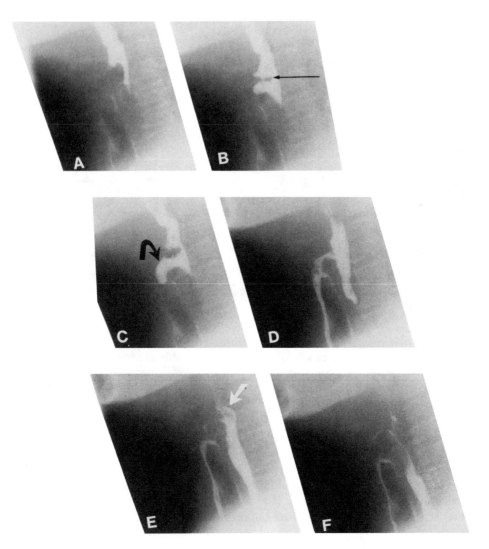

Figure 7.9 (A–F) Sequence from a cineradiographic examination in lateral projection during barium swallow. Late closure of the laryngeal vestibule. The liquid barium reaches into the pharynx while the vestibule is still open. Part of the barium bolus reaches into the vestibule (C, bent arrow), the epiglottis is halted in a horizontal position (B, thin arrow). (E) Late during swallowing the laryngeal vestibule is closed. (F) Pharyngeal constrictor activity clears the barium from the pharynx. (With permission from Ekberg O, Wahlgren L: Pharyngeal dysfunctions and their interrelationship in patients with dysphagia. Acta Radiol Diagn 1985; 26:659–64.)

matter of chance whether it is expelled or reaches the trachea (Ekberg and Hilderfors 1985). Defective closure of the subepiglottic portion of the laryngeal vestibule is usually interpreted as delayed closure. A majority of these patients propel the bolus into the pharynx beyond the superior inlet of the laryngeal vestibule too early in relation to its closure. In these patients, it is more appropriate to identify the abnormality as an oral propulsion disorder instead of a laryngeal closure deficiency. Closure of the subepiglottic portion often is normal, but delayed. However, in half of the patients in whom contrast medium reaches into the subepiglottic portion, closure is never complete (Curtis et al. 1984). In patients with nonclosure of the subepiglottic space, it is obvious that when they inspire after swallowing the retained contrast medium might be aspirated.

Pharyngeal Constrictors

Pharyngeal constrictors play a crucial role in swallowing (Ekberg and Nylander 1981). If constrictor muscles are paretic, the pharyngeal chamber undergoes an abnormal expansion during the compression phase of swallow. This lack of compliance may result in impaired transit of bolus from the oral cavity into the esophagus, even if the tongue acts normally (Figure 7.10). Defective action of the pharyngeal constrictors leads to retention of barium in the pharynx. This constrictor activity is best evaluated in the frontal projection. As the middle pharyngeal constrictor is the most commonly involved, retention characteristically occurs at the level of the superior laryngeal inlet and may lead to aspiration after swallowing. Unilateral constrictor paresis is rare (Donner and Siegel 1965). Since the barium is assymmetrically transported (in the anteroposterior view), it may mimic a pharyngeal tumor on the normal side (Thulin and Welin 1954).

Discovery of misdirection of the barium into the larynx and/or trachea should not lead to the interruption of the study. However, there are patients with massive penetration into the trachea in whom a very limited study is sufficient for answering the clinician's immediate question apropos of possible oral feeding. It is important to elucidate the underlying pathophysiology in these patients. Therefore, a few swallows should be obtained in the lateral projection, even following aspiration of the first swallow. The hazard for acquiring bronchopneumonia secondary to a misdirected barium bolus carries little morbidity.

Pharyngoesophageal Segment

Failure of the PE segment to open may be seen in neurologic disease, but generally is not accompanied by abnormal pharyngeal bolus transport (Curtis et al. 1984; Ekberg 1986a). Failure of the cricopharyngeal muscle to open or elongate may be due to (1) defective relaxation, (2) defective distensability, (3) hypertrophy/hyperplasia, or (4) fibrosis. The posterior bar intruding into the barium that is created by contraction of the cricopharyngeus muscle is seldom

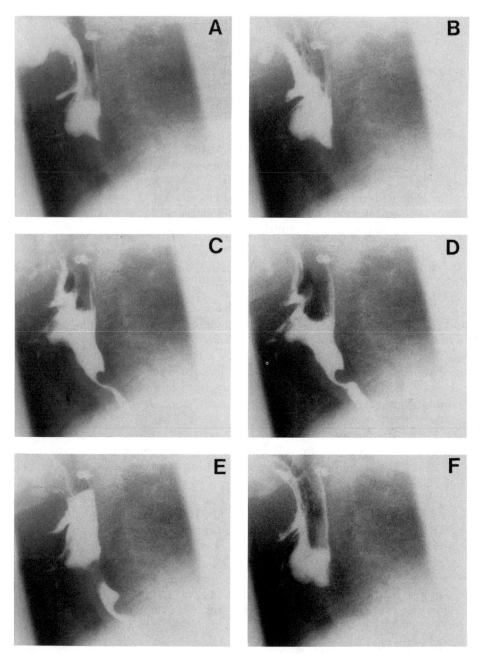

Figure 7.10 (A–F) Cineradiographic examination in lateral projection during barium swallow. Multiple pharyngeal dysfunction. There is paresis of the middle and inferior pharyngeal constrictors. The epiglottis is not tilting down, allowing the contrast medium to reach the laryngeal vestibule and trachea. There is defective opening of the cricopharyngeal muscle.

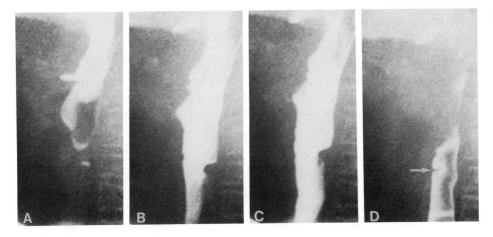

Figure 7.11 (A–D) Delayed opening of the PE segment. The cricopharyngeal muscle is seen as a posterior inbulging. There is also a small cervical esophageal web (D, white arrow).

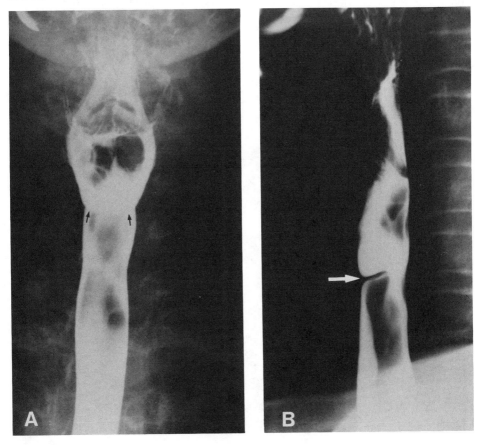

Figure 7.12 (A) Anteroposterior view. (B) Lateral view of the pharynx during barium swallow. There is a deep web in the anterior wall (arrow).

an isolated dysfunction. It commonly is associated with abnormal motor function in the segment above (i.e., the inferior pharyngeal constrictor) and/or in the segment below (i.e., the cervical esophageal region) (Figure 7.11). Therefore, even though the cricopharyngeal indentation is the most conspicuous, it may be only one aspect of severe motor dysfunction in the adjacent PE segment (Ekberg 1986a).

In dysphagic patients, cervical esophageal webs are relatively common (Ekberg et al. 1986; Clements et al. 1974) and often are present together with cricopharyngeal indentation (Ekberg and Wahlgren 1985b). However, webs may be the only abnormality (Figure 7.12). The web is easy to dilate during endoscopy.

Less common are diverticula in the PES. A Zenker's diverticulum is located in the posterior midline, superior to the cricopharyngeus muscle (Figure 7.13). When large, they regularly protrude to the left of midline. A Killian-Jamieson type diverticulum is located laterally and inferior to the insertion of the crico-pharyngeus muscle on the cricoid cartilage (Ekberg and Nylander 1983) (Figure 7.14).

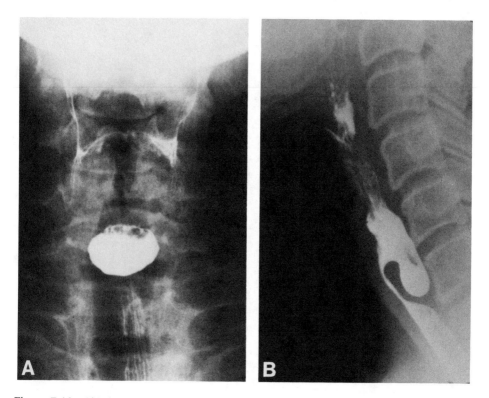

Figure 7.13 (A) Anteroposterior projection. (B) Lateral projection. Zenker's diverticulum.

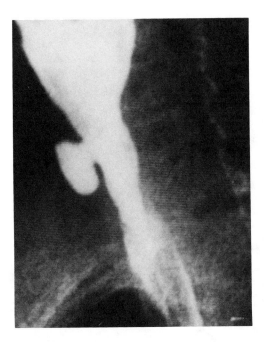

Figure 7.14 Cine frame from an examination during a barium swallow in the oblique projection. There is a 2-cm diverticulum of the Killian-Jamieson type that protrudes obliquely and anteriorly to the right.

Structural abnormalities in the pharynx and PES are common. When suspected following radiography, endoscopy should be done. The importance of double-contrast technique in this circumstance is emphasized as superficial lesions are likely to be obscured without it. Benign tumors in the pharynx include cysts in the vallecula, that usually are asymptomatic unless large or infected. Carcinoma of the epiglottis and piriform sinus may be of considerable size before producing symptoms. Laryngeal carcinoma often spreads beyond the larynx into the pharynx. The latter are likely to have produced hoarseness well before dysphagia.

Adapted and compensated swallow may have the same radiologic appearance. In the majority of patients it is difficult to demonstrate. Therefore, a normal radiologic study may not rule out pharyngeal dysfunction (Buchholz et al. 1985).

Esophagus

Abnormal motor function of the esophagus is radiologically demonstrated as absent or defective primary peristalsis or as increased or vigorous contractions (see Chapter 4). The opening of the lower esophageal sphincter may be abnormal, either in closing or opening. Therefore, radiographic dysfunction falls into one of five major categories. Achalasia is seen as absence of peristalsis with defective opening of the lower esophageal segment. The latter is seen as a "bird-beak" narrowing (Figure 7.15). The esophagus is often dilated and sometimes tortuous.

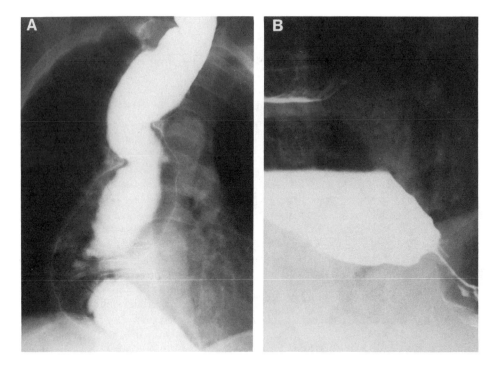

Figure 7.15 (A) Thoracic esophagus. (B) Lower esophageal sphincter segment. In a patient with achalasia the esophagus can be dilated and tortuous. During swallowing the barium accumulates in the distal esophagus above the lower esophageal sphincter.

The etiology is unknown, but seems to imply defective innervation of the esophageal musculature.

In scleroderma, a disease of smooth muscle, there is absence of primary peristalsis; however, the lower esophageal segment is open and gastroesophageal reflux may be severe.

Diffuse esophageal spasm is seen as nonpropulsive vigorous contractions, as well as weak or absent primary peristalsis. Nutcracker esophagus is one variety of diffuse esophageal spasm and has a pathognomonic manometric appearance with very high pressures. However, the radiologic appearance may be that of normal bolus transit.

Gastroesophageal reflux may commonly cause cervical dysphagia (Jones et al. 1985). Ekberg (1986a) found that 12 percent of patients without gastroesophageal reflux and 40 percent of patients with reflux had cricopharyngeal indentation. Other pharyngeal dysfunctions were not common among patients with gastroesophageal reflux. This finding supports the assumption of a possible relationship between gastroesophageal reflux and cricopharyngeal function. The pathogenesis of this relationship, however, is unclear. Peptic strictures are com-

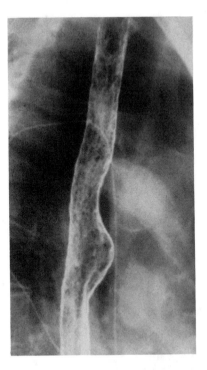

Figure 7.16 *Candida* esophagitis. There are multiple millimeter protrusions from the esophageal mucosa. These protrusions are arranged in rows. The distension of the esophagus is limited.

mon and may be severe. Peristalsis is weak or absent in the distal esophagus, and this causes prolonged contact between the acid and the mucosa.

Morphologic abnormalities of the esophagus include inflammatory lesions that may be caused by infections such as *Candida* (Figure 7.16) or by chemicals such as acid reflux. It has been suggested that dysphagia should be produced during gastroesophageal reflux only if the pH is below four and in the presence of esophagitis (Triadafilopoulos 1989). Benign (leiomyoma) and malignant tumors (squamous cell carcinoma) (Figure 7.17) also must be considered.

The immunocompromised patient with oral and pharyngeal candidiasis is seen with increasing frequency. During double-contrast examination, *Candida* appear as a mottled and/or nodular mucosal surface.

Structural abnormalities in the esopohagus are important to detect in these patients. Infectious esophagitis secondary to *Candida* or herpes may be the cause of dysphagia. However, they may occur in patients with other functional abnormalities of the swallowing apparatus and therefore be overlooked if the potential of the radiologic study is not fully used.

A distal esophageal ring (Schatzki's type) is another cause of intermittent dysphagia, particularly during solid bolus swallow. A ring with a diameter of more than 20 mm is rarely symptomatic. A diameter less than 13 mm nearly always causes dysphagia. Radiologic demonstration of this mucosal ring requires distention of the esophagogastric region above or beyond the caliber of the ring.

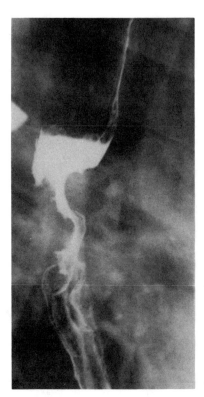

Figure 7.17 Carcinoma of the esophagus. In the midesophagus there is a short irregular stricture with overhanging edges. During endoscopy adenocarcinoma was revealed.

Course of Swallowing Disorders

The course of dysphagic symptoms and their consequences on function often do not correlate. Deterioration or progression of dysphagia is, as a rule, well compensated. Only by attempting to decompensate swallow can one reveal the progression, as when the radiologist intentionally elicits decompensation by extension of the neck or by giving a large bolus at a faster rate (Buchholz et al. 1985).

It is important to remember that repeat studies of pharyngeal function in patients suspected of progressive disease can be very important. Disability might go undetected if a repeat study is not considered.

REFERENCES

Ardran GM, Kemp FH. The protection of the laryngeal airway during swallowing. Br J Radiol 1952; 23:406–16.

Ardran GM, Kemp FH. Closure and opening of the larynx during swallowing. Br J Radiol 1956a; 29:205–8.

Ardran GM, Kemp FH. Radiologic investigation of pharyngeal and laryngeal palsy. Acta Radiol Diagn 1956b; 46:446–57.

Ardran GM, Kemp FH, Wegelius C. Swallowing defects after poliomyelitis. Br J Radiol 1957; 30:169–89.

Ardran GM, Kemp FH. The mechanism of the larynx II: the epiglottis and closure of the larynx. Br J Radiol 1967; 40:372–89.

Bosma JF, Brodie DR. Disabilities of the pharynx in amyotrophic lateral sclerosis as demonstrated by cineradiography. Radiology 1969a; 92:97–103.

Bosma JF, Brodie DR. Cineradiographic demonstration of pharyngeal area myotonia in myotonic dystrophy patients. Radiology 1969b; 92:104–9.

Buchholz DW, Bosma JF, Donner MW. Adaption, compensation and decompensation of the pharyngeal swallow. Gastrointest Radiol 1985; 10:235–9.

Calne DB, Shaw DG, Spiers AS, et al. Swallowing in parkinsonism. Br J Radiol 1970; 43:456–7.

Clements JL, Cox GW, Torres WE, et al. Cervical esophageal webs—a roentgen-anatomic correlation. AJR 1974; 121:221–31.

Curtis DJ, Cruess DF, Berg T. The cricopharyngeal muscle: a video-recording. AJR 1984; 146:497–500.

Curtis DJ, Cruess DF, Dachman AH. Normal erect swallowing: normal function and incidence of variations. Invest Radiol 1985; 20:717–26.

Curtis DJ, Cruess DF, Willgress ER. Abnormal solid bolus swallowing in the erect position. Dysphagia 1987; 2:46–49.

Curtis DJ, Sepulveda GV. Epiglottic motion: Video recording of muscular dysfunction. Radiology 1983; 148:473–7.

Dantas RO, Dodds WJ, Massey BT, et al. The effect of high- vs low-density barium preparations in the quantitative features of swallowing. AJR 1989; 153:1191–5.

Dodds WJ. The physiology of swallowing. Dysphagia 1989; 3:171–8.

Donner MW, Siegel L. The evaluation of pharyngeal neuromuscular disorders by cine-fluorography. AJR 1965; 94:299–307.

Donner MW, Silbiger ML. Cineradiofluorographic analysis of pharyngeal swallowing in neuromuscular disorders. Am J Med Sci 1966; 251:600–16.

Ekberg O, Nylander G. Pharyngeal constrictor paresis in patients with dysphagia: a cineradiographic study. Clin Radiol 1981; 33:253–8.

Ekberg O, Nylander G. Cineradiography of the pharyngeal stage of deglutition in 150 individuals without dysphagia. Br J Radiol 1982; 55:253–7.

Ekberg O, Sigurjonsson SV. Movement of the epiglottis during deglutition: a cineradiographic study. Gastrointest Radiol 1982; 7:101–7.

Ekberg O. Defective closure of the laryngeal vestibule during deglutition. Acta Otolaryngol 1982; 93:309–17.

Ekberg O. Cineradiography in 45 patients with acute dysphagia. Gastrointest Radiol 1983a; 8:295–302.

Ekberg O. Epiglottic dysfunction during deglutition in patients with dysphagia. Arch Otolaryngol 1983b; 109:376–80.

Ekberg O, Nylander G. Lateral diverticula from the pharyngoesophageal junction area. Radiology 1983; 146:117–22.

Ekberg O, Nylander G. Double contrast examination of the pharynx. Gastrointest Radiol 1985; 10:263–71.

Ekberg O, Wahlgren L. Dysfunction of pharyngeal swallowing: a cineradiographic investigation in 854 dysphagic patients. Acta Radiol Diagn 1985a; 26:389–95.

Ekberg O, Wahlgren L. Pharyngeal dysfunctions and their interrelationship in patients with dysphagia. Acta Radiol Diagn 1985b; 26:659–64.

Ekberg O, Hilderfors H. Defective closure of the laryngeal vestibule: frequency of pulmonary complications. AJR 1985; 145:1159–64.

Ekberg O. The cricopharyngeus revisited. Br J Radiol 1986a; 59:875–9.

Ekberg O. Posture of the head and pharyngeal swallow. Acta Radiol Diagn 1986b; 27:691–6.

Ekberg O, Hillarp B. Radiologic evaluation of the oral stage of swallow. Acta Radiol Diagn 1986; 27:533–7.

Ekberg O, Lindgren S. Gastroesophageal reflux and pharyngeal function. Acta Radiol Diagn 1986; 27:421–3.

Ekberg O, Malmquist J, Lindgren S. Pharyngeal webs in dysphageal patients. Fortschr Rontgenstr 1986; 146:75–80.

Ekberg O, Lindgren S, Schultz T. Pharyngeal swallowing in patients with paresis of the recurrent nerve. Acta Radiol Diagn 1986; 27:697–700.

Ekberg O, Olsson R, Sundgren-Borgstrom P. Relation between bolus-size and pharyngeal swallow. Dysphagia 1988; 3:69–72.

Feinberg M. Aspiration and the elderly. Dysphagia 1990; 5:61–71.

Fink BR, Martin RW, Rohrman CA. Biomechanism of the human epiglottis. Acta Otolaryngol 1979; 87:554–9.

Ginai AZ, Lenkate FJW, ten Berg RGM, et al. Experimental evaluation of various available contrast agents for use in the upper gastrointestinal tract in case of superficial leakage effects on lung. Br J Radiol 1984; 57:895–901.

Goldstein HM, Zornoza J. Association of squamous cell carcinoma of the head and neck with cancer of the esophagus. AJR 1978; 9:791–4.

Gray C, Sivaloganathan S, Simpkins KC. Aspiration of high-density barium causing pulmonary inflammation: report of two fatal cases in elderly women with disordered swallowing. Clin Radiol 1989; 40:397–400.

Halpert RD, Spickler E, Feczko PJ. Dysphagia in patients with gastric cancer and a normal esophagram. Radiology 1985; 154:589–91.

Hamlet SL, Stone M, Shawker TH. Posterior tongue grooving in deglutition and speech: preliminary observations. Dysphagia 1988; 3:65–68.

Horner J, Massey EW, Riski JE, et al. Aspiration following stroke: clinical correlates and outcome. Neurology 1988; 38:1359–62.

Jones B, Donner MW. Examination of the patient with dysphagia. Radiology 1988; 167:319–26.

Jones B, Ravich WJ, Donner MW, et al. Pharyngoesophageal interrelationships: observations and working concepts. Gastrointest Radiol 1985; 10:225–33.

Kahrilas PJ, Dodds WJ, Dent J, et al. Upper esophageal sphincter function during deglutition. Gastroenterology 1988; 95:52–62.

Kelly JE Jr. The marshmallow as an aid to radiologic examination of the esophagus. N Engl J Med 1961; 265:1306–7.

Kim WS, Buchholz D, Kumar AJ, et al. Magnetic resonance imaging for evaluating neurogenic dysphagia. Dysphagia 1987; 2:40–45.

Levine MS, Rubesin SE. Radiologic investigation of dysphagia. AJR 1990; 154:1157–63.

Linden P, Siebens AA. Dysphagia: predicting laryngeal penetration. Arch Phys Med Rehabil 1983; 64:281–4.

McAlister WM, Askin FB. The effects of some contrast agents in the lung: an experimental study in the rat and dog. AJR 1983; 14:245–51.

McConnel FMS, Cerenko D, Mendelsohn MS. Manofluorographic analysis of swallowing. Otolaryngol Clin North Am 1988a; 21:625–35.

McConnel FMS, Cerenko D, Jackson RT, et al. Clinical application of the manofluorogram. Laryngoscope 1988b; 98:705–11.

Murray JF. Deglutition in myasthenia gravis. Br J Radiol 1962; 35:43–52.

Ott DG. Radiologic evaluation of esophageal dysphagia. Curr Problem Diagn Radiol 1988; 17:1–33.

Palmer JB, Tanaka E, Siebens AA. Motions of the posterior pharyngeal wall in swallowing. Laryngoscope 1988; 98:414–17.

Richter JE, Castell JA. Esophageal manometry. In: Gelfand DW, Richter JE, eds. Dysphagia: diagnosis and treatment. New York: Igaku-Shoin 1989; 83–114.

Robbins J, Levine RL. Swallowing after unilateral stroke of the cerebral cortex: preliminary experience. Dysphagia 1988; 3:11–17.

Robbins JA, Logemann JA, Kirschner HS. Swallowing and speech production in Parkinson's disease. Ann Neurol 1986; 19:283–7.

Rubesin SE, Glick SN. The tailored double-contrast pharyngogram. CRC Critical Reviews in Diagn Radiol 1988; 28:132–79.

Rubesin SE, Jessurun J, Robertson D, et al. Lines of the pharynx. Radiographics 1987; 7:217–37.

Silbiger M, Pikielney R, Donner MW. Neuromuscular disorders affecting the pharynx. Invest Radiol 1967; 2:442–8.

Somers S, Stevenson GW, Thompson G. Comparison of endoscopy and barium swallow with marshmallow in dysphagia. J Can Assoc Radiol 1986; 37:72–75.

Splaingard ML, Hutchins B, Sutton LD, et al. Aspiration in rehabilitation patients: videofluoroscopy vs. bedside clinical assessment. Arch Phys Med Rehabil 1988; 69:637–40.

Thompson WM, Oddson TA, Kelvin F, et al. Synchronous and metachronous squamous cell carcinoma of the head, neck, and esophagus. Gastrointest Radiol 1978; 3:123–7.

Thulin A, Welin S. Radiographic findings in unilateral hypopharyngeal paralysis. Acta Otolaryngol 1964; 116(suppl):288–93.

Triadafilopoulos G. Nonobstructive dysphagia in reflux esophagitis. Am J Gastroenterol 1989; 84:614–8.

Veis SL, Logeman JA. Swallowing disorders in persons with cerebrovascular accident. Arch Phys Med Rehabil 1985; 66:272–5.

8

General Treatment of Neurologic Swallowing Disorders

Robert M. Miller
Michael E. Groher

An early and accurate diagnosis and evaluation of patients suspected of having dysphagia secondary to neurologic disease is essential for the design of safe and effective treatment. The neurogenic causes for dysphagia are numerous (see Chapter 2) and it is important that the dysphagia specialist become familiar with the clinical pathologic mechanisms of certain disease processes. This should include a thorough understanding of effects on the neuromuscular system, clinical course and expected prognosis, changes that medical or surgical intervention might bring, and potential effects on the patient's learning skills. The interaction of these factors should determine the proper approach to management.

The most challenging aspect of neurologically based swallowing disorders is that patients with similar pathologic processes develop swallowing disorders which differ in severity and in schedule. For instance, all patients with amyotrophic lateral sclerosis (ALS) will not develop similar patterns of dysphagia and therefore require identical therapy. In some ALS patients, dysphagia is a significant problem at first diagnosis. In others it is not evident until the later stages of the disease, and even then, its clinical manifestations may differ among individuals. Even though dysphagia with significant aspiration may be part of a well-known set of clinical signs for a particular neurologic disease, it may not manifest itself in an identical manner, and may be demonstrated at unpredictable times. And when dysphagia becomes apparent, patients with identical causative conditions require different treatment approaches due to disease severity, previous medical history, willingness to cooperate and/or learn, and present state of health. Successful management is dependent on an awareness of such disparities.

These introductory comments alert the reader to the fact that the treatment concepts presented in this chapter should not be generalized. The approaches described are to be used only as guidelines for treatment. Overgeneralization may result in inflexibility in dealing with patients who require a great deal of adaptation of treatment. Unfortunately, each patient will not benefit from our suggestions; however, with continued investigation and the application of individualized clinical problem solving, those with neurogenic dysphagia can be managed effectively. Specific neurofacilitative approaches to deglutition management that often are used as precursors to oral intake are covered in detail in Chapter 9.

TREATMENT OF DYSPHAGIA PARALYTICA

Diseases that affect the lower motoneurons of the brain stem or their peripheral connections to the swallowing muscles may render the musculature needed for swallow either weak or paretic. There may be several disorders of cranial innervation so that the ability to swallow is incapacitated. Facial and/or hypoglossal nerve involvement may be present. The cough reflex, which is mediated by the ninth and tenth cranial nerves, may be so impaired that the patient is unable to expel accumulated secretions or a bolus that has penetrated the larynx. Cineradiography may demonstrate failure of the cricopharyngeus muscle to relax, thus incapacitating pharyngeal swallow. The principal causes of dysphagia secondary to lower motoneuron involvement are discussed in Chapter 2.

Because the respiratory centers are located in the brain stem, and because of patients' failure to adequately control their own secretions, those with dysphagia paralytica may require a tracheostoma. Increased respiratory rates (greater than 30) also may interfere with the time requirement for airway closure during swallow. The critical medical condition in the acute stages often requires intravenous and subsequent nasogastric, or bypass feeding to support life.

Although one of the goals of a swallowing management program is to avoid the prolonged use of nasogastric tube feedings, these are particularly important in the initial stages of medical management because they supply the nutrients that may eventually give the patient the strength to begin receiving nutrition orally. As metabolic balance is achieved, critical protective reflexes may return and a swallowing treatment plan can be implemented.

Such a feeding program should not begin until the physician feels the patient's acute medical status warrants it. The swallowing evaluation must demonstrate that the patient has an adequate protective and productive cough reflex and can elevate the larynx during a swallow (see Chapter 6). Ideally, the cannula will be removed, as the tracheostoma tube may interfere with normal laryngeal elevation and cricopharyngeal relaxation (Bonanno 1971). The presence of the tube also may alter the pressure gradient needed in a normally closed system to move a bolus rapidly from the mouth to esophagus.

Swallowing management and treatment of patients with dysphagia paralytica is based on five major concepts: (1) establish an effective means of communication; (2) use a safe and stimulating diet in an effort to trigger a weak reflex; (3) capitalize on intact voluntary cortical drive to facilitate swallowing; (4) strengthen weakened oral and pharyngeal musculature; and (5) attempt surgical intervention.

Communication

Before consideration can be given to diet and muscle strengthening exercises, the clinician's work will be greatly facilitated if a viable communication system is established between patient and staff. Due to the weakened articulatory muscles, patients with dysphagia paralytica often cannot produce intelligible speech even though their mental abilities with respect to language remain intact. Electronic communication aids, silent spokesman boards and yes/no question strategies are all commonly employed modes of communication that aid in the patient's treatment. More elaborate computer interface systems can be employed if recovery is prolonged. It is very beneficial to the clinician if the patient can express difficulties and successes that occur during swallowing remediation.

Diet

If the swallow reflex is absent or very weak, patients with brain stem pathology need maximal dietary stimulus to give the reflex the best chance to respond. Rather than recommending the traditional pureed foods, a diet that enhances the sensations of taste, temperature, texture, and pressure is recommended (Curran and Groher 1990). Purees appeal to none of these, and in fact, they might be more difficult to swallow because of their bland taste, unappealing appearance, lack of temperature and texture, and minimal pressure requirements for chewing (Figure 8.1). Purees are difficult to control in the oral cavity when the musculature is weakened, and the patient with lower motoneuron weakness finds it difficult to form the necessary bolus to trigger a swallow. For the same reason, fluids often are harder to control than semisolids. Some patients with dysphagia paralytica who also have accompanying cricopharyngeal dysfunction may find that if the reflex is elicited, softer foods and liquids pass into the esophagus more easily, while solids are obstructed at this level due to failure of the sphincter to relax or because of premature sphincter closure. In selected cases, larger boluses may improve the function of this sphincter.

In general, patients with lower motoneuron dysphagia should avoid foods such as applesauce that falls apart as it passes through the pharynx, fresh white bread or bananas that are sticky and tend to hang up, and chocolate or ice cream that increases heavy mucus retention, which can in itself become an interference.

Muscle Strengthening

If patients demonstrate that they are unable to take liquids safely, and solids fail to reach the esophagus, they perhaps can be taught to swallow a nasogastric feeding tube orally (Campbell-Taylor et al. 1988) (Figure 8.2). We prefer a red rubber urinary catheter because of its ease of insertion and tolerance in the oropharynx. Its length will not penetrate the lower esophageal sphincter, which minimizes reflux, but should only be used for patients with known competent

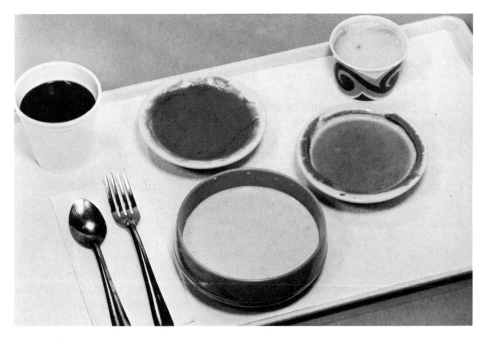

Figure 8.1 Typical pureed food consisting of strained vegetables, thinned applesauce, soup, and coffee. All items are liquid and appear unappetizing in addition to their bland flavoring.

distal esophageal function. Because the gag reflex already is diminished or absent, the patient may find this easy to do. Stimulation of the tongue and pharyngeal muscle bundles by the tube during oral passage may activate contraction of weakened muscles. By reciprocal action, enhancement of contraction of the inferior constrictor allows the cricopharyngeus to relax. The patient will not only be able to self-administer nutrition, but at the same time will receive the added benefit of strengthening the muscles needed for swallowing with an easily retrievable bolus. Intermittent passage of the tube allows the patient to receive nutrition, water, and medication and avoids the constant irritation of a naso-gastric tube. With recovery, sensation and active reflexes in the pharynx may return. If the patient reports nausea during orogastric tube passage or while the tube is in place, the procedure should be discontinued until the cause is determined. Emesis must be avoided because of the potential for aspiration of stomach contents.

Passage of an oral tube can be used as an exercise for swallowing in which the patient uses the tongue and facial muscles to move the tube back and attempts to elevate the larynx. In patients with paralysis of swallowing due to progressive degenerative neurologic diseases such as ALS or exacerbation of myasthenia

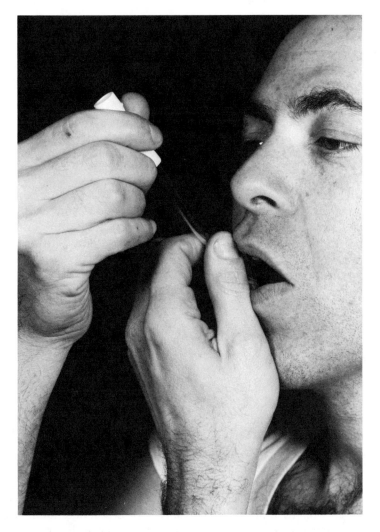

Figure 8.2 Patient passing a feeding tube through his mouth. This serves as a convenient way to take nutrition and helps to exercise weakened oral and pharyngeal musculature.

gravis, exercises for strengthening are contraindicated. For them, the feeding tube can be passively inserted and used as a tool for nutritional management.

For those with swallowing reflex delay, thermal stimulation may enhance the swallowing reflex. In 25 patients with pharyngeal swallow reflex delay, thermal stimulation at that anterior faucial arch prior to swallow improved total transit time in 82 percent while ingesting liquid and in 100 percent while ingesting a paste consistency (Lazzara et al. 1986). Rosenbek et al. (1991) studied the long-term consequences of thermal application on the reduction of oropharyngeal dysphagic symptoms in seven neurologically impaired subjects using a single-subject withdrawal (ABAB) paradigm. Measures of improvement were taken from descriptions of videoradiographs and actual timed sequences. They concluded that the efficacy of thermal stimulation with this design could not be denied or supported, but could positively change some aspects of swallow performance.

Intellectual Controls

Since most of the patients with dysphagia paralytica retain intellectual functions and some voluntary (upper motoneuron) control of the swallowing musculature, this can be used to advantage during feeding. Once the treatment plan has advanced to the point of using food and liquid to stimulate swallowing, the patient's attention can be focused on fully appreciating the taste, feel, and temperature of the bolus. Once the bolus has moved posteriorly in the oral cavity, the patient should concentrate on swallowing. This often will trigger a reflex when the bolus alone fails to activate the weakened muscles (Larsen 1976). Some patients can be taught to hold a full breath consciously during each swallow and produce a gentle voluntary cough on completion of the swallow. This procedure may assist in protecting the airway.

Surgical Alternatives

At times it is appropriate to consider surgical intervention either to improve the chances of the patient swallowing and protecting the airway, or to provide an alternative route by which the patient can receive food and water. If radiography demonstrates that the cricopharyngeus has failed to relax, the patient may be a candidate for a myotomy of this sphincter. If the problem is unilateral vocal cord paralysis and associated ineffectiveness of cough, the patient may be considered for Teflon injection of the paralyzed cord to improve glottic closure and thereby enhance the strength of the cough. Following these procedures, the patient may be able to continue successfully with oral intake (Shin et al. 1990).

It is important to remember that many patients with brain stem pathology such as those with end-stage demyelinating diseases will not improve or show increased strength in the swallowing musculature. As a consequence, their nutritional intake will not be through the oral route and a surgical alternative must be considered. In most cases we favor the feeding esophagostomy (English et al. 1970) over the gastrostomy because the patient can sit in an upright position while eating, which aids in proper digestion; the tube can be removed between feedings, which is to the patient's psychologic advantage; skin care is minimal; and the procedure is easily reversible should the patient's neurologic status improve. Percutaneous endoscopic placement also should be considered, although patients with bulbar pathology may be at respiratory risk when the esophagoscope is in place.

If a patient is incapable of protecting the airway from aspiration, and recurrent aspiration pneumonia is a problem, considerations for surgery might include laryngeal closure (Montgomery 1975), tracheoesophageal anastomosis (Lindemann 1975), or even laryngectomy (Smith et al. 1965). With each of these procedures voice is sacrificed, but aspiration is eliminated. Alternative forms of communication then become a primary consideration. (See Chapter 13 for a full discussion of surgical issues and procedures.)

TREATMENT OF PSEUDOBULBAR DYSPHAGIA

Of the patients with neurologic disease whom we have examined for dysphagia, the majority have pseudobulbar dysphagia. Typically, this is the result of bilateral upper motoneuron involvement. The patient frequently has had bilateral capsular infarctions, the first of which may cause transitory dysphagia, and successive infarcts cause further dysphagia. This is not unusual when we are reminded of the distinctive bilateral representation of swallow coordination. In the acute stages of single hemispheric stroke, dysphagia also may be present, and its effects are hemisphere specific (Robbins and Levine 1988). Following the acute phase, most patients can expect improvement (Barer 1989). Pseudobulbar dysphagia also can be an effect of diffuse cerebrocortical disease. In older patients there may be no other demonstrable neurologic deficits, but there is usually a pattern of "soft signs" of central nervous system disintegration together with decompensation in meeting daily needs. Cineradiologic swallows in such patients may be similar to those in patients who have specific demonstrable neurologic deficits. The overall pattern shows occasional penetration of swallowed material into the pharyngolaryngeal spaces with varying degrees of aspiration and reflex delay.

In pseudobulbar dysphagia, the musculature for swallowing may be somewhat weak and uncoordinated. This condition is distinguished from dysphagia secondary to involvement of the lower motoneurons in that patients retain a swallowing reflex even though it may be difficult to stimulate or initiate voluntarily (Table 8.1). On physical examination, signs such as positive bilateral extensor movements of the great toe (Babinski's sign) are found and are consistent with involvement of the upper motoneurons. There is considerable disinhibition of oral reflexes as evidenced by active rooting, sucking, and biting reflexes that frequently interfere with feeding. Palatal and gag reflexes may be present and may be hyperative. Speech may be harsh and unintelligible, and language expression and comprehension may be impaired. Because pseudobulbar dysphagia frequently results from bilateral damage to upper motoneurons, patients may lose the cortical controls of swallowing. Loss of learning potential and a reduced ability to make sound judgments may also be found in clinical testing. Disorientation and perceptual deficits may also be present. Part of therapeutic management is directed toward compensating for these deficits (Miller and Groher 1982).

The loss of intellectual control over swallowing may be superimposed upon

Table 8.1 Differences Between Pseudobulbar Dysphagia and Paralytic Dysphagia

Factor	Paralytic Dysphagia	Pseudobulbar Dysphagia
Pathology	Lower motoneuron	Upper motoneuron
Swallow reflex	Absent or very weak	Present, slow, or uncoordinated
Intellect	Intact	May be impaired
Oral strength	Poor	May be normal or uncoordinated
Affect	May be labile	Lability is common
Speech	Flaccid dysarthria	Spastic, hypokinetic, or hyperkinetic dysarthria

uncoordinated performance. Because of the wide variance in the contribution of each of these factors, the clinician must be able to use different combinations of treatment strategies. The challenge is to employ the proper combination of intellectual controls in an effort to give the swallow reflex a maximal chance of triggering.

Loss of these intellectual controls translates behaviorally into: (1) forgetting to chew and swallow, usually secondary to reduced environmental awareness and/or distractability; (2) poor judgment characterized by excessive bite sizes or a rapid eating rate, making it most difficult to swallow an overly large bolus; (3) failure to adequately clear the oral cavity before the next bite (the phenomenon of squirreling or pouching of food contents may be related to sensory loss); (4) failure to understand feeding directions secondary to aphasia; (5) different degrees of parietal and frontal lobe pathology that interfere with the patient's perception of the food tray or result in inability to sequence the motor act for feeding; (6) an attempt to eat and talk simultaneously, risking aspiration; (7) generalized failure to appreciate the importance of eating that often is interpreted as lack of motivation, as depression, or as failure to cooperate; and (8) inability to organize and initiate a volitional swallow (Miller and Groher 1982).

Patients with pseudobulbar dysphagia frequently will have a nasogastric tube already in place when a feeding plan is initiated. As stressed earlier, before beginning the program, it is desirable to have the patient in an optimal state of nutrition and hydration. The decompensating effects of nutritional deficiency and dehydration on bilaterally brain-damaged patients can be marked. Some become so decompensated that once they are fed by nasogastric or intravenous routes their ability to swallow improves dramatically. A team should include a physician and dietitian to monitor progress to give the patient the best chance to succeed when oral feeding trials begin.

The First Feeding Trial

As soon as the patient is medically stable, appropriately alert, and cooperative, the first trial feeding can begin. Ideally, this is attempted with the nasogastric tube out, although there is no evidence that patients are not decompensated by small-bore nasoenteric feeding tubes. It should not be attempted immediately after a nasogastric feeding, as this would take away the advantage of the hunger drive as an important motivator. The presence of a large (greater than 14 French) tube during oral feeding has four negative effects: (1) it is a mechanical interference in a neurologically impaired system; (2) it partially blocks normal nasal airflow, which makes it more difficult to swallow; (3) its presence in the nasal cavity often forces the patient to mouth-breathe, which dries the oral mucosa and interferes with swallowing; and (4) it can cause food to adhere to it and fall off at an unexpected time, and perhaps be aspirated.

Some patients with pseudobulbar dysfunction may swallow well enough to protect the airway, but fail to maintain an adequate nutritional state. Fatigue, distractions, and dietary factors may contribute to inadequate intake. Intermittent use of the nasogastric tube in the evening can supplement intake. Clinicians should watch for evidence of irritation of the nasal mucosa that can occur with frequent passage of a feeding tube.

Selection of Foods

As with dysphagia paralytica, the principle of maximal stimulation to trigger the reflex should be applied to patients with pseudobulbar dysphagia. "Easy to chew does not mean easy to swallow" (Larsen 1976). We recommend using foods that maximally stimulate sensory receptors and are of such consistency that they can be swallowed as a single bolus.

Patients with pseudobulbar dysphagia typically report that liquids are more difficult to swallow than solids. A problem with controlling liquids is a most believable complaint for the patient whose swallowing mechanism lacks the proper timing and reflex elicitation due to neurologic impairment. Liquids that unpredictably spill into the pharynx make them particularly bothersome. Fruit juices are somewhat better because they are flavorful. We have had greater success with liquids if they are first frozen into slush form. The slush consistency provides temperature and texture and helps to form a more predictable and therefore more manageable bolus. Another medium for facilitating intake of liquids is gelatin desserts, particularly when they are prepared with less water than usual (finger Jello), or blenderized to the consistency of whipped cream. Food in these forms does not melt rapidly and is moderately manageable in the mouth and pharynx. Additionally, commercially prepared thickeners that can be added to any fluid may be used to control fluids. Some alter fluid texture significantly and may be rejected by the patient. None have been tested for tolerance by the lungs following aspiration.

Most of these patients do best with solid foods that are of soft consistency. If possible, it helps to select foods in this category that the patient enjoys. If this information is unavailable from the patient, a family member or friend usually can provide it. Foods that are the most enjoyable serve as motivators and are easier to swallow because of their appeal. The clinician always should be cognizant of making the first few bites significant, and using favorite foods can be of assistance. Selecting the proper semisolid and thickening fluids in those with pseudobulbar dysphagia significantly reduced the occurrence of aspiration pneumonia in patients with known histories of this complication (Groher 1987).

Food items that have proved to be effective in eliciting swallowing are medium-soft boiled eggs, cottage cheese, and sliced canned peaches (Larsen 1976). Bergman (1982) listed foods that are tolerated best in the early stages of treatment: mildly sweet and salty foods; gelatin; poached, boiled, or scrambled eggs; clear soups; broccoli, beets, carrots, peas, and beans; egg and tuna salad; and gravy. She goes on to list foods that are difficult to eat, including such items as hamburger patties, plums, prunes, mashed potatoes, cola-flavored carbonated beverages, all crackers except biscuits, and onions. We recommend that medications should be given in custard, jelly, or blenderized flavored gelatin rather than in an applesauce mixture because of the latter's tendency to fall apart during swallowing. Sticky foods, dry substances, mucus producers, and boluses that fall apart should be avoided.

The patient may tend to use poor judgment by attempting to wash down a solid bolus with liquids. This practice can lead to aspiration if the bolus has either been inadequately masticated or has become lodged in the valleculae. Even mixing liquids with solids in a single bite can confuse the sensory receptors of brain-damaged patients and result in a choking episode.

Intellectual Controls

Selecting the correct diet must be combined with providing the intellectual controls the patient may lack. Therefore, all beginning feedings will require direct assistance aimed at providing the necessary cortical inputs to get a patient swallowing safely.

The first step in providing these controls is to reduce the number of environmental distractions that tend to draw the patient's attention from eating. The first set of distractions is patient-generated. For instance, discomfort due to an improperly positioned arm can serve as enough distraction to focus attention away from eating. If the patient is in pain, prescribed analgesics should be taken well before the meal so that their comforting effect is felt by mealtime. All prosthetic aids should be working and fitting properly, otherwise they are a constant source of distraction. Patients with heavy mucous secretions should have thorough suctioning before meals. Papain, found in most meat tenderizers or in tablet form at health food stores, can be used on a swab to thin thickened secretions. The oral cavity may need to be cleaned with a fresh swab or toothbrush to stimulate saliva flow and provide needed moisture. In short, the patient should be as comfortable as possible before eating.

The second set of distractions comes from outside sources such as other patients, staff, televisions, and radios. Turning off the television and radio, pulling curtains, and closing doors or facing the patient toward the wall all help the dysphagic individual concentrate on swallowing. The importance of minimizing these distractions in preparation for swallowing should not be overlooked. We have seen patients who complain at initial feedings about discomfort from leg braces, hand splints, condom catheters, or intravenous apparatus. It was impossible to focus their attention on feeding because of these distractions. Clinicians who have made the effort to rehabilitate patients with bilateral brain pathology can attest to the importance of reducing distractions as a prerequisite for learning.

The Feeding Process

After the patient has been properly settled in an upright position, head slightly forward with neck flexed, the feeding process can be initiated (Figure 8.3). (See Chapter 9 for additional detail.) The clinician should avoid long explanations of what is to be expected and accomplished, as these often serve to add confusion to brain-damaged patients, particularly those with language deficits. For the same reason, excessive verbal and gestural cueing by the clinician during feeding should be avoided. In most cases, the patient will know this person is there to assist with feeding and that is sufficient.

The feeding process begins with the patient or feeder loading the utensil with a medium-sized bite (about 15 cc). Bites smaller than this may not create enough pressure to trigger the reflex easily. It often helps to let the patient see and smell the bolus before placing it midway into the oral cavity. This helps to

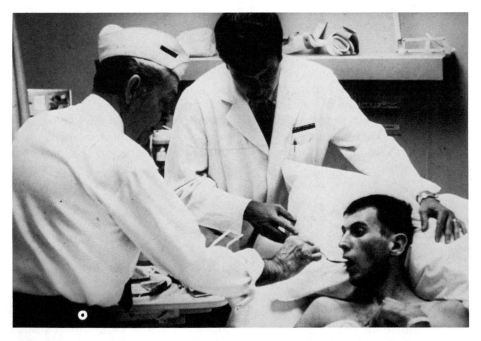

Figure 8.3 Bedridden patient is positioned properly for oral intake with the assistance of a trained volunteer.

prepare the mechanism for swallowing and is not unlike what happens with normal eating. Immediate assessment of what the patient does with the bolus should be made including the elicitation of a swallow reflex (by palpation or auscultation), postswallow residuals and phonatory integrity, and attention to change in the respiratory baseline. Determination of the proper bolus size and amount can be made with dynamic radiography that samples the effect of these variables on the pharyngeal swallow. There is no evidence to suggest, however, that the successful ingestion of one bolus size is predictive of an effective swallow of larger or smaller boluses.

Cognitive cues will have to be provided as necessary. Some patients need verbal or gestural cueing to chew; some need to be told when to swallow; others need to be reminded that food has remained in their mouth and that it must be swallowed before another bite is taken. At this point, it is important to let the patient know when the desired sequence of motor behaviors have been performed (Hargrove 1980). Constant reinforcement of correct behaviors assists the patient in retaining what has been learned.

The clinician should carefully observe each swallow, paying particular attention to the moment of laryngeal elevation. If the patient prematurely tires or loses interest, there must be no attempt to force feed as it will only frustrate both clinician and patient (Hargrove 1980). If the patient progresses satisfactorily, the clinician should begin to eliminate specific cues and observe for evidence of compensations in behavior and improved judgment while eating. Some patients will not make these generalizations, and family members or other attendants must be trained to provide the proper input at each meal.

Patients who demonstrate active biting and rooting reflexes that can interfere with placement of utensils often do well if they are allowed to feed themselves. If motor control does not allow this, we recommend a trial with finger foods in measured bites that can be placed in the mouth without utensils or reflex inhibition techniques as described in Chapter 9.

Many patients need an excessive amount of time to complete a meal. Because of the time factor, foods tend to become cold and unappetizing and therefore less stimulating. Patients in this stage of swallowing management benefit from smaller portions given more frequently, or from early tray scheduling.

MYASTHENIA GRAVIS

Because myasthenia gravis involves the striated musculature, it may compromise swallowing. Its predilection for the bulbar nuclei and accompanying dysphagia are common.

An estimated 33 percent of patients with myasthenia have significant deglutitory disorders due to fatigue following mastication (Murray 1962; Silbiger et al. 1967).

Because of this tendency for the musculature to fatigue easily after repeated exercise, patients typically do well at the beginning of a meal, but tire at the end (Merritt 1967). Mastication and swallowing may be normal and then deteriorate to the point at which there is total loss of the ability to chew and swallow. Continued attempts at feeding past this point can lead to significant aspiration.

Murray (1962) demonstrated by cinefluoroscopy that tongue movements were slow and weak and continued to weaken with additional attempts at swallowing. Holding the bolus on the tongue was particularly troublesome. He studied 23 with disease ranging from mild to severe. Most had barium residual in the oropharynx and valleculae because the tongue failed to arch backward and down into the pharynx. Patients with moderate to severe disease could not clear the valleculae on repeated attempts. There was no evidence of myasthenia affecting the cricopharyngeal sphincter, a finding that Silbiger and colleagues (1967) and Donner and Siegel (1965) supported. Kramer et al. (1957), however, reported on two patients whose cricopharyngeus tired as quickly as their tongue and pharynx. Using cinefluorography, Donner and Siegel (1965) noted the marked fatigability of the tongue and pharyngeal musculature on repeated swallowing attempts. The pharyngeal walls showed prolonged barium coating with pharyngeal recess pooling and loss of tone. Repeated swallowing in some patients produced nasal regurgitation because the pharynx failed to rise adequately to seal the nasopharyngeal port.

The observation that myasthenics have difficulty holding a bolus on the tongue suggests that patients may do better if they are given foods that do not fall apart easily during mastication. Such foods require more lingual effort and hasten fatigue.

Typically, patients with myasthenia are given anticholinesterase-producing drugs that, when administered in the proper doses, greatly facilitate muscle movement. It is important that these medications be coordinated with feeding times so as to facilitate swallowing. If possible, patients should be reminded to limit physical activity before a meal in an effort to maintain sufficient strength to complete it. Such activity can range from strenuous physical therapy to excessive talking. Conservation of energy in the early stages of dysphagia often can be the difference between oral or nasogastric feeding.

AMYOTROPHIC LATERAL SCLEROSIS

Amyotrophic lateral sclerosis (ALS) is a progressive disease of the upper and lower motoneurons of unknown cause and without known treatment. In a significant number of patients, bulbar muscles are involved and the patient experiences serious difficulties with swallowing. In other cases, the deterioration of ALS is confined to muscles supplied by the spinal cord, and dysphagia, if present, is related to the loss of respiratory muscle support.

Clinical findings in the ALS patient with bulbar involvement show a combination of spasticity and flaccidity. In the bulbar muscles specifically, the muscles of mastication (particularly the pterygoids) develop weakness that is experienced as chewing fatigue. The facial muscles (particularly the orbicularis oris) may become weak and drooling is common. The lingual muscles are frequently the first bulbar muscles affected (Hillel and Miller 1989) and may look like a "bag of worms" because of muscle fasciculations (Blount et al. 1979). As atrophy continues, the tongue weakens and may eventually be paralyzed. Palatal and pharyngeal weakness is common. Nasal regurgitation is possible when swallowing, but is not a common finding. The gag reflexes may range from hyperactive in one patient to absent in another. An intact gag can disappear during the course of the disease. The suprahyoid muscles that elevate the larynx may develop weakness and/or cramping, and the cricopharyngeus may fail to open during swallowing. Impairment of vocal fold function is a frequent complication. Vocal cord adduction may be incomplete and the folds may appear bowed as they meet. More commonly, vocal cord abduction is impaired, causing restriction of breathing due to incomplete or even paradoxical movement (Hillel and Miller 1989). Progressive respiratory insufficiency and weakness of abdominal muscles lead to a poor protective cough. Loss of sensation is infrequently reported and most patients retain good cognitive function.

Since the dysphagia of ALS generally is progressive and the symptoms variable, establishing a baseline of function and following the patient throughout the course of the disease is recommended. The baseline data should include a thorough clinical examination for dysphagia (see Chapter 6) and a scaled assessment of bulbar and spinal muscle functions. The ALS Severity Scale is a reliable, easily administered ordinal instrument that can be used to measure speech, swallowing, upper extremity, and lower extremity functions for staging the disease (Hillel et al. 1989). On follow-up examinations the physician should obtain an accurate weight, a current diet and fluid intake record, a pulmonary vital capacity measure, and a functional staging of the disease. Some centers advocate following patients with a series of cineradiographic studies (Bosma and Brodie 1969). However, such studies are costly and not easily tolerated by patients with advanced disease.

Management of dysphagia should begin early in the course of the disease. Initial emphasis is on patient education and the prevention of complications associated with dysphagia and nutritional or fluid deficiencies. Patients will need to be instructed to eat in an upright posture with the neck flexed (DeLisa et al. 1979). Foods that cause problems should be noted so that the consistency of the diet can be controlled. As expected, thin fluids are more easily aspirated than solids. Blenderized foods may act like liquid and fall apart in the mouth and pharynx. Soft, cohesive food boluses such as macaroni casseroles and custard tend to be tolerated well in early stages. As with other dysphagic patients, sticky food and dry, crumbly substances should be minimized in the diet. Optimal calorie and fluid intake requirements should be defined and the patient's progress toward these goals measured.

As the disease progresses, the management of nutrition by oral feeding may become unsafe and inefficient. In our experience, aspiration pneumonitis is not a common complication in ALS until the patient reaches end-stage disease. The progressive nature of the dysphagia and difficulties with self-feeding commonly result in a loss of enjoyment, fear, and even dread of eating. The identification of these feelings is imperative.

It is the dysphagia specialist's role to recommend procedures that may improve swallowing or alternative methods of providing nutrition. The alternative of choice for nutritional management is percutaneous endoscopic gastrostomy (PEG) performed under local anesthesia. This procedure does not interfere with swallowing functions and can be used either to supplement oral feedings or for primary nutritional intake. A nonsurgical feeding tube alternative that can be used when the patient's gag reflex permits is intermittent orogastric placement. A nasogastric tube may be used for patients in end-stage disease when other alternatives are not feasible.

Timing is very important when recommending surgical alternatives to swallowing. While many patients desire to maintain oral intake of food and liquid for as long as possible, those who quit eating and drinking for even short periods of time may become too weak to withstand surgical intervention. Others have severely compromised respiratory systems, predisposing them to surgical complications (Short and Hillel 1989). Even a PEG cannot be safely performed after pulmonary vital capacity falls below 1 L. Therefore, continuous monitoring of patients' ability and desire to eat and their nutrition and hydration status is necessary for optimal management.

Clinicians who offer symptomatic management for patients with progressive motoneuron disease should realize that the clinical course is highly variable and, so far, unpredictable. Although the primary symptoms cannot be arrested or prevented, the support offered by the dysphagia specialist may go far in preventing secondary complications of malnutrition, dehydration, and aspiration, and improving the quality of the patient's remaining life.

HUNTINGTON'S CHOREA

Some of the feeding problems of patients with Huntington's chorea are unique to this disease, while others are typical of patients with pseudobulbar dysphagia. The characteristic choreatic movements of Huntington's disease eventually severely compromise feeding and swallowing. At the time of diagnosis, feeding and swallowing disorders are infrequent. As the disease progresses, however, and the involuntary movements become more frequent and uncontrollable, dysphagia emerges as a significant problem. The constant movements cause a significant number of calories to be burned, and patients frequently have appetites that are difficult to satisfy; their focus on food and eating becomes paramount. Difficulty with oral intake conflicts with their unsatisfied hunger and creates a significant feeding management problem. For some patients, their frustrations are compounded by documented changes in mental status that interfere with the ability to learn compensatory feeding and swallowing strategies. The majority are not cognizant of their swallowing deficits, but with treatment can learn to make necessary compensations (Kagel and Leopold, 1992).

Typically, patients first lose the ability to manipulate utensils for self-feeding and require direct assistance in food transport. Once food and liquids are placed in the mouth they usually are managed without great difficulty. At this stage, some patients prefer to remain independent in feeding and therefore exercise the option of increasing the number of food items that can be consumed without utensils such as sandwiches, fruits, and selected vegetables.

As the choreatic movements intensify, there is marked involvement in the coordination of swallowing. In addition, unpredictable, sudden gulps of air during the inspiratory cycle open the glottis at irregular intervals, compromising protection of the airway. The head may suddenly be thrust back, exposing the airway. Because of the characteristic writhing tongue, lateralization and posterior transportation of food toward the pharynx are difficult. Forming the posterior bolus needed to trigger a swallowing reflex becomes an obstacle in completing a normal swallow (Kilman 1977). Foods and liquids reach the oropharynx with unpredictable speed. We can postulate that such irregular control may create abnormal timing sequences that invite laryngeal penetration and aspiration. Kagel and Leopold (1992) gathered diagnostic and treatment data on the behavioral and swallowing characteristics of 35 patients with Huntington's disease of a mean duration of 6.6 years. All but one had moderately advanced disease with dysphagia. Following videoradiographic and clinical evaluation, the patients fell into two categories: those with primary hyperkinetic features (30), and those with rigid and bradykinetic symptoms. Those with hyperkinetic features were not as liable to pharyngeal decompensation with aspiration as those with bradykinesia and rigidity. Interruption of normal esophageal peristalsis coincident with respiratory chorea resulting in distal-to-proximal bolus redirection was a finding in 14 patients with a hyperkinetic component and in none of those with bradykinesia.

Initial treatment for both groups (Kagel and Leopold 1992) focused on proper trunk and leg support, with below-the-waist food presentation to maintain neck flexion. The hyperkinetic group was trained in incentive spirometry to control respiratory patterns prior to attempts at oral feeding. Oral chorea was managed with precedent iced-lemon stimuli followed by a textured bolus with iced-lemon impregnation. For this group crisp substances in textured foods enhanced mastication. For those with bradykinetic features, swallow was enhanced by lateral and dorsal tongue tapping, with training in a negative suck transfer focusing on labial closure. Iced-lemon stimuli were effective in clearing pharyngeal residue after each swallow. With a median reevaluation period of 5 years, patients in both groups continued to eat by mouth. Some needed periodic treatment sessions to reinforce compensatory strategies.

Over a 5-year period, Groher had the opportunity to follow six patients with advanced Huntington's disease and swallowing complaints. All patients were hospitalized, nonambulatory, and could not meet most of their daily needs, including self-feeding. Four of the six had accompanying changes in mental status such as poor judgment, uncontrollable outbursts of temper, and disorientation. Their mean age was 47.6 years. All patients had had the disease for 12 years or more.

The patients were evaluated for their dysphagic complaints. At the time of the evaluation, all were receiving their nutrition orally; however, fluoroscopic evidence of increased laryngeal penetration suggested they should receive a complete dysphagia work-up. None had demonstrable aspiration pneumonia, although the nurses reported considerable choking, sputtering, and prolonged coughing at mealtimes. All six were eating pureed foods and not one was satisfied with this diet. The swallowing evaluation consistently revealed the following: (1) the nursing assistant who was feeding the patient had great difficulty placing the food in the patient's mouth due to marked choreatic movements of the head and trunk; (2) once the food was placed, the tongue often pushed the bolus anteriorly out of the mouth; (3) oral mastication was labored and the time between oral placement and a swallow reflex was not consistent, frequently being either too fast or delayed; (4) laryngeal elevation during swallowing was normal; (5) solids were managed better than liquids; (6) all had protective coughs; (7) all swallowed a soft mechanical diet without difficulty; and (8) all swallowed more efficiently when the environment was free of distraction (measured by less coughing and shorter total mealtime).

The evaluation revealed that the most crucial phase of swallowing management in patients with Huntington's disease took place in the preparatory stages of swallowing. For instance, two of six patients could not maintain a proper position for effective swallowing. This was managed as well as possible by providing head and trunk restraints during meals. Such restraints, of course, did not reduce the choreatic movements, but did help patients to maintain upright posture. Spoon feeding was accomplished best when the feeder did not try to introduce the spoon at his or her will, but rather held the spoon in front of the patients waiting for them to take the food from it. Allowing the patient to take the food voluntarily resulted in fewer incidents of the tongue pushing the bolus out of the oral cavity. Finally, all patients were more motivated to eat because they received a diet that was more pleasing to their senses and equally as easy to swallow.

PARKINSON'S DISEASE

Another variant of pseudobulbar symptomatology is seen in patients with Parkinson's disease. The clinical features of tremor and rigidity may precipitate swallowing dysfunction. Like those with Huntington's chorea, patients with Parkinson's disease become progressively handicapped and are frequently not aware of their swallowing disability (Robbins et al. 1986; Bushmann et al. 1989). When rigidity is the prominent feature, dysphagia becomes a significant management problem (Lieberman et al. 1980).

Lieberman and associates (1980) contended that some degree of dysphagia may be present in 50 percent of cases, but is rarely so severe as to require gastrostomy. Eadie and Tyrer (1965) reported a similar figure, and our clinical experience suggests that most patients are able to take nutrition orally, even in the end stages of disease. Eadie and Tyrer (1965) found no correlation between severity of disease and dysphagia. In 25 percent of these patients dysphagic complaints began within 2 years of diagnosis. Their findings are supported by Lieberman and his colleagues (1980) who studied two cases with end-stage disease; one had adequate voice and tongue mobility but aspirated, and one had poor voice and tongue movement but did not aspirate. After studying six patients radiographically with varying stages of disease, Robbins and colleagues (1985) did not find correlative evidence between swallowing disability and disease stage, although the most severe did have the largest number of videoradiographic abnormalities.

The results of cineradiography are conflicting. Silbiger and associates (1967) found swallowing abnormalities in all 11 patients studied. Abnormalities were described as poor bolus formation, misdirected swallow, abnormal pharyngeal motility, pharyngeal stasis, and abnormal cricopharyngeal function. Eadie and Tyrer (1965a) questioned 107 patients and postulated that dysphagia existed secondary to faulty control of the pharyngeal constrictors. Palmer (1974) reported that the dysphagia associated with Parkinson's disease usually was due to hypopharyngeal dysfunction, and recommended relief with posterior cricopharyngeal sphincterotomy. Calne and associates (1970) studied 20 patients and found no pharyngeal pathology. They attributed the differences between their studies and Silbiger's to the fact that the latter studied patients in the prone position rather than sitting upright. Calne et al. (1970) concluded that parkinsonism dysphagia was more related to oral and/or esophageal disorders, as they had noted lingual hesitancy and piecemeal deglutition in the oral stages. They presented fluoroscopic evidence of excessive mastication time, limited tongue and mandibular excursion, and poor posterior bolus formation. Once a swallow reflex was triggered, the larynx rose normally. Robbins et al. (1986) described both oral (most prominent) and pharyngeal stage abnormalities, but did not find isolated impairment in the pharyngoesophageal segment. Of particular importance in their study was the prevalence of aspiration without cough in patients who had no dysphagic complaints, a finding supported by the work of Bushmann et al. (1989). Logemann et al. (1977) presented cineradiographic evidence showing that regardless of the stage of disease, patients have slowed oral and esophageal transit times.

Other investigators have noted the presence of esophageal symptoms in patients with Parkinson's disease. Eadie and Tyrer (1965b) compared a group of 72 patients with parkinsonism with matched controls, finding a higher incidence of esophageal abnormalities in those with parkinsonism including esophageal spasm, hiatal hernia, and gastroesophageal reflux. They speculated that some disorders of esophageal motility may be secondary to involvement of the dorsal vagal nucleus.

We can conclude from these investigations that swallowing disorders in parkinsonism may be present in varying degrees and combinations in the mouth, pharynx, and esophagus, and that the severity of the movement disorder probably does not correlate with the severity of the dysphagia.

Because of the excessive time taken for oral mastication, it is more advantageous for patients to eat smaller portions more frequently, especially if feeding times are restricted. Changing the portions and increasing the length of mealtimes have two distinct psychologic advantages. First, patients feel they do not need to finish a large portion in a short time and therefore enjoy their meals more. Second, they are aware they will not be left hungry if they do not finish one large meal in a fixed time segment. These facilitators are important motivators for swallowing.

In our experience, patients with Parkinson's disease generally do well with regular diets. In the end stages of disease, they find it easier to eat soft foods that require less effort to masticate. Teaching a more posterior spoon placement often is helpful in reducing oral transit times, but patients must avoid bypassing sensory receptors that help trigger the swallow reflex.

The timing of dopaminergic medications should coincide with mealtimes so that their effect can facilitate oral and pharyngeal movements. Such an effect will vary from patient to patient depending on drug dosage and individual metabolic rates. Lieberman and associates (1980) pointed out that it is important to have patients swallow their medications because parenteral anticholinergics are not as effective as levodopa taken orally. However, ingestion of solid forms of medication may be problematic, with retention of pills in the valleculae leading to irregular absorption and subsequent lack of a clinical response (Bushmann et al. 1989). Esophageal dismotility may compromise absorption further. In our experience, discontinuance of medications to manage parkinsonism in order to evaluate a clinical response to new drugs or dosage levels may put the patient at risk for aspiration. As the drug is withdrawn, patients should be monitored closely for signs of aspiration and/or changes in the physical and mental status examination that might predispose to increased inability to protect the airway. The usefulness of levodopa in alleviating dysphagic symptoms remains controversial, however. Some patients have benefited, while others have not (Cotzias et al. 1969; Calne et al. 1970; Lieberman et al. 1980). Bushmann et al. (1989) found general improvement in swallow for those patients on oral levadopa and carbidopa, but no improvement in swallow after increasing the dosage.

SUMMARY

This chapter contains some general treatment guidelines for patients who suffer from dysphagia secondary to neurologic impairments. Specific treatment and pretreatment considerations for this group are covered in the following chapter.

The clinician must remain cognizant of the fact that signs and symptoms of neurologic pathology may change over time. In addition, well described disease entities and processes affect patients in differing ways. Therefore, we should not lose sight of the fact that dysphagia management with this group of patients is predicated on individualized plans.

REFERENCES

Bergman K. Dysphagia in the adult patient. Conference on rehabilitation of dysphagia in adults. Detroit, Michigan, July 29 and 30, 1982.

Blount M, Bratton C, Luttrell N. Management of the patient with amyotrophic lateral sclerosis. Nurs Clin North Am 1979; 14:157–71.

Bonanno PC. Swallowing dysfunction after tracheostomy. Ann Surg 1971; 174:29–33.

Bosma JF, Brodie DR. Disabilities of the pharynx in ALS as demonstrated by cineradiography. Radiology 1969; 92:97–103.

Bushmann M, Dobymeyer SM, Leeker L, et al. Swallowing abnormalities and their response to treatment in parkinson's disease. Neurology 1989; 39:1309–14.

Calne DB, Shaw DG, Spiers ASD, Stern GM. Swallowing in parkinsonism. Br J Radiol 1970; 43:456–7.

Campbell-Taylor I, Nadon GW, Schlacter AL, et al. Oro-esophageal tube feeding: an alternative to nasogastric or gastrostomy tubes. Dysphagia 1988; 4:220–2.

Cotzias GC, Papavalilion PS, Gellene R. Modification of parkinsonism—chronic treatment with L-dopa. N Engl J Med 1969; 280:337–45.

Curran J, Groher ME. Development and dissemination of an aspiration risk reduction diet. Dysphagia 1990; 5:6–12.

DeLisa JA, Mikulic MA, Miller RM, Melnick RR. Amyotrophic lateral sclerosis: comprehensive management. Am Fam Physician 1979; 19:137–42.

Donner MW, Siegel CI. The evaluation of pharyngeal neuromuscular disorders by cinefluorography. Am J Roentgenol 1965; 94:299–307.

Eadie MJ, Tyrer JH. Radiological abnormalities in the upper part of the alimentary tract in parkinsonism. Aust Ann Med 1965; 14:23–7.

Eadie MJ, Tyrer JH. Alimentary disorders in parkinsonism. Aust Ann Med 1965; 14:13–22.

English GM, Morfit HM, Ratzer ER. Cervical esophagostomy in head and neck cancer. Arch Otolaryngol 1970; 92:335–9.

Groher ME. Bolus management and aspiration pneumonia in patients with pseudobulbar dysphagia. Dysphagia 1987; 1:215–6.

Hargrove R. Feeding the severely involved patient. J Neurosurg Nurs 1980; 12:102–7.

Hillel AD, Miller RM. Bulbar amyotrophic lateral sclerosis: patterns of progression and clinical management. Head and Neck 1989; 11:51–9.

Hillel AD, Miller RM, Yorkston K, et al. Amytrophic lateral sclerosis severity scale. Neuroepidemiology 1989; 8:142–50.

Kagel MC, Leopold NA. Dysphagia in Huntington's disease: a 16 year retrospective. Dysphagia 1992; 7:106–14.

Kilman WJ. Diseases of the pharynx and larynx. Curr Probl Diagn Radiol 1977; 7:1–43.

Kramer P, Atkinson M, Wyman SM, Ingelfinger FJ. The dynamics of swallowing. II. Neuromuscular dysphagia of the pharynx. J Clin Invest 1957; 36:589–95.

Larsen GL. Rehabilitating dysphagia: mechanica, paralytica, pseudobulbar. J Neurosurg Nurs 1976; 8:14–17.

Lazzara GD, Lazarus C, Logemann JA. Impact of thermal stimulation on the triggering of the swallowing reflex. Dysphagia 1986; 1:73–7.

Lebo CP, Sang UK, Norris FH. Cricopharyngeal myotomy in amyotrophic lateral sclerosis. Laryngoscope 1976; 86:862–8.

Lieberman AM, Horowitz L, Redmond P, Pachter L, Lieberman I, Leibowitz M. Dysphagia in Parkinson's disease. Am J Gastroenterol 1980; 74:157–60.

Lindeman RC. Diverting the paralyzed larynx: a reversible procedure for intractable aspiration. Laryngoscope 1975; 85:157–80.

Logemann JA, Boshes B, Blonsky RE, Fisher HE. Speech and swallowing evaluation in the differential diagnosis of neurologic disease. Neurologica-Neurocirugia-Psiquiatria 1977; 18:71–8.

Logeman JA, Bytell DE. Swallowing disorders in three types of head and neck surgical patients. Cancer 1979; 44:1095–1105.

Merritt HH. A textbook of neurology. Philadelpha: Lea & Febiger, 1967.

Miller RM, Groher ME. The evaluation and management of neuromuscular and mechanical swallowing disorders. Dysarthria, Dysphonia, Dysphagia 1982; 1:50–70.

Montgomery WW. Surgery to prevent aspiration. Arch Otolaryngol 1975; 101:679–82.

Murray JP. Deglutition in myasthenia gravis. Br J Radiol 1962; 35:43–52.

Palmer ED. Dysphagia in parkinsonism. JAMA 1974; 229:1349.

Robbins J, Levine RL. Swallowing after unilateral stroke of the cerebral cortex: preliminary experience. Dysphagia 1988; 3:11–17.

Robbins JA, Logeman J, Kirshner A. Swallowing and speech in Parkinson's disease. Ann Neurol 1986; 19:283–7.

Rosenbek JC, Robbins J, Fishback B, Levine RL. Effect of thermal application on dysphagia after stroke. J Speech Hear Res 1991; 34:1257–68.

Shin T, Tadatsugu M, Umezaki T, et al. Surgical rehabilitation for dysphagia caused by neuromuscular disorders. In: Inouye T, Fukuda H, Sato T, Hinohara T, eds. Recent advances in bronchoesophagology. Amsterdam: Excerpta Medica, 1990.

Short SO, Hillel AD. Palliative surgery in patients with bulbar amyotrophic lateral sclerosis. Head and Neck 1989; 11:364–9.

Silbiger ML, Pikielney R, Donner MW. Neuromuscular disorders affecting the pharynx: cineradiographic analysis. Invest Radiol 1967; 2:442–8.

Smith AC, Spanling JM, Ardran G, Livingstone G. Laryngectomy in the management of severe dysphagia in nonmalignant conditions. Lancet 1965; 2:1094–6.

9

Management of Neurologic Disorders: The First Feeding Session

Wendy Avery-Smith

Evaluation of a patient with neurogenic dysphagia reveals whether the patient is alert enough for a feeding trial, the areas of oral and pharyngeal impairment that may interfere with swallowing, and the risk factors that may be associated with aspiration. Although a preliminary estimation of swallowing prognosis can be made based on clinical evaluation and radiographic studies, only implementation of a course of treatment will determine the patient's ultimate potential for safe eating. The goal for the patient with potential for dysphagia rehabilitation may range from independent consumption of a full oral diet to limited oral feeding with compensatory techniques and nonoral supplements. Prefeeding therapy also may reveal whether a patient requires a permanent nonoral feeding route.

Due to the changes in status that accompany many neurologic disorders, reevaluation is an inherent part of the initial and all subsequent feeding sessions. Patients with neurogenic dysphagia may have a safe but compensated swallow; decompensation caused by the natural course of disease may lead to an unsafe swallow (Buchholz et al. 1985). The clinician must keep in mind that changes in the care plan are an important and integral part of treatment.

This chapter presents a program for prefeeding management, the initial feeding trial, and swallowing training. Because dysphagia in the neurologically impaired population is often accompanied by cognitive, perceptual, physical, and functional problems that influence swallowing, interventions for these deficits are discussed as well.

PREFEEDING MANAGEMENT
Cognitive and Perceptual Status

Alertness and cooperation on the part of the patient are prerequisites for a safe feeding trial because lethargy and unwillingness to eat may increase the risk of aspiration. For patients who are sleepy but easily roused, stimulation techniques may be used to improve the patient's level of arousal. Loud verbal and gentle physical stimulation, such as rubbing the patient's arm, may suffice. Occupational or physical therapy may have a beneficial effect on arousal level,

219

postural control, and swallowing skills; it may be therapeutic to schedule feeding sessions after other rehabilitative procedures. The room should be well lit and the patient positioned properly, as these factors have a stimulating effect on the central nervous system.

Some patients may need a more vigorous program of multisensory stimulation to improve alertness. This includes rhythmic music, variation in the therapist's tone of voice, and a cheerful environment. Stimulation must be planned and orderly and sensory stimuli applied in a regular manner. A noisy environment with many interruptions can be overstimulating and have a disorganizing effect on the patient's performance (Ayres 1973; Trombly 1989). Feeding sessions for patients who need intensive stimulation in order to attend for even brief periods should be deferred until the patient demonstrates a sufficient level of arousal.

Various strategies will be helpful in working with the cognitively impaired or aphasic patient. Because eating is such a familiar and overlearned behavior, minimal orientation to the activity may be necessary. Even a very confused and distracted patient may demonstrate the attention span to eat, especially if he or she is hungry. Mere presentation of a serving of food will provide a strong cue as to the activity at hand. Providing foods that are normally eaten at the time of day they are presented, such as oatmeal at breakfast, will have an orienting effect on the patient. A quiet room with a minimum of distractions will help to direct the patient's attention to the food. Self-feeding will help to direct attention as well. For patients with unilateral inattention, a colorful "anchor," such as a piece of red construction paper, will help to draw the attention to the neglected side of the meal tray. Feeding sessions should not occur when a patient is fatigued, such as after test procedures. If a patient's overall endurance is reduced, time spent out of bed should be during mealtime. Because continuous drip and bolus tube feedings may suppress appetite and thus reduce motivation to eat, arrangements should be made to halt or delay these for several hours prior to the feeding session.

Sensory Impairment

When oral or facial sensation is impaired, the patient or care giver must be educated as to the type and extent of impairment. Safety techniques for alterations in sensation may be done by the patient who is intellectually capable of remembering and carrying out techniques or by the care giver. Such precautions must be emphasized to prevent injury from hot foods, biting, or other injury. Abnormal sensation may result from sensory loss or from heightened sensation.

In patients with severe hyposensitivity, food should be placed initially in the most sensitive area of the mouth for protection, as well as to receive maximal sensory stimulation. Taste, temperature, texture, shape, weight, and size define the sensory qualities of a bolus (Coster and Schwarz 1987). These characteristics stimulate swallowing, and the therapist may wish to experiment with these components to find the best bolus type for the patient. If there is food retention in sensory impaired areas, the use of verbal cues, a mirror, and frequent observation of the oral cavity will be helpful. As the patient progresses, food should be placed at midline so that sensory retraining and normal oral patterns are encouraged. As they improve, compensatory techniques may be gradually withdrawn.

Hyersensitivity to touch may be noted in brain-injured patients. This may be observed in aversive reactions such as grimacing or backing away from sensory stimuli. To treat this Farber (1982) recommends applying continuous pressure with a finger to the perioral area across the maxilla between the nose and the upper lip. Once this is tolerated, pressure to the lips and the dorsum of the anterior third of the tongue may be maintained with a tongue blade and lip mold (Figure 9.1). This device is fabricated by molding lip-shaped thermoplastic splinting material around a padded tongue blade. The patient may then progress to a graded program of application of sensory stimuli. Firm touch with a hard object is more easily tolerated, so the program starts with harder objects, such as eating utensils, and then progresses to softer objects, such as toothbrushes and moistened swabs. Touch is gradually reduced in pressure. The patient may be better able to tolerate self-application of stimuli (O'Sullivan 1990).

Oral Hygiene

Extra care must be taken in providing oral hygiene to dysphagic patients. Because of diminished sensation, the patient may not feel residual food particles in the oral cavity. Mouth breathing may cause additional drying of oral structures, secretions, and residual food. Dried food and secretions further inhibit sensation and promote growth of bacteria. Oral care should be done after each feeding session and may need to be done before feeding. Lemon glycerine swabs or a swab dipped in diluted mouth wash may be used to clean around the teeth and gums. Secretions that are thick or hardened in the oral cavity should be moistened and removed with a damp washcloth. If the patient has the oral control and airway protection to do so, he or she should brush the teeth and rinse the mouth, with assistance and supervision as needed.

Dentures and partial plates should be worn. If muscle tone has been affected by neurologic illness, oral prostheses may be loose or fall out. It may be difficult for the patient to insert dentures due to reduced intraoral pressure. This can be remediated by use of a dental adhesive. The wearing of oral prostheses will lend contour to the mouth and support oral structures, permitting more normal movement. If dentures or partial plates cause pain or lacerations, they should be removed and their fit checked by a dentist.

Muscle Tone

Patients with upper motoneuron disease may demonstrate abnormalities in muscle tone proximally in the body, and distally in the head, neck, and extremities. Both proximal and distal tone abnormalities may interfere with the move-

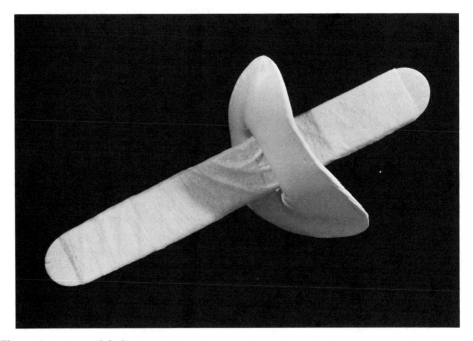

Figure 9.1 A modified tongue depressor can be used to apply pressure to the tongue dorsum to inhibit hypersensitivity.

ments needed for eating and swallowing. Muscle tone may be increased or spastic, or decreased or flaccid. A combination of spasticity and flaccidity is often seen, and compensatory or substitution movements are observed as the patient tries to move. Pathologic reflexes also may be seen. Mood, stress, discomfort, and effortful activities all influence muscle tone. Various techniques are useful in eliciting normal tone and movement. The treatment techniques outlined here are used with both acutely and chronically impaired neurologic patients. The treatment program for acute patients changes frequently as the patient progresses; while chronic patients may progress, but at a slower rate (Helfrich-Miller et al. 1986). Therefore, they may benefit from an established, ongoing program. These techniques should be applied by a trained occupational, physical, or speech therapist because of their complexity as well as their consequences to overall movement. Many techniques such as stretching, when applied in different ways, have an opposite effect.

Treatment techniques that reduce spasticity are termed "inhibitory"; techniques that increase muscle tone or movement are "facilitory." Sustained pressure, slow stretch, slow rocking, and prolonged icing are inhibitory; quick touch, quick pressure, quick stretch, and quick icing are facilitory (Stockmeyer 1967; Farber 1982; Voss et al. 1985). Treatment should begin proximally as in the trunk because establishing improved proximal control facilitates improved distal control (Stockmeyer 1967; Davies 1985; Voss et al. 1985; Bobath 1990). Facilitation of a neutral neck position (Figure 9.2) and the ability to flex the neck and tuck the chin are important to emphasize, because these movements are critical for airway protection and as a compensatory swallowing technique. Once improved trunk posture and movement have been achieved, the patient is then positioned and ready to work on self-feeding and oral-pharyngeal skills.

A variety of inhibition and facilitation techniques may be used to improve oral and pharyngeal movement (Silverman and Elfant 1979; Farber 1982; Davies 1982; Langley 1987; O'Sullivan 1990). Excessive spasticity in the cheek can be relieved by stretching it slowly from inside with the back of a spoon or a gloved finger. Vibration is facilitatory; an electric toothbrush can be used to activate tone in the cheeks and stimulate lip closure (Davies 1985). A quick touch with ice to the lips stimulates lip movement (Stockmeyer 1967). Gustatory stimuli can be used to stimulate movement as well; bitter tastes stimulate tongue protrusion, while sweet tastes stimulate tongue retraction and sucking (Stockmeyer 1967). Flavored water may be applied on the tongue with a cotton swab or an eye-dropper if the patient is not yet able to manage a bolus.

For patients whose movement is slow, poorly coordinated, or ataxic, treat-

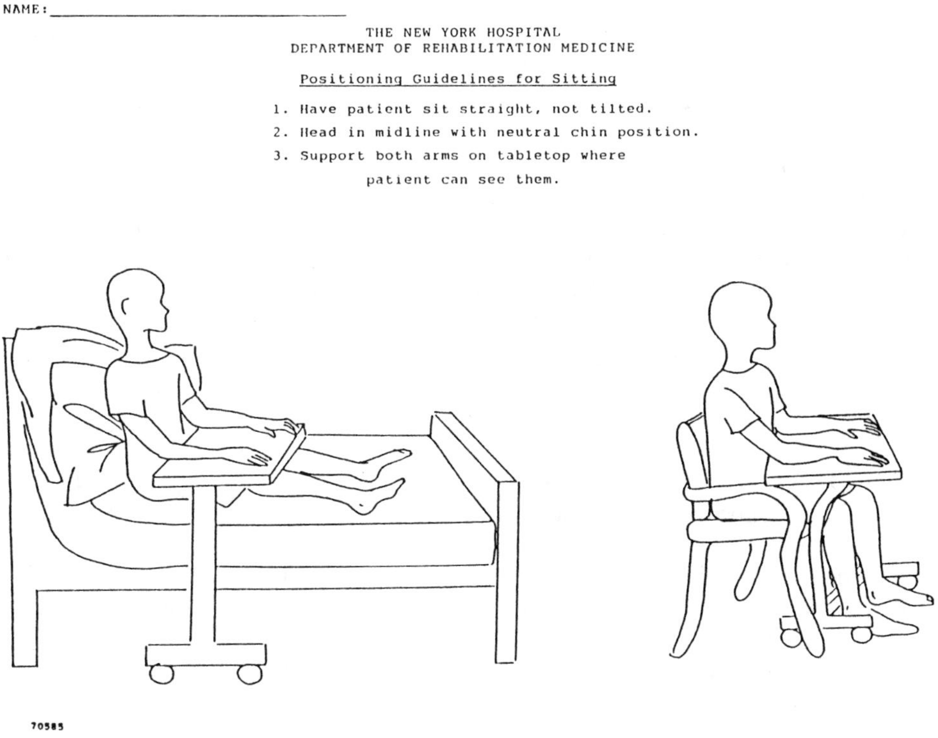

NAME: _____

THE NEW YORK HOSPITAL
DEPARTMENT OF REHABILITATION MEDICINE

Positioning Guidelines for Sitting

1. Have patient sit straight, not tilted.
2. Head in midline with neutral chin position.
3. Support both arms on tabletop where
   patient can see them.

70585

Figure 9.2 Proper sitting position. (Reprinted by permission of the Department of Rehabilitation Medicine, The New York Hospital-Cornell Medical Center.)

ment focuses on developing coordination between opposing muscle groups and on developing speed. This is done through direct exercises that focus on speed and timing or using games such as blowing bubbles or blow darts. Lip, tongue, cheek, and jaw movements may be retrained using "retrievable boluses" such as lifesavers on a string, or food wrapped in gauze.

Oral and Pharyngeal Reflexes

Reflexes may be categorized as abnormal, such as bite and rooting, or normal, such as cough and gag. Treatment focuses on inhibiting abnormal reflexes and facilitating normal ones. Proper positioning is critical in both reducing abnormal reflexes and in promoting normal movement. While not a true reflex, the sensory and motor events that promote swallowing may be used therapeutically to elicit a swallow reflex.

Abnormal Reflexes

Abnormal reflexes include the bite reflex, rooting, mouth opening, tongue thrust, sucking, and hyperactive gag. A distinction is made between those reflexes that are abnormal at any age, such as the bite reflex, and those that are seen early in development, such as rooting. Developmental reflexes may not interfere with swallowing as much as pathologic reflexes. Diminution of all abnormal reflexes may be a goal in feeding training.

Abnormal reflexes may be indirectly inhibited by avoiding the stimuli that elicit them (Silverman and Elfant 1979). Not touching the teeth, gums, or cheeks will minimize occurrence of the bite reflex. If the bite reflex is elicited, the therapist should wait until it relaxes and not force the jaws open, as this will further elicit the reflex. Applying direct pressure at the temporomandibular joint may inhibit this reflex. Avoiding tactile stimulation of the lips and cheeks will prevent accidental triggering of the rooting reflex. The mouth opening reflex is elicited by the visual stimulus of food on a utensil coming toward the mouth and may be used to overcome a tonic bite reflex. Asking the patient to open the mouth before visual presentation of food may help to control this reflex at the cortical level. These reflexes will often diminish as neurologic recovery occurs.

Tongue thrust is reduced by facilitating tongue retraction (Silverman and Elfant 1979; Farber 1982). Fixation of the tip of the tongue on the hard palate behind the upper teeth is associated with neck flexion (Stockmeyer 1967). Thus, neck flexion may be useful in conjunction with other maneuvers to stimulate retraction. Retraction may be facilitated by applying manual vibration on either side of the frenulum under the tongue to the muscles of tongue retraction, or by quick stretch to the tongue in the direction opposite the desired movement (Farber 1982). Sucking activities reduce tongue thrust by promoting stabilization of the tongue in a retracted position, an important skill that permits movement of the posterior portion of the tongue during swallowing.

Sucking is considered a primitive reflex if the patient is unable to control it, or it may be dependent on the presence of a stimulus on the tongue and/or lips, such as a straw or lollipop. Reflexive sucking may be observed as part of a suck-swallow sequence. The sucking reflex may be used to elicit a reflexive swallow when a volitional swallow is absent. Both reflexive (Farber 1982) and volitional sucking (Ramsey 1986) have been used therapeutically to elicit a swallow for nutritional purposes. Farber (1982) recommends a simple device to promote swallowing that can be constructed from a plastic squeeze bottle, fish tank tubing, and thermoplastic material (Figure 9.3). The mouthpiece and tube extending into the mouth provide pressure over the tongue and lips, which stimulates the reflex. The fish tank tubing must be bonded to the mouthpiece with a heat gun, and optimally the mouthpiece is molded on the individual patient, with a "shelf" in between the lips.

An abnormal hyperactive gag reflex may be seen in the brain-injured adult. To inhibit the gag reflex, pressure is applied on the dorsum of the tongue using a padded tongue depressor, maintaining pressure for several seconds and then gradually moving back (Stockmeyer 1967; Farber 1982).

Normal Reflexes

Normal reflexes include the gag, palatal, and cough reflexes. Silverman and Elfant (1979) advocate stroking the posterior tongue, uvula, and anterior and posterior faucial arches to elicit a depressed or absent gag reflex. The palatal reflex may be stimulated by stroking the soft palate with a cotton swab followed by attempts to phonate (Sullivan et al. 1982; Davies 1985). Activities that encourage palatal movement through nasopharyngeal closure, such as sucking through a straw, also may be done provided a Valsalva maneuver is not contraindicated. Both volitional and reflexive cough are important for airway protection during swallowing. Volitional cough may be strengthened by performing deep breathing exercises and vocal cord adduction, followed by active attempts at coughing, and by applying manual pressure to the abdominal musculature while trying to cough (Kisner and Colby 1985). A "tracheal tickle," which is done by pressing posteriorly toward the trachea at the sternal notch with a circular movement, will help to stimulate a reflexive cough (Frownfelter 1978; Kisner and Colby 1985).

The swallowing reflex can be facilitated if the dry swallow is observed to be weak or absent. Swallowing is facilitated by stroking the anterior faucial arches with a cold stimulus, such as an iced laryngeal mirror, followed by active attempts at swallowing (Logemann 1983; Helfrich-Miller et al. 1986; Lazzara et al. 1986). Silverman and Elfant (1979) describe the use of other maneuvers, including icing the sternal notch for several seconds during attempts to swallow, upward stroking under the chin, and manual vibration under the chin and lateral to the larynx. Stockmeyer (1967) notes that contraction of the orbicularis oris provides a facilitory quick stretch to the buccinator, which in turn provides stretch to the pharyngeal constrictors. Activities aimed at improving oral skills will also improve swallowing. As consecutive dry swallows are difficult to achieve, these techniques may be more successful using a retrievable bolus such as a lollipop, ice slush, or a few drops of fruit juice. Because of the many sensory

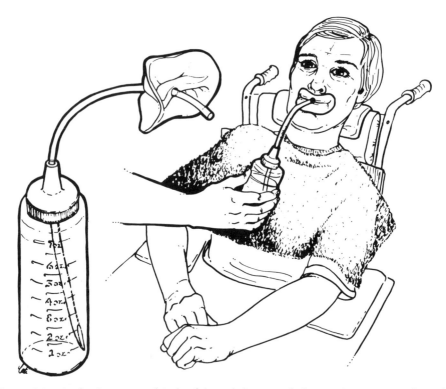

Figure 9.3 A plastic squeeze bottle, fish tank hose, and thermoplastic material can be used to promote swallowing behavior. (Reprinted by permission of the publisher, from Farber SD. Neurorehabilitation: a multisensory approach. Philadelphia: WB Saunders, 1982.)

and motor stimuli that facilitate swallowing, each patient should be evaluated individually to determine the success of the maneuvers attempted.

Weakness

Patients with weakness caused by lower motoneuron involvement require a treatment program that focuses on strengthening weakened structures. Strengthening activities may be contraindicated in some diagnoses, such as amyotrophic lateral sclerosis, in which exercise produces further weakness. A complete muscle test assists the clinician in developing an exercise program for specific muscles or muscle groups. Compensatory movements are often seen, as stronger muscles attempt to take over for weakened muscles. Prefeeding treatment may involve reducing the activity of these muscles before proceeding with exercises and strengthening activities. The facilatory techniques described in the section on muscle tone are useful with those with lower motoneuron impairment (Sullivan et al. 1982). Movement in weakened cheek and lip musculature due to a peripheral facial nerve palsy may be facilitated with quick icing and quick stretch, followed by active smiling and sucking exercises. Once active movement is possible, resistive exercise such as sucking or blowing on a pinched straw should begin. In order to improve strength, the appropriate amount of resistance must be supplied (Farber 1982). It is important not to overfatigue weak muscles, especially prior to a meal.

FEEDING TRAINING

When the patient is alert and has been deemed a candidate for attempts at eating, feeding training may begin. Feeding training is differentiated from nutritional feeding; if the patient is not able to swallow safely, the training session is rehabilitative, and the patient receives complete nutrition through an alternative route (Logemann 1983). During feeding the patient should be observed for signs and symptoms of aspiration, which may include changes in respiratory or heart rate, color, voice quality, or coughing. It is also helpful to auscultate with a stethoscope at the neck, to assess whether audible pooling develops in the upper airway. Auscultation of the lungs before and after swallowing will help to assess pulmonary integrity. During initial feeding sessions, suctioning equipment should be available in the circumstance of suspected aspiration.

Positioning and Environment

Appropriate positioning is critical for safe and maximally independent eating and swallowing. Upright position allows optimal functioning of oral and pharyngeal structures (Farber 1982). The ability to keep the airway clear by coughing is stronger in an upright position (Frownfelter 1978). A flexed position is physiologically associated with swallowing success (Farber 1982) and prevents mass extension through the trunk and limbs that may be seen in the neurologically impaired patient. The seated position illustrated in Figure 9.2 incorporates flexion at the hips, knees, and shoulders; the arms are supported on the table and flex toward the body as the patient self-feeds. The head should be neither flexed nor extended, but in a neutral position with a slight chin tuck. This position minimizes the possibility of food entering the airway. For patients with difficulty maintaining position, repositioning may be necessary during the feeding session. Patients should remain upright for 15 to 30 minutes following eating, longer if there is an accompanying esophageal dysphagia.

The first feeding sessions should be conducted in a quiet room that allows for concentration on eating activity. If possible, the therapist should sit directly in front of the patient, as this promotes postural symmetry. If the patient has cognitive or perceptual problems, the therapist may wish to present one food item at a time. Conversation should be kept at a minimum in order to discourage simultaneous eating and talking, although brief conversation between swallows may help the therapist to assess changes in the patient's voice quality that may indicate compromise to the airway.

Food Selection and Administration

Patients with neurogenic dysphagia should first be evaluated with a soft, semiformed bolus that requires a minimum of oral preparation, such as applesauce or jello. Cold boluses, such as sherbet, can be highly facilitory for swallowing. Ice pops may facilitate sucking behaviors (Farber 1982). Liquids should be avoided initially as they can be easily aspirated, although they may be easier to manage for tracheostomized patients or those with cricopharyngeal dysfunction. Crumbly or solid textures are difficult because they require more oral preparation, dropping prematurely into an unprepared pharynx.

There are two positions illustrated in Figure 9.4 that the therapist may use to facilitate eating and swallowing (Davies 1985). In Figure 9.4A, the therapist stands at the patient's side and the arm is used to maintain the correct head position by reinforcing a neutral position of the neck with a gentle upward force. The head should never be pushed forward from behind (Farber 1982), as this will trigger an extension response. The position depicted in Figure 9.4B is used when the patient has adequate head control. In both positions the therapist's hand is used to monitor tone and control and to facilitate movement in the lips, cheeks, and tongue. To administer food, the therapist should bring the utensil toward the mouth, allowing the patient to see and smell it. Presenting the spoon

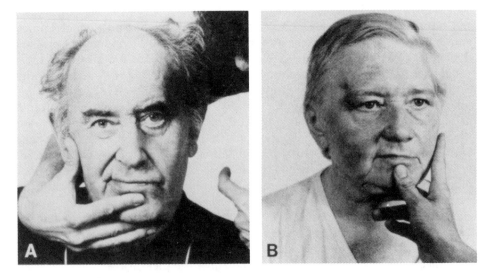

Figure 9.4 Hand placement to facilitate oral-pharyngeal movement during swallowing. (A) Facilitation for the patient with poor head and neck control. (B) Facilitation for the patient with primarily oral-pharyngeal control problems. (Reprinted by permission of the publisher, from Davies PM. Steps to follow: a guide to treatment of adult hemiplegia. Berlin: Springer-Verlag, 1985.)

from below the level of the mouth will help to maintain head position. If the patient is being fed, the spoon should be placed firmly on the tongue in order to stimulate removal of food from the spoon by the oral structures (Mueller 1975). The bolus should be placed at midline on the tongue. If the patient is unable to mobilize it from this position, it may initially be placed toward the stronger or more sensitive side of the mouth. The first few spoonfuls should be considered test swallows and the patient monitored for signs and symptoms of aspiration. The mouth should be inspected, and residual food removed if the patient is unable to clear it. For patients at high risk for aspiration, initial attempts at feeding should be done under videofluoroscopy to assess whether prefeeding treatment with an alternative nutritional route is necessary.

Verbal cues, if needed at all, should be short and simple to avoid confusing patients with cortical lesions. Some patients, because of reduced safety judgment and attention, may not be safe when eating and will require supervision and/or assistance at mealtime indefinitely. Patients who need to use more complex swallowing maneuvers, as described in the following section, must be able to follow directions and remember to use such techniques.

Once test swallows have been successful, several ounces of a trial food should be attempted. Different soft foods should be tried because of varying tolerance for subtle changes in texture; for instance, some patients may tolerate pudding but not applesauce. Once soft foods are tolerated, other textures should be attempted. A frequently used continuum of foods is soft chewables (canned fruit, well cooked vegetables), thick liquids (fruit nectars), thin liquids (fruit juice and water), chewables (raw vegetables and cooked meat), foods that require biting (rolls), and finally mixed textures (pills and water). Progression through this continuum is individualized, and may take from days to months. Some patients may never be able to safely manage certain textures, particularly thin liquids, chewables, and mixed textures. Individual food preferences as well as cultural attitudes toward types of foods and eating habits should be taken into consideration.

Special swallowing techniques may be appropriate for the patient with neurogenic dysphagia. Linden (1989) has outlined various compensatory swallowing techniques and indications for their use, e.g., neck flexion or supraglottic swallow when the patient has difficulty protecting the larynx, head rotation in the presence of unilateral weakness, and clearing the throat and reswallowing if there is intermittent wet-hoarseness. Logemann et al. (1989) noted that head rotation during swallowing in patients with unilateral pharyngeal weakness facilitated bolus propulsion by the pharyngeal musculature on the stronger side and enhanced relaxation of the cricopharyngeus muscle. Voluntarily prolonging the rise of the larynx by prolonging tongue contraction, the "Mendelsohn maneuver," also may help to improve opening of the pharyngoesophageal segment (Logemann and Kahrilas 1990). Compensatory swallowing maneuvers should be verified radiographically with the use of relevant food textures to assess their usefulness for the individual patient (Linden 1989).

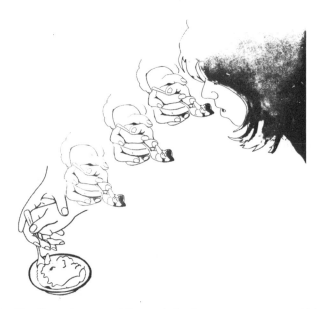

Figure 9.5 Tactile cueing or guiding to help the apraxic patient self-feed.

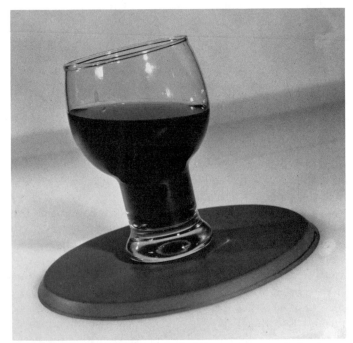

Figure 9.6 Use of a nonslip rubberized disk for holding eating utensils in place to prevent sliding. (Reprinted by permission of Maddak, Inc. Pequannock, NJ.)

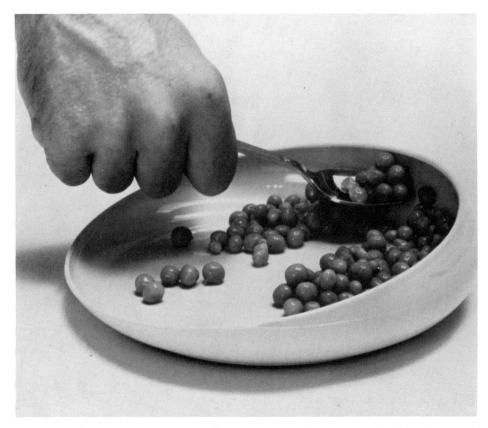

Figure 9.7 Example of a high-rimmed dish that assists the patient in loading the utensil for self-feeding. (Reprinted by permission of Fred Sammons, Inc.)

Apraxia

Apraxia is defined as the inability to plan and execute a skilled movement in the absence of sensory and motor deficits. The apraxic patient is not able to demonstrate a movement on verbal request. Both oral and limb apraxias may be observed. Therefore, the patient with oral apraxia is unable to smile when asked. Similarly the patient with limb apraxia is unable to demonstrate how to bring a spoon to the mouth. In treatment, the apraxic patient benefits from a natural setting, with food as the focus of activity. Demonstrating movements in addition to giving verbal cues will enhance the patient's ability to execute oral movements. The patient may be able to self-feed in the context of the actual activity, even though demonstration of self-feeding out of context was impossible. If the patient is unable to initiate or follow through with movements, tactile cueing or guiding will help to organize available movements into self-feeding. Figure 9.5 demonstrates the sequence of movements as the therapist gently guides

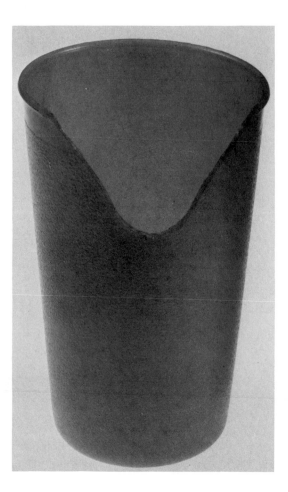

Figure 9.8 Example of a nose cutout cup to avoid neck extension while drinking. (Reprinted by permission of Fred Sammons, Inc.)

the patient during self-feeding. Often, guiding is necessary at the beginning of a session, but after several mouthfuls the patient is able to continue independently. Oral movements that were not elicited with verbal cues and demonstration may be observed during eating.

Adaptive Equipment

Adaptive feeding equipment may be useful in increasing eating independence and safety. There is a wide range of equipment available. Such equipment should be chosen with care by the occupational therapist, who can assess patient needs and skills and train the patient or care giver in their use. Nonskid pads (Figure 9.6) or a wet cloth under a dish prevents slipping. A high-rimmed plate allows the patient to load food onto the utensil more easily (Figure 9.7). A cup

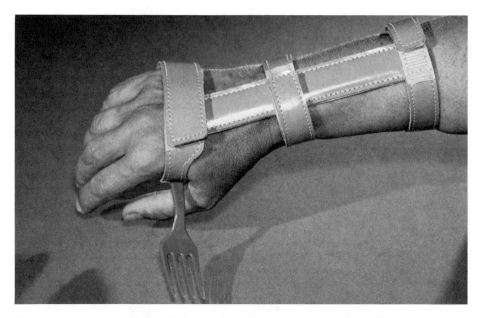

Figure 9.9 The universal cuff fits over the hand, pictured here with a wrist support splint; it requires only arm motion for feeding. (Reprinted by permission of Fred Sammons, Inc.)

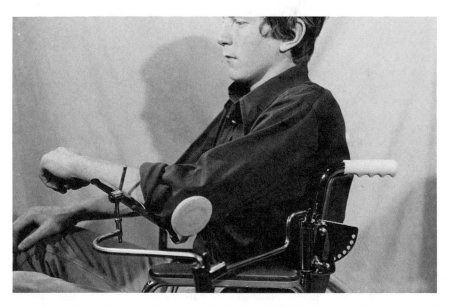

Figure 9.10 The Michigan ball-bearing feeder is useful for patients with large muscle or proximal weakness. (Reprinted by permission of the publisher, from Trombly CA. Occupational therapy for physical dysfunction. Baltimore: Williams & Wilkins, copyright 1989. Photographer, Judith LaDrew.)

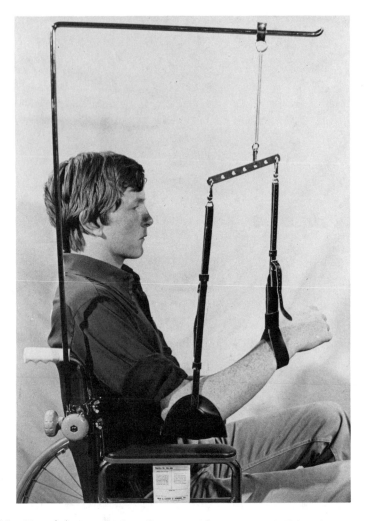

Figure 9.11 Use of the suspension sling can aid patients in self-feeding. (Reprinted by permission of the publisher, from Trombly CA, Scott AD. Occupational therapy for physical dysfunction. Baltimore: Williams & Wilkins, copyright 1977. Photographer, Judith LaDrew.)

with a nose cutout helps to prevent neck extension during drinking (Figure 9.8). For patients with distal upper extremity weakness, a universal cuff fitted with a utensil allows increased independence in eating (Figure 9.9). There are many types of equipment available for patients with proximal weakness, such as ball-bearing feeders (Figure 9.10) and overhead slings (Figure 9.11), as well as complex electronic and computerized devices for the more disabled patient.

SUMMARY

In this chapter the swallowing clinician was provided with a prefeeding and feeding program for use with the neurogenically dysphagic patient following diagnostic evaluation. Intervention that addresses the patient's cognitive, perceptual, physical, and functional abilities will maximize safe and independent eating and swallowing. Some patients may require prefeeding treatment before intake may begin. Modifications in both environmentally manipulated variables, such as how food is administered, and internal or patient-manipulated variables, such as specific swallowing methods, help to compensate for swallowing disorders (Linden 1989). Treatment should be designed for the individual patient, and effectiveness of treatment strategies should be reevaluated frequently.

REFERENCES

Ayres AJ. Sensory integration and learning disorders. Los Angeles: Western Psychological Services, 1973.

Bobath B. Adult hemiplegia: evaluation and treatment. Oxford, England: Heinemann Medical Books, 1990.

Buchholz DW, Bosma JF, Donner MW. Adaptation, compensation, and decompensation of the pharyngeal swallow. Gastrointest Radiol 1985; 10:235–9.

Coster ST, Schwarz WH. Rheology and the swallow-safe bolus. Dysphagia 1987; 1: 113–8.

Davies PM. Steps to follow: a guide to treatment of adult hemiplegia. Berlin: Springer-Verlag, 1985.

Farber SD. Neurorehabilitation: a multisensory approach. Philadelphia: WB Saunders, 1982.

Frownfelter D. Chest physical therapy and pulmonary rehabilitation: an interdisciplinary approach. Chicago: Year Book Medical, 1978.

Helfrich-Miller KR, Rector KL, Straka JA. Dysphagia: its treatment in the profoundly retarded population with cerebral palsy. Arch Phys Med Rehabil 1986; 67:520–5.

Kisner C, Colby LA. Therapeutic exercise: foundations and techniques. Philadelphia: FA Davis, 1985.

Langley, J. Working with swallowing disorders. Bicester, Oxon, England: Winslow Press, 1987.

Lazzara GD, Lazarus C, Logemann JA. Impact of thermal stimulation on the triggering of the swallow reflex. Dysphagia 1986; 1:73–77.

Linden P. Videofluoroscopy in the rehabilitation of swallowing dysfunction. Dysphagia 1989; 3:189–91.

Logemann JA. Diagnosis and treatment of swallowing disorders. San Diego: College Hill Press, 1983.

Logemann JA, Kahrilas PJ. Relearning to swallow after stroke—application of maneuvers and indirect biofeedback: a case study. Neurology 1990; 40:1136–8.

Logemann JA, Kahrilas PJ, Kobara M, et al. The benefit of head rotation on pharyngoesophageal dysphagia. Arch Phys Med Rehabil 1989; 70:767–71.

Mueller H. Feeding. In: Finnie NR, ed. Handling the young cerebral palsied child at home. New York: EP Dutton, 1975.

O'Sullivan N. Dysphagia care: team approach with acute and long term patients. Los Angeles: Cottage Square, 1990.

Ramsey WO. Suckle facilitation of feeding in selected dysphagia patients. Dysphagia 1986; 1:7–12.

Silverman EH, Elfant IL. Dysphagia: an evaluation and treatment program for the adult. Am J Occup Ther 1979; 33:382–92.

Stockmeyer SA. An interpretation of the approach of Rood to the treatment of neuro-muscular dysfunction. Am J Phys Med 1967; 46:900–61.

Sullivan PE, Markos PD, Minor MAD. An integrated approach to therapeutic exercise. Reston, VA: Reston Publishing Co., 1982.

Trombly CA. Occupational therapy for physical dysfunction. Baltimore: Williams & Wilkins, 1989.

Voss DE, Ionta MK, Myers BJ. Proprioceptive neuromuscular facilitation: patterns and techniques. Philadelphia: Harper & Row, 1985.

10

Treatment of Mechanical Swallowing Disorders

Susan M. Fleming

Although deglutition has been studied for many years, it has been only in the last decade that there has been such an interest in the subject, particularly in approaches to treatment (Kasprisin et al. 1989). Most clinicians and researchers appreciate the range of intrasubject and intersubject variability in the normal swallow (Christrup 1964; Ekberg and Nylander 1982; Hamlet 1989). At some point on this continuum of deglutition variability, the normal swallow becomes decompensated, with resultant dysphagic symptomatology. Dysphagia itself is also on a continuum, with the extent of abnormal variability influencing the degree of severity.

Some clarification of problems associated with dysphagia is provided to establish a clearer concept of subsequent management suggestions. This description of disorders is followed by suggestions for treating postsurgical patients with difficulties of bolus transport during the oral and pharyngeal stages of swallowing. Esophageal performance also may be influenced by some of these suggestions (e.g., upright versus supine positioning). The astute clinician will want to remember that although, by convention, we often speak in terms of the three stages of swallowing, the normal swallow is a rapid, synchronous process that is the sum of its representative parts.

DESCRIPTION OF DISORDERS

When dysphagia is present, swallowed contents do not traverse the normal route of deglutition in a timely fashion. Rather, one or more of the following events occurs: drooling, nasoregurgitation, aspiration, esophageal regurgitation or reflux, or the swallowed contents remain as residual that eventually may follow four alternative routes. These routes include anteriorly past the lips, into the nasal cavity, into the airway, or from the esophagus or stomach into the mouth or pharynx. Dysphagia, therefore, is not a disease, but a sign or symptom of another underlying disease or disorder that may be debilitating or life-threatening.

Forces of swallowed materials such as increased viscosity may negatively influence bolus flow. When this occurs, a mechanical dysphagia will become more apparent. The problems associated with mechanical dysphagia are multifaceted and allow an array of management possibilities. Consequently, determining the optimal plan can be challenging.

Aspiration is of greatest concern since it is life-threatening (Weiss 1988). At one time or another, most people have aspirated food or liquid into their airway. In healthy persons this results in a cough to expel the substance. In dysphagic patients whose overall physical status may be deteriorated, aspiration may be tolerated poorly (Kirsch and Sanders 1988).

Aspiration may be caused by unilateral incompetence of the hypoglossal nerve. In this circumstance the process of swallowing is out of control, the tongue no longer able to regulate the passage of the bolus. The pharynx receives the bolus prematurely, threatening the unprotected airway. Considering also that the laryngeal elevators may be impaired with hypoglossal nerve dysfunction, care must be taken in assessing potential risk of aspiration. In other words, disruption of tongue control is not the only factor in hypoglossal nerve dysfunction.

Involvement of the soft palate alone does not result in aspiration. In many neurologic disorders, however, problems of the soft palate accompany problems of the pharynx because of common innervation by the vagus and glossopharyngeal nerves. If peristalsis is disrupted, aspiration is possible since swallowing is such a rapid, synchronous process. Bolus stasis in the pharynx indicates that once the structures assume an at-rest or nonswallowing position, food may enter the unprotected airway. Further down the alimentary tract, a stricture of the cricopharyngeus or upper esophagus could result in reflux of swallowed substance that might then be spilled into the unprotected airway. Aspiration of this refluxed material, particularly if it contains hydrochloric acid, a normal constituent of gastric juice, may further compromise pulmonary status.

Problems of bolus transport can occur anywhere along the feeding route. For example, a person with unilateral involvement of the hypoglossal nerve with resection of portions of the tongue would have difficulty lateralizing a bolus for mastication and transport into the oropharynx to initiate the second stage of swallowing. Resection or paralysis of the soft palate may result in nasal regurgitation of the bolus, especially if the bolus is liquid (Kilman and Goyal 1976). Pharyngeal involvement results in disrupted peristaltic activity of the pharyngeal constrictors. Stenosis or narrowing of the alimentary tract at the level of the cricopharyngeus may prevent a food bolus from moving beyond that point. Esophageal transit may be disrupted in a similar manner.

Prior to deciding which mechanical devices to use in aiding bolus transport, the clinician must have medicolegal clearance to work with the dysphagic patient. Presuming legal consent such as clinical privileges and medical clearance have been obtained, the clinician must completely review the patient's chart as a beginning to a thorough assessment. If the patient appears to be at risk for aspiration (e.g., frequently coughs, has a "wet" sounding voice, or is unable to clear secretions well), the clinician must discuss this with the attending physician. Assuming that the patient is not at significant risk of aspiration, mechanical devices can be considered to enable the patient to eat more easily and more conveniently, and most importantly, to maintain nutrition and hydration.

POSITIONING

The position taken while eating affects bolus transport. If the head is lowered and there is incomplete lip closure, drooling may occur. In patients with insufficient velopharyngeal closure, lowering the head, as when drinking from a water fountain, may result in nasoregurgitation. With some esophageal disorders, reflux is greater in the supine rather than the upright position. Depending on the manifestation of the swallowing disorder, aspiration secondary to pharyngeal incompetence may be reduced by turning the head to the involved side (Logemann et al. 1989). Turning the head toward the involved side eliminates that side of the pharynx from its participation in bolus transit, allowing the nonimpaired side to propel the bolus. This is demonstrated both clinically and radiographically. Flexing the neck so that the head tilts forward improves the protection of the laryngeal vestibule (Ekberg 1986). This chin tuck maneuver frequently is seen as a compensation made by patients in the absence of any deglutition training. Apparently, experience has taught these patients that this compensatory technique improves their swallow efficiency.

The size of the bolus ingested is related to positioning. Tracy et al. (1989) found that as bolus volume increased, the oral transit time of the bolus head decreased and the duration of the cricopharyngeal opening increased. Significant changes in swallow coordination were reported by Castell et al. (1990) when comparing the factors of upright versus supine, wet versus dry swallows, and varying textures.

Collectively, there are many factors that alter patterns of deglutition in both normal individuals and in those with swallowing impairment. Variations in performance suggest that there are no equations or recipes for solving dysphagic complications, even for those who present with what appear to be similar problems. One must integrate what is known in the laboratory about the normal swallow with one's clinical experience in managing the disordered mechanism to formulate the most appropriate treatment program.

FEEDING DEVICES
Glossectomy Feeding Spoons

Glossectomy feeding spoons provide a means of transporting the bolus of food to the oropharynx. Not all patients with a partial or total glossectomy are candidates for the device. There are two criteria for use of the spoon. First, the patient should not be considered a high risk for aspiration. Significant resection of the base of the tongue or problems at the pharyngeal stage of swallowing might render the larynx vulnerable to the oncoming bolus. In addition, swallowing may be compromised severely in patients with resection of the hyomandibular complex (Summers 1971). Second, the patient can use the glossectomy feeding spoon with greatest ease if at least 50 percent of the tongue has been resected. The presence of more tongue actually interferes with placement of the device.

Pureed (blenderized) or finely chopped food is placed in the bowl of the spoon. The food should be ground to a consistency that eliminates the need for mastication. If lubrication is a problem, gravies, juices, and the like can be mixed in with the food. Holding the spoon level to keep the bolus from falling off, the bowl is placed as far back into the oral cavity as possible (avoid eliciting a gag reflex). Placement should be on the side where the patient has greater tongue mass remaining and/or better sensation. Sliding the triggering mechanism on the handle will cause the push plate on the bowl of the spoon to move and deposit the food onto the base of the tongue.

The glossectomy feeding spoon is useful because it gives patients an opportunity to enjoy something besides liquids that are transported by way of other devices. It is also more esthetically acceptable than a tube since it closely resembles commonly used flatware. There are at least two types of metal glossectomy feeding spoons available today (Figure 10.1). The one shown on the bottom of the figure is available through Maddock, Inc. Developed at the VA Medical Center, Allen Park, Michigan, the device has been used by several patients and found quite acceptable. Shown in the middle of Figure 10.1 is a measuring spoon

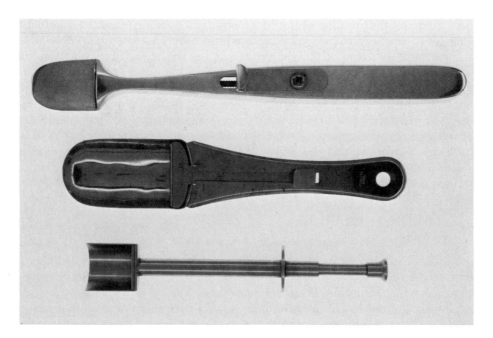

Figure 10.1 (Top) Commercially available glossectomy feeding spoon. (Middle) Cooking measuring spoon that should not be used for feeding. (Bottom) Glossectomy feeding spoon originally available for eligible military veterans, but now commercially available.

used for cooking. It is included here only to show what should not be used for feeding patients; other than being somewhat unwieldly, it is risky to use, as the push plate easily slides out from the spoon's handle and may be inadvertently deposited into the patient's oropharynx.

If funding is not available to purchase the commercially available spoon, a glossectomy feeding spoon can be constructed readily by the clinician (Fleming and Weaver 1983). It may not be as esthetically pleasing or as easy to use (particularly if trismus is present) as the one described, but it will be economical and based on the same principles. It is made from a 20-cc plastic syringe (Figure 10.2). Using a medium-fine hacksaw blade, a horizontal cut is made to one side of the protruding tip at the distal end of the syringe. A second cut is made perpendicular to the first cut so that the larger portion of the distal tip may be removed and discarded. A beveled 45 degree third cut is made on the cylinder wall about 3 cm from the distal end of the cylinder. This cut should continue only to the midpoint of the cylinder. Finally, two parallel cuts are made into the cylinder from the distal end toward the proximal end, intercepting the third cut. The portion of the cylinder that is sectioned by the third and fourth cuts is discarded. The inner portion of the cylinder is then ground down enough so that the piston can move freely. Fine sandpaper is used to remove bits of plastic and to smooth rough edges. The entire process takes less than ten minutes. At the top of Figure 10.3 is a glossectomy feeding device made from a plastic syringe in the manner described.

Syringes

Patients with lingual paresis or those having less than 50 percent tongue resection also may have difficulty with transport of an oral bolus. For them, use of the glossectomy feeding spoon is impractical because of the presence of tongue mass. For these patients, a 50- or 60-cc catheter-tipped syringe (Bakamjian and

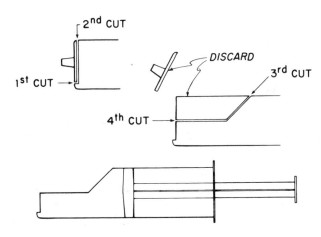

Figure 10.2 Steps used in making a glossectomy feeding spoon from a 20-cc plastic syringe. See the top of Figure 10.3 for the finished product.

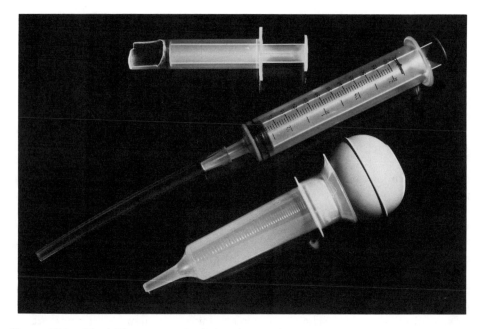

Figure 10.3 (Top) Glossectomy feeding spoon made from a 20-cc plastic syringe. (Middle) Catheter-tipped 60-cc syringe with tubular extension device for feeding. (Bottom) Bulb type syringe sometimes used for feeding.

Cramer 1960) with a 15-cm extension of pliable connecting tubing can be used (Figure 10.3, middle). The syringes can be made of glass, but they are more expensive (approximately 30 dollars each) and more easily broken than the plastic ones. They do have advantages, however, in that they are easy to clean and pistons slide easily within them. Plastic syringes are more difficult to keep clean and the washerlike tip at the distal end of the piston demonstrates wear by sticking, particularly if very warm foods are used. The major advantages of the plastic syringes are that they cost about one-twentieth the amount of the glass syringes and they are unbreakable. Individual circumstances suggest which type of syringe to use, but in most settings it is probably better to start with a plastic model and progress to a glass one when the patient is able to manage the device handily.

Prior to issuing a catheter-tipped syringe with a tubular extension, the risk of aspiration must be considered. Again, it is incumbent upon the clinician to obtain medical clearance before attempting to use the device with a patient. In addition, the clinician must consider the patient's overall ability to handle the syringe. For example, although only a few patients manage syringe feedings with only one hand, the majority require use of both hands (one to support the device and the other to regulate the piston). The bottom of Figure 10.3 shows a bulb type syringe. Most patients find this difficult to control, complaining that it squirts food into their mouths, resulting in a startle or recoil response.

The patient must fill the catheter-tipped syringe by slowly withdrawing the piston as the distal tip of the tubular extension is submerged into a liquid or thin puree. The object is to fill the syringe with food, but not pockets of air. Practice enables most patients to acquire this skill within the first session. To make the task easier, the puree should be strained and not too thick. Once the syringe is filled with food, the patient places the distal tip of the tubular extension at the place in the mouth where there is greatest sensation and ability to move the bolus with the tongue. For patients with surgical excision that is usually on the back of the unresected portion of tongue. For those with cerebrovascular accident or other neuromuscular problem, the distal tip should be placed where the bolus can be most easily handled.

Connecting tubing is the most convenient tubular extension to use since it is available in most settings and its large diameter (approximately 6 mm or 18 French) allows pureed foods to pass. Smaller-diameter tubing (e.g., 3 mm or 10 French) may have at least two applications. First, it allows more precise placement, which is beneficial in stimulation exercises. Second, some patients, such as those with severe trismus, may be unable to open their mouths wide enough for even the 6-mm connecting tube extension. For them a narrower tube may be more easily tolerated.

Finally, there are those patients who, through trauma or elective surgery, must have their teeth wired to prevent jaw opening. For them the problem is usually only a mechanical one—getting liquid food into the oral cavity. A small-gauge feeding tube can be threaded behind the third molar into the oral cavity. Feeding may then proceed with syringe or gavage bag, that is, the pliable plastic container used to hold the tube feeding, commonly referred to as the feeding bag. The attending physician must be informed of intended method of feeding and be assured that the patient can handle the feedings without aspiration.

The optimal position for feeding dysphagic patients is upright, with head support if necessary (Buckley et al. 1976). The head should not be tilted back, as such a posture only increases the chances of aspiration. The one exception to the upright position is when the patient has a problem transporting an oral bolus compounded by drooling and intraoral pooling, but does not have significant risk of aspiration. Eating may be easier if the patient assumes a semireclining position (e.g., 50 degrees), but with the head and body on the same plane. The goal is to decrease aspiration (head remains on plane with the body, not tilted) while increasing oral transport of the bolus (gravity helps the patient move the bolus to the oropharynx).

The patient with a supraglottic laryngectomy should not extend the head posteriorly in an effort to swallow. There is no reason to do so since transport of the bolus is not a problem. Extending the head posteriorly only increases aspiration because the laryngeal inlet becomes more accessible to the oncoming bolus.

Sometimes it is necessary to remind or train these patients to learn the supraglottic swallow. This technique, also known as the "controlled" or "safe" swallow, can be applied to many patient populations. It is just an extension of what one normally does when swallowing, i.e., masticate the food, assemble it as a collecting mass-bolus, position it on the tongue, inhale, hold breath, swallow, exhale, swallow again, and exhale again. This sequence of events is almost normal and should be reinforced since it serves to protect the airway and to clear pooled food from the laryngeal aditus. There are two points to emphasize when teaching this normal sequence. First, exhalation, not inhalation, must follow the swallow. If one were to inhale immediately following a swallow, aspiration would probably occur. Second, the swallow must occur at the beginning, not the end, of the exhalation phase of respiration. This allows an adequate amount of pulmonary air to help clear the laryngeal aditus. Another swallow must follow to clear any materials pooled in the pharyngeal recesses.

Nasogastric Tubes

Unfortunately, in spite of efforts to rehabilitate dysphagic patients, there are times that adequate oral nutrition and hydration are not possible. Although problems associated with patients handling their own secretions persist, those problems associated with aspiration of food and fluids can be circumvented through other means. Surgically, an altered feeding route, such as a feeding gastrostoma, jejunostoma, percutaneous endoscopic gastrostoma (PEG), or esophagostoma, can be created. These procedures are reserved for patients whose eating problems are considered long term (see Chapter 13). Parenteral feeding is one method of supplying nutrition (Hegedus and Pelham 1975) (see Chapter 12). Another option is the use of a nasogastric (NG) feeding tube (Figure 10.4). Although feeding tubes come with a variety of features, perhaps the most important one is their diameter. From the standpoint of patient comfort and fewer complications, the smaller size (10 French) is preferred; it also achieves a slower rate of feeding. Patients with larger feeding tubes (16 to 18 French) tend to feed themselves too rapidly, which causes gastric distress (Cataldo and Smith 1980). Also, esophageal ulceration increases with larger tubes, especially if they are employed for an extended period of time. The only advantages to larger feeding tubes are that they are easier to insert and do not clog as easily as the smaller ones. (See Chapter 12 for additional discussion of NG tubes.) These are staff conveniences that do not necessarily improve the patient's comfort and tolerance.

For patients who abhor the thought of being seen outside the hospital setting with a nasogastric feeding tube in place, there is an alternative. They can be taught to carefully insert a shorter feeding tube, take the feeding, withdraw the tube, and clean it properly after use (Donaldson et al. 1968) (Figure 10.5). If they so desire, they can become accustomed to the procedure. The obvious risk is, of course, incorrect insertion of the tube. The objective is to place the distal tip of the reusable tube into the upper esophagus so that it bypasses the level of the pharynx where food might be aspirated into the larynx. The decision

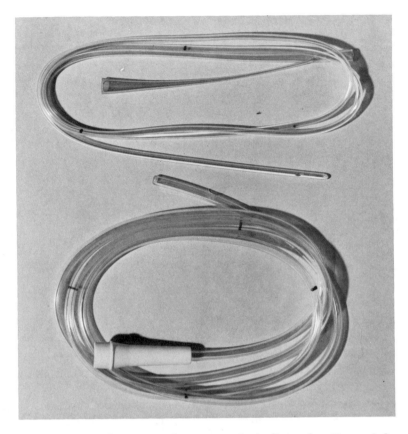

Figure 10.4 (Top) Small (10 French) nasogastric feeding tube. (Bottom) Large (16 French) nasogastric feeding tube.

to use this device rests with the physician and dysphagia team members and is based on their perception of how adequately the patient can adapt to the method.

TRACHEOSTOMA TUBES

Many patients with mechanical dysphagia have a tracheostoma tube in place, especially in the acute stage of their illness. While tracheostoma tubes assure an airway, they do interfere with swallowing (Feldman et al. 1966; Nash 1988). In a retrospective study, Arms et al. (1974) demonstrated increased risk of aspiration with their presence. Normally, when one swallows, the larynx is lifted in an anterosuperior direction to protect the laryngeal inlet from the oncoming bolus. The presence of a tracheostoma tube may anchor the larynx and make it more accessible to the bolus (Bonanno 1971). Another problem concerns pulmonary air, which cannot be used to clear the larynx if obstructions

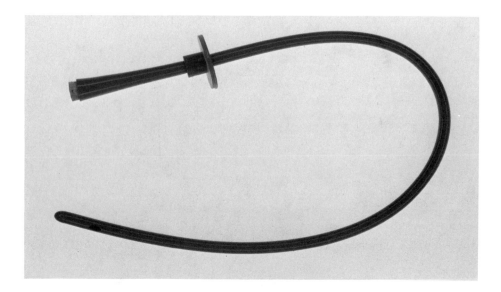

Figure 10.5 Nasoesophageal feeding tube with safety retention flange.

impede the flow of air. Normally, immediately following a swallow we exhale to clear the laryngeal aditus of foreign substance. With a tracheostoma tube, pulmonary air is shunted out via the tube. Evidence, including scintigraphic data, indicate that aspiration usually increases when a tracheostomy tube is not occluded (Fleming et al. 1989; Muz et al. 1989). Figure 10.6 illustrates how most of the pulmonary air is shunted out of the tracheostoma tube when the outer cannula takes up such a large portion of the inner diameter of the trachea. The

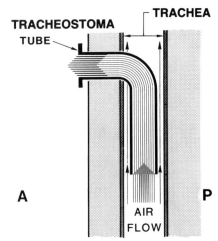

Figure 10.6 The large arrow within the tracheostoma tube indicates a significant proportion of air shunted out of the tracheostoma tube. Smaller arrows show a relatively small proportion of pulmonary air available for clearing the laryngeal aditus.

usual manner of clearing the larynx is not available. Nothing can be done about the presence of the tracheostoma tube limiting anterosuperior laryngeal elevation, but there are some things to consider about improving the flow of pulmonary air through the larynx.

The most practical way to effect passage of air through the larynx instead of out the tracheostoma tube itself is to plug or cover the opening of the tube. The patient can do this with the index finger, which is effective for the immediate purpose, but it is not convenient since it necessitates the continued use of one hand. Full closure plugs (Figure 10.7) can be used to occlude the port. These (Pilling Co.) are tapered and fitted by size so that there is no danger of their being drawn into the trachea. Another means of closing the opening of the tracheostoma tube is by use of a one-way Kistner valve (Figure 10.8). The Kistner valve opens on inhalation and closes when the user exhales. Exhaled air passes upward through the larynx. It should be noted that if a tracheostoma tube diameter is so large that it occludes much of the inner tracheal diameter, no amount of plugging at the open end of the tube will allow pulmonary air to reach the larynx. This is a mechanical blockage that must be dealt with. The simplest solution is to reduce the tracheostoma tube by two sizes. For example, if a patient with a number 8 tube cannot get adequate air to the larynx for phonation or coughing when the tracheostoma opening is plugged, a number 6 tube should be used.

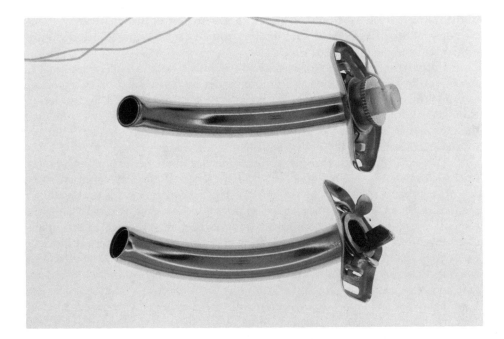

Figure 10.7 (Top) Full closure plugs can be used to occlude the tracheostoma. (Bottom) Unplugged tracheostoma tube.

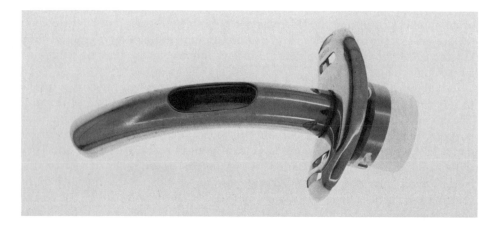

Figure 10.8 A one-way valved tracheostoma tube.

Another way to get pulmonary air to pass upward into the larynx is by use of a fenestrated tracheostoma tube (Figure 10.9, top). Some of these also are provided with a valve for the fenestration. These work well unless the patient has copious secretions that could impede the functioning of the fenestration and its valve. Their use may be limited because of problems associated with irritation of the tracheal wall. To eliminate this irritation no part of the fenestration should be adjacent to the tracheal wall. Verification of fenestration location may be done radiographically.

Cuffed tracheostoma tubes present problems such as infection, tracheal stenosis, esóphageal erosion, and innominate artery fistualization (Cooper and Grillo 1969; Sasaki 1980). The cuff is inflated to keep food, liquid, and secretions from getting into the lungs. The top of Figure 10.10 shows a cuff that is inflated; the cuff in the bottom of the figure is not inflated. The cuff should be inflated to the specifications of the physician (Nahum and Harris 1981).

There are, however, three reasons for not feeding patients orally while their tracheostoma cuffs are inflated. First, if a patient's medical condition is so precarious that a cuffed tracheostoma tube is warranted, perhaps oral feeding is premature. It has been demonstrated radiographically that a liquid bolus may get past the cuff and enter the lower trachea. Second, presence of an inflated cuff prevents pulmonary air from clearing the larynx; this mechanical blockage is not desirable. Third, if a patient is aspirating the food bolus it is vital to know when it occurs so that suctioning can be done immediately. With an inflated cuff that knowledge is delayed.

There are guidelines for working with these patients. Once medical clearance has been obtained, the tracheostoma should be suctioned, the cuff deflated, and suctioning repeated. Then the patients may be fed. Adding blue food coloring to the food will help verify aspiration. Once the patients have been fed they should be suctioned again and the cuff inflated to the physician's specifications.

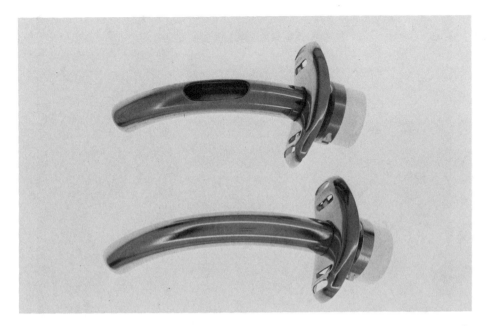

Figure 10.9 (Top) Fenestrated and one-way valved tracheostoma tube. (Bottom) Unfenestrated and one-way valved tracheostoma tube.

SYNTHETIC SALIVA

Patients taking certain medications, those with salivary gland dysfunction, and those patients receiving irradiation to the oral or pharyngeal areas will experience xerostomia or dry mouth (Shedd 1976; Dreizen et al. 1977; Sobol et al. 1979; Caruso et al. 1989). In addition to physical discomfort, this causes at least two other problems. First, there is the loss of saliva that normally serves to cleanse and protect the teeth. Without the protection provided by saliva, dental caries increase (Trowbridge and Carl 1975). Second, with decreased saliva there is reduction in the ability to moisten food and facilitate mastication and deglutition (Mansson and Sandberg 1975). This leads to weight loss in many patients.

Although saliva cannot be replaced, artificial saliva is available to provide lubrication. Presently, there are several commercially available synthetic saliva products from which to choose. They are not alike, however. They differ in terms of viscosity, preference, and performance. Ideally, the synthetic saliva should lubricate both hard and soft oral tissues (Aguirre et al. 1989). Usually patients are directed to take the synthetic saliva as needed. Most rinse with a spoonful of the synthetic saliva just prior to eating. Some of these products contain fluoride needed to deter caries formation (Dudgeon et al. 1980). Unfortunately, some may have a drying effect (Daeffler 1981); therefore their use must be assessed on an individual basis.

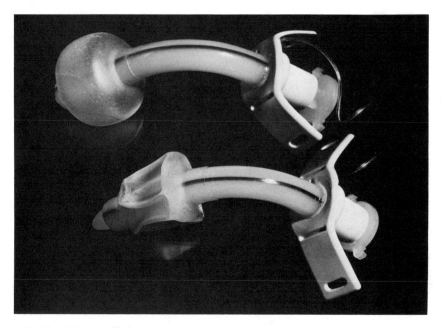

Figure 10.10 (Top) Cuffed tracheostoma tube with cuff inflated. (Bottom) Cuffed tracheostoma tube with cuff somewhat deflated.

Lemon-glycerin swabs are available for the patient to cleanse and freshen the mouth. Although for many patients these special swabs provide relief, others find that they add to oral dryness with long-term use. Thus patient preference will help determine the amount and frequency of use of lemon-glycerin swabs.

In addition to synthetic saliva, a surface anesthetic applied just prior to eating may help reduce the pain associated with deglutition. Surface anesthesia should be used carefully in those patients at high risk for aspiration, since the swallowing mechanism should not be further compromised by reduced sensation.

FOOD BLENDERS

Perhaps the most a clinician can do for the patient is to provide the food consistency that is best tolerated. Unfortunately, most people assume that liquid consistency is best. This is not necessarily so. Many patients with mechanical disorders leading to dysphagia do better with food of puree consistency (Ardran and Kemp 1952; Summers 1971; Edwards 1973; Paavolainen 1977; Silverman and Elfant 1979). Pureed material is less mobile than liquid, and with an impaired oropharyngeal mechanism it is important to minimize aspiration. This is especially true of the patient who has undergone a supraglottic laryngectomy. Evidence of this is supported by our clinical experience and radiographic observations. Fluids are more easily tolerated by patients who demonstrate an organic stenosis (Hellemans et al. 1981).

Dentition status will influence masticatory performance. Additionally, patient perceptions about actual texture acceptability will affect anxiety associated with chewing and swallowing performance (Garcia et al. 1989). Consequently, offering easy to chew foods or foods that have been blenderized to a patient's optimal texture may facilitate deglutition (von Branchitsch and May 1968).

Food consistency is of such importance that some facilities make food blenders available to patients. An added benefit of blenders is that the cost of purchasing specially prepared products can be reduced as patients are able to puree items that are consumed by the rest of the family (Farrior and Kelly 1979).

Just as food blenders are available for altering the rheologic characteristics of solid foods, there are commercially available food thickeners to modify the viscosity of liquids. A significant concern for the dysphagic patient is not only calories and nutrition, but hydration. For the patient who is quite compromised with liquids, the use of food thickeners may well determine whether or not a feeding tube (nasogastric or surgical) is necessary. Caution dictates, however, that in patients who are severely dysphagic, the use of food thickeners still may not be sufficient. Some patients who have been taking artificially thickened fluids on a long-term basis complain that they fail to quench their thirst. As with many treatment and management techniques, the problem may be ameliorated but not eliminated.

SUMMARY

Mechanical swallowing disorders in the mouth, pharynx, and esophagus usually result from a combination of structure loss and/or rearrangement and potential peripheral nerve involvement secondary to removal of cancerous lesions. Such lesions in the mouth and pharynx may require glossectomy, partial pharyngectomy, and partial laryngectomy resulting in difficulty transporting and channeling a bolus. Decisions concerning the appropriate mechanical device and diet needed to obviate mechanical disorders are based on the type and amount of resection, concomitant medical complications, and patient acceptance and cooperation. Alternatives to regular dietary intake via nasogastric tube feeding, surgically created feeding routes, and blenderized textures need to be considered.

REFERENCES

Aguirre A, Mendoza B, Reddy MS, et al. Lubrication of selected salivary molecules and artificial salivas. Dysphagia 1989; 4:95–100.

Ardran GM, Kemp FH. The protection of the laryngeal airway during swallowing. Br J Radiol 1952; 23:406–16.

Arms RA, Dines DE, Tinstman TC. Aspiration pneumonia. Chest 1974; 65:136–39.

Bakamjian V, Cramer L. Surgical management of advanced cancer of the tongue. Ann Surg 1960; 152:1058–66.

Bonanno PC. Swallowing dysfunction after tracheostomy. Ann Surg 1971; 174:29–33.

von Branchitsch H, May W. Deaths from aspiration and asphyxiation in a mental hospital. Arch Gen Psychiat 1968; 18:129–36.

Buckley JE, Addicks CL, Maniglia J. Feeding patients with dysphagia. Nurs Forum 1976; 15:69–85.

Caruso AJ, Sonies BC, Atkinson JC, et al. Objective measures of swallowing in patients with primary Sjogren's syndrome. Dysphagia 1989; 4:101–5.

Castell J, Dalton C, Castell D. Effects of body position and bolus consistency on the manometric parameters and coordination of the upper esophageal sphincter and pharynx. Dysphagia 1990; 5:179–96.

Cataldo CB, Smith L. Tube feedings: clinical applications. Columbus, Ohio: Ross Laboratories, 1980.

Christup J. Normal swallowing of foodstuffs of pasty consistence. Dan Med Bull 1964; 11:79–91.

Cooper JD, Grillo HC. The evolution of tracheal injury due to ventilatory assistance through cuffed tubes: a pathologic study. Ann Surg 1969; 169:334–48.

Daeffler R. Oral hygiene measures for patients with cancer. Cancer Nurs 1981; 4:29–35.

Donaldson RC, Skelly M, Paletta FX. Total glossectomy for cancer. Am J Surg 1968; 116:585–90.

Dreizen S, Daly TE, Drane JB, Brown LR. Oral complications of cancer radiotherapy. Postgrad Med 1977; 61:85–92.

Dudgeon BJ, DeLisa JA, Miller RM. Head and neck cancer, a rehabilitation approach. Am J Occup Ther 1980; 34:243–51.

Edwards H. Neurological disease of the pharynx and larynx. Practitioner 1973; 211: 729–37.

Ekberg O. Posture of the head and pharyngeal swallowing. Acta Radiologica Diag 1986; 27:691–6.

Ekberg O, Nylander G. Cineradiography of the pharyngeal stage of deglutition in 150 individuals without dysphagia. Br J Radiol 1982; 55:253–7.

Farrior JB III, Kelly MT. Home nutrition for patients with head and neck tumors. Ear Nose Throat J 1979; 58:84–85.

Feldman SA, Deal CW, Urquhart W. Disturbance of swallowing after tracheostomy. Lancet 1966; 1:954–55.

Fleming S, Nelson R, Muz J, et al. Scintigraphy in the dysphagic patient. National Conference, American Speech-Language-Hearing Association, St. Louis, MO, November 1989.

Fleming SM, Weaver AW. Glossectomy feeding device readily adapted from a plastic syringe. Arch Phys Med Rehabil 1983; 64:183–5.

Garcia RI, Perlmutter LC, Chauncey HH. Effects of dentition status and personality on masticatory performance and food acceptability. Dysphagia 1989; 4:136–45.

Hamlet S. Dynamic aspects of lingual propulsive activity in swallowing. Dysphagia 1989; 4:136–45.

Hegedus S, Pelham M. Dietetics in a cancer hospital. J Am Diet Assoc 1975; 67:235–40.

Hellemans J, Pelemans W, Vantrappen G. Pharyngoesophageal swallowing disorders and the pharyngo-esophageal sphincter. Med Clin North Am 1981; 65:1149–71.

Kasprisin A, Clumeck H, Nino-Murcia M. The efficacy of rehabilitative management of dysphagia. Dysphagia 1989; 4:48–52.

Kilman WJ, Goyal RK. Disorders of pharyngeal and upper esophageal sphincter motor function. Arch Intern Med 1976; 136:592–601.

Kirsch CM, Sanders A. Aspiration pneumonia: medical management. Otolaryngol Clin North Am 1988; 21:677–90.

Logemann J, Kahrilas P, Kobara M, et al. The benefit of head rotation on pharyngoesophageal dysphagia. Arch Phys Med, 1989; 70:767–71.

Mansson I, Sandberg N. Salivary stimulus and swallowing reflex in man. Acta Otolaryngol 1975; 79:445–50.

Muz J, Mathog RH, Nelson R, et al. Aspiration in patients with head and neck cancer and tracheostomy. Am J Otolaryngol 1989; 10:282–6.

Nahum AM, Harris JP, Davidson TM. The patient who aspirates—diagnosis and management. J Otolaryngol 1981; 10:10–16.

Nash M. Swallowing problems in the tracheotomized patient. Otolaryngol Clin North Am 1988; 21:701–9.

Paavolainen M. Rehabilitation of eating after supraglottic laryngectomy. Minerva Otorhinolaryngol 1977; 27:91–5.

Sasaki CT. Paralysis of the larynx and pharynx. Surg Clin North Am 1980; 60:1079–92.

Shedd DP. Rehabilitation problems of head and neck cancer patients. J Surg Oncol 1976; 8:11–21.

Silverman EH, Elfant IL. Dysphagia: an evaluation and treatment program for the adult. Am J Occup Ther 1979; 33:382–92.

Sobol SM, Conoyer JM, Sessions DG. Enteral and parenteral nutrition in patients with head and neck cancer. Ann Otolaryngol 1979; 88:495–501.

Summers GW. Physiologic problems following ablative surgery of the head and neck. Otolaryngol Clin North Am 1971; 7:217–50.

Tracy J, Logemann J, Kahrilas P, et al. Preliminary observations on the effects of age on oropharyngeal deglutition. Dysphagia 1989; 4:90–94.

Trowbridge JE, Carl W. Oral care of the patient having head and neck irradiation. Am J Nurs 1975; 75:2146–9.

Weiss MH. Dysphagia in infants and children. Otolaryngol Clin North Am 1988; 21:727–35.

11

Nutritional Considerations

Jean E. Curran

The importance of early recognition of patients who are at risk for developing protein-calorie malnutrition in both acute and chronic care settings, with subsequent provision of appropriate therapy and nutritional support, has only recently begun to receive the attention it deserves. The distressingly prevalent incidence of hospitalized patients found to be malnourished, and the deleterious effect malnutrition has on clinical outcome, has heightened health care professionals' awareness of the need for timely nutrition intervention in a manner comparable to other medical or surgical treatment (Bistrian et al. 1976). The assessment of nutritional status, implementation of a care plan, and continuous monitoring and evaluation of individual patients to determine the effectiveness and appropriateness of the nutritional care plan must take precedence to correct nutrient imbalances and restore nutritional well-being.

Patients presenting with dysphagia and the inability to take adequate food and fluid by mouth, whether due to neurologic disease or surgical resections involving any part of the alimentary tract, should be considered at high nutritional risk. Only recently has this population been identified as a group for whom optimal patient care is dependent on adequate nutritional support (Jones and Altschuler 1987). The consequence of untreated dysphagia is protein-calorie malnutrition (Hynak-Hankinson 1984). This may lead to life-threatening conditions due to increased susceptibility to infection secondary to compromise of the immune system (Goodhart and Shils 1980).

ASSESSMENT OF NUTRITIONAL STATUS

The registered dietitian in a clinical setting is the primary allied health professional responsible for ensuring that all patients are adequately nourished, either by provision of nutrients, appropriate in both quality and quantity based on individual needs, and by counseling patients and/or their families in their own food choices (Zeman 1983). Dietitians are uniquely trained not only in the fields of biochemistry, anatomy and physiology, food science, and diet therapy, but also in behavioral sciences and counseling skills as well as institutional management. They are, therefore, qualified to assume the role of nutrition specialist, taking greater responsibility in preventing the problems associated with malnutrition by identifying patients with predisposing factors who are at nutritional risk, planning and implementing the appropriate route and mode of nutrient delivery, and monitoring and evaluating the whole process (Kamel 1990).

Based on the patient population and specific needs of an institution, a standardized nutritional screening form with a set of valid guidelines should be developed. This provides either the dietetic technician or registered dietitian with a simple and expedient way of determining whether a patient requires routine nutritional care or an in-depth work-up and assessment by a dietitian who specializes in the particular nutritional problems of a specific medical and/or surgical population.

Identification and Screening

The initial step in preventing complications of malnutrition is being able to identify those patients with predisposing factors who are at risk and who are likely to benefit from nutritional support. Malnutrition generally results from factors that affect ingestion, digestion, and impaired absorption or utilization of nutrients (Lang and Cashman 1989). Table 11.1 lists the variety of factors, including physiologic, psychological, and psychosocial, that suggest a patient might be at nutritional risk. Nutritional care procedures in an acute care facility should include such a list as a way of assisting dietitians in identifying patients at risk by noting the number and severity of risk factors present in each patient screened. The routine screening process normally includes recording the initial diagnosis, medical and surgical history, height and weight, dental status, medication orders, and serum albumin concentration. Weight, in the absence of edema, is the most useful clinical parameter employed in both the initial nutritional assessment and in evaluating the process of nutritional repletion. Although serum albumin concentration is an important prognostic indicator of nutritional status, specifically visceral protein, it may be affected by hydration status, hepatic disease, and ongoing losses and stress. Therefore, it generally should be interpreted more critically (Lang and Cashman 1989). Other variables, such as transferrin and total iron-binding capacity may be useful in determining protein status as well as acute responses to changes in nutritional status (Kamel 1990).

Dietary Interview

A dietary interview, conducted by a dietetic technician or registered dietitian should seek to obtain additional information regarding usual body weight and any recent significant weight change, changes in appetite, usual eating habits, chronic or acute problems that may affect food intake, such as nausea, vomiting, diarrhea, or constipation, food allergies, food preferences, compliance to therapeutic diet regimens when applicable, and use of vitamin and mineral preparations or commercial nutritional supplements. Observation of patients at mealtime, or "meal rounds" is then done on a daily basis. It is an invaluable way of obtaining first-hand information on any problems in chewing, swallowing, self-feeding ability, or overall food intake.

Table 11.1 Factors Suggesting Nutritional Risk

Diagnosis indicative of nutritional risk
  Alcoholism and/or drug abuse
  Acquired immunodeficiency syndrome
  Cancer
  Coronary heart disease
  Dehydration
  Diabetes
  Gastrointestinal tract disease
  Liver disease
  Lung disease
  Malnutrition
  Neurologic disorders
  Obesity
  Infection, trauma, burns
  Psychiatric illness

Physical findings indicative of nutritional risk
  Cachexia
  Involuntary weight loss
  Poor dentition, ill-fitting dentures
  Inability to feed self
  Anorexia from illness, drugs, therapy
  Dysphagia
  Losses via diarrhea, draining wounds, and fistulas

Hospital treatment indicative of nutritional risk
  Chemotherapy
  Radiation therapy
  Surgical resections of head and neck or gastrointestinal tract
  Dental
  Drug-nutrient interactions
  Chronic use of medications that affect digestion, absorption, or utilization
  Prolonged use of inadequate diets (i.e., clear liquids)
  Nothing by mouth for more than 3 days

Psychosocial factors
  Fear, anxiety, depression about illness
  Isolation, inability to shop or cook for self
  Dislike of hospital food and/or therapeutic diet
  Food idiosyncrasies or concern about the side effects or after effects of eating specific foods (i.e., milk)

Determining Nutritional Risk

Once screening information is obtained and the patient is interviewed and observed at meal rounds, the level of nutritional risk can be determined. Common indices for malnutrition include nonvolitional weight loss of more than 10 percent of total body weight or a weight below 90 percent of the ideal (Kamel

1990), the presence of hypoalbuminemia (serum albumin concentration of less than 3.5 g/dL) (Ciocon 1990), a statement from the patient regarding recent change in appetite, complaints of chewing and swallowing problems (unremedied by a standard diet texture change), and observation of poor intake at meal rounds. These patients should be referred to the registered dietitian for an in-depth nutritional assessment. It is important to note that there is no single specific test or laboratory value that can be used to determine whether or not a patient is malnourished (Blackburn et al. 1977). Collection of the previously mentioned data, gross evidence of protein-calorie malnutrition noted on physical examina-tion, and good clinical judgment in interpreting the data based on their overall relationship to the patient's medical and/or surgical status will allow the clinician to formulate a feasible and appropriate nutritional care plan.

DIETITIAN'S ROLE

Dietetic clinicians working specifically with populations at risk for swal-lowing disorders should be familiar with the principal causes of dysphagia, such as neurologic disease, cerebrovascular disease, demyelinating disorders, end-stage dementia, comatose state, late-stage Parkinson's disease (Ciocon 1990), impair-ment from surgical resections of the head and neck (glossectomy, hemilaryngec-tomy, supraglottic laryngectomy), acute inflammatory processes (pharyngitis, tonsillitis, thrush), and the potential side effects of radiation therapy that impact on normal deglutition (Fleming et al. 1977). The medical and surgical history should be reviewed, taking into account those previously mentioned problems and any history of aspiration pneumonia, lung disease, or esophageal disorders. As the dietitian's involvement with identifying and preventing potential drug-nutrient interactions has expanded greatly in recent years (Murray and Healy 1991), a review of the patient's current medication orders may identify the use of a drug or drugs that frequently cause xerostomia (Table 11.2) and subsequent problems with chewing and/or swallowing. Familiarity with the symptoms of dysphagia that are observed at mealtime (reduced attention, distractibility, ab-normal head and body position, drooling of liquid bolus, pocketing, coughing, choking, changes in vocal quality, slow eating), and observation of a patient's inability to feed independently and use eating utensils can alert the dietitian to the possibility of a problem patient. Finally, the dietitian's expertise in eliciting subjective information about usual eating habits, sometimes difficult or impos-sible in patients with swallowing disorders secondary to altered mental status and/or impaired speech (Miller 1992), may be a key factor in identifying a patient in need of a thorough swallowing evaluation. The patient and/or care giver may initially deny having problems with swallowing; however, further investi-gation may reveal a diet history suggestive of avoidance of solid and/or liquid food items, food preparation methods such as mashing, chopping, or blender-izing, reliance on nutritional supplements, and/or the use of commercial baby food. Dietitians, therefore, play an important role in identifying patients with

Table 11.2   Classes of Drugs with Xerostomic Side Effects

Analgesic mixtures
Anticonvulsants
Antiemetics
Antihistamines
Antihypertensives
Antinauseants
Antiparkinsonism agents
Antipruritics
Antispasmodics
Appetite suppressants
Cold medications
Decongestants
Diuretics
Expectorants
Muscle relaxants
Psychotropic drugs
   Central nervous system depressants
   Benzodiazepine derivatives
   Monoamine oxidase inhibitors
   Phenothiazine derivatives
   Tranquilizers, major and minor
Sedatives

Reprinted with permission from Bahn SL. Drug-related dental destruction. Oral Surg 1972; 33:50.

swallowing problems and can be instrumental in initiating referrals to the swallowing team.

FEEDING CONSIDERATIONS

Although nasoenteric feedings in patients with dysphagia due to upper aerodigestive tract dysfunction has its associated risks (Sitzmann 1990), nasogastric tube feeding is routinely used in patients as a temporary means of providing nutrition.

Tube feeding to provide total nutritional requirements is indicated for patients with protein-calorie malnutrition with inadequate oral intake for 5 days and for those with normal nutritional status with less than 50 percent of required nutritional intake for 7 to 10 days (Ciocon 1990). Dysphagic patients presenting in a weakened and debilitated state due to poor intake may require enteral feeding to improve nutritional status before dysphagia therapy can be initiated successfully. Enteral feeding also is initiated for patients who have undergone surgical procedures for head and neck cancer and for those with severe neurologic impairments that compromise the mechanism and cognitive integrity needed to protect the airway during swallow. For these patients, an oral diet is contraindicated due to the high risk of aspiration and its life-threatening consequences. However, when the primary physician, in consultation with the speech/language pathologist, considers the patient able to ingest an oral diet, the choice of the appropriate food and fluid consistency becomes a critical factor in subsequent management. A dysphagia evaluation tray, provided by the department of nutrition services and containing a variety of food and fluid textures, can be used during a bedside evaluation to determine the food and fluid consistency best tolerated by the patient. A systematic way of preparing and delivering these foods and fluids from kitchen to bedside should be developed and implemented, taking into account the kitchen and food production/service schedule, availability of certain food items at specific times during the day, and available manpower needed to deliver as well as pick up food trays postevaluation (Table 11.3). Based on the results of the food texture evaluation and, if necessary, the modified barium swallow, the speech/language pathologist and dietitian must coordinate efforts to determine the oral diet most suitable for the patient.

Liquid and/or pureed food often is the only type of consistency safely tolerated by patients with mechanical disorders leading to dysphagia or oral mucosa changes that frequently accompany other concurrent treatment modes

Table 11.3 Food Texture Order (Dysphagia Team, VA Medical Center, New York, NY)

A dysphagia team evaluation/ treatment is currently in progress for inpatient/ outpatient _____ SS#: _____ on _____ at _____ a.m./p.m. Please assemble the items circled and deliver tray to _____: Specify flavor when applicable.

Level 1 thick juice	Ground meat with gravy
Level 2 thick juice	Mashed potatoes w/gravy
Level 3 thick juice	Cream soup
Level 2 thick milk	Rice
Regular juice	Peas or corn
Coffee or Tea	Vegetable soup
Milk	Crackers or cookies
Sustacal® Pudding _____	Bread
Sustacal® HC or Ensure® Plus _____	Hot cereal
Regular pudding _____	Pureed tray
Canned peaches or fruit cocktail	Mechanical tray
Applesauce	Aspiration reduction tray
Jello	Other _____

Requested by:	Reviewed by:
Joyce F. West, Ph.D.	Jean Curran, R.D.
Chief, Speech Pathology & Audiology	Clinical Dietitian

Assembled by:

_____
Food Service Foreman

such as radiation or chemotherapy (Fleming et al. 1977). However, for patients with suspected oropharyngeal pathologic conditions that would put them at risk for aspiration of food and fluid, pureed and liquid diets are often contraindicated (Groher 1987). Such patients have more difficulty with fluids and thinned foods (pureed) because the disordered mechanism cannot respond in time with sufficient control to protect the airway. Studies have demonstrated that, in general, substances that are easy to chew (pureed consistency) are not always easy to swallow, especially for those with neurogenic oropharyngeal pathologic conditions (Groher 1987). Instead, for patients with decreased laryngeal elevation, a weak or uncoordinated swallow, or poor oral muscular control or reduced oral sensation, semisolid consistencies that do not easily disperse in the mouth and can be swallowed as a single bolus are more palatable and better tolerated than pureed foods. Unlike purees, textured soft foods with high moisture content and flavor can assist in triggering a weak reflex. Table 11.4 lists examples of food items and prepared dishes that are suitable for dysphagic diet menus.

Many institutions offer a dysphagia diet in stages during the early phases of swallowing retraining. For instance, a dysphagia I diet may include starter foods such as thick pureed fruit, ice cream, frozen yogurt, mashed popsicles, or frozen juice. Based on individual patient tolerance, the diet is gradually advanced to stages II and III, where additional food items such as custard, pureed vegetables, canned fruit, and chopped whole food are served. Based on the patient's overall progress with swallowing rehabilitation, the diet may be advanced to semisolid or regular textured foods. Frequently, early stage diets omit thin liquids and, since small amounts of a limited variety of foods are offered, these regimens are inadequate to meet caloric, protein, and fluid requirements. Therefore, enteral feedings and, if necessary, intravenous fluids are normally required as adjunct therapy.

Mindful of financial constraints in any facility, as well as shortages in manpower needed for preparation and serving, diets for the swallowing impaired do not necessitate the procurement of additional food items or food supplies. A dysphagic diet can easily be adapted from the institution's regular diet. If meat chunks are set aside for cooks to dice into smaller pieces for mixed dishes, and extra gravy, sauces, and binders such as mayonnaise are included in the dysphagic entrees to ensure moist, well-lubricated food, most of the food items on the dysphagic menu can be served on standard mechanical or geriatric diets. Foods that fall or break apart (Table 11.5) or sticky food such as plain mashed potatoes, peanut butter, and white bread should not be served on the dysphagic diet. Omission of these food items reduces the risk of small pieces of food entering the airway, increasing the risk of respiratory compromise.

The importance of serving a diet to the dysphagic patient that provides contrasting color, flavor, texture, size, shape, and temperature cannot be over-emphasized. However, recent studies have shown that a high percentage of elderly residents in nursing homes receive pureed or blenderized food. Pureed food is ordered most often for behavioral feeding problems such as a patient's reluctance to eat, confusion and lack of cooperativeness during mealtime, and the patient's

Table 11.4 Dysphagia Menu Items

Scrambled, poached, or soft cooked eggs
French toast (crust removed) and pancakes with syrup
Dry cereal (without raisins, dried fruit, or nuts) softened in milk
Hot cereal
Corned beef hash
Soft rolls, firm-textured bread without crust
Omelets or quiche
Moist, boneless fish
Sliced, tender meat or poultry with gravy
Cottage cheese
Macaroni and cheese
Meatloaf
Stew made with diced or chopped ingredients
Chopped tuna, egg, or potato salad made without celery or onion pieces
Cheese blintzes
Souffles or aspics
Tender Salisbury steak
Chopped beef burgundy
Shepherd's pie made with diced or chopped meat
Swedish meatballs with gravy
Ground beef and noodle or macaroni casserole
Noodles Alfredo
Ala kings
Tuna noodle casserole
Turkey tetrazzini
Lasagna, ravioli, or spaghetti
Whipped or mashed potatoes with gravy
Boiled or baked white or sweet potatoes (or yams) without skin
Moist bread dressing made without celery or onion pieces
Noodles or pasta with sauce or gravy
Pudding or custard
Ice cream or sherbet
Custard and cream pies
Plain, soft cake, donuts, or graham crackers, softened in milk
Yogurt
Canned fruit without pits
Soft fresh fruit such as orange and grapefruit sections, bananas, ripe melon, and pitless stewed prunes
Well-cooked vegetables, chopped, diced, or mashed
Sliced carrots or beets, squash, or asparagus tips

Table 11.5 Foods That Fall or Break Apart

Dry muffins
Pound cake
Plain rice
Peas
Corn, mixed vegetables
Chili con carne
Minestrone and vegetable soup
Coconut
Fruit cocktail
Items containing celery, nuts, or raisins

---

inability to self-feed (Cluskey 1989). If one must resort to the use of a blenderized diet for patients whose swallowing disorder severely limits their individual diets, care must be taken in creating a palatable pureed diet that has eye as well as taste appeal, through the use of food processors, garnish, and attractive serving dishes (Mayes 1985).

Patients who are unable to tolerate thin liquids are at increased risk for aspiration and dehydration. Commercial thickeners that thicken both hot and cold liquids without cooking are now available for institutional use. Fluids can generally be thickened to several consistency levels, determined by the speech/language pathologist and dependent on the amount of thickener used. During the process of digestion, starch-based thickeners, as opposed to vegetable gum thickeners, release the fluid back into the gastrointestinal tract so that almost all of the water in the thickened liquid is available for free water absorption (Vartan 1989). Despite their ease of use and availability, issues such as cost, patient acceptance, and personnel responsible for preparing the thickened liquids need to be addressed. The use of rice, tapioca, instant or mashed potatoes, unflavored gelatin, or baby cereal can be used for thickening purposes, especially for patients discharged home (Table 11.6); however these mediums may mask or alter food flavor and/or texture.

Often, the most difficult challenge the dysphagic patient faces is consuming adequate quantities of thickened liquids to meet fluid needs. Therefore, the incorporation of high fluid content foods such as pureed fruit, custards, gelatin desserts, and frozen juice will assist in increasing the overall fluid content of the diet. Also, the addition of extra margarine, cream, half-and-half, powdered or evaporated milk, and whipped topping to recipes can add extra calories to the diet without substantially increasing the volume of food the patient is required to consume to meet caloric needs.

Commercial nutritional supplements served with meals or as between-meal nourishment are generally available in most institutions for those patients who are unable to meet nutrient needs. These may be given for those with poor appetites, difficulty swallowing, increased requirement secondary to illness, or excessive fatigue during the feeding process, rendering them unable to complete

Table 11.6 Food Preparation Suggestions

Hot liquids: Milk-based liquids: add rice cereal (baby product) or plain gelatin. Other liquids: add potato flakes, mashed potatoes, or flaked baby cereal

Cold liquids: May be thickened by adding plain gelatin or jello, pureed fruits, banana flakes

Pureed fruits: May be thickened with flaked rice cereal (baby product), gelatin or jello, cooked cream of rice or wheat cereal

Pureed vegetables: May be thickened with mashed white or sweet potatoes, potato flakes, plain sauces

Pureed soups: may be thickened with potato flakes, mashed potatoes, thick sauces or gravies, or canned pureed or strained baby meat, i.e., chicken noodle soup, pureed and thickened with strained baby meat

Specific measurements for thickening agents are not given due to the variety of thicknesses desired. Reprinted with permission from Dereiko B, Stout PM. Swallowing Safely, Swallowing Nutritiously. Portland, OR, 1986.

meals. Multivitamin and mineral preparations also can be ordered by physicians for those patients requiring extradietary supplementation due to suboptimal intake.

As most texture-modified diets contain low levels of fiber, constipation often becomes problematic, especially for elderly bedridden residents who are unable or unwilling to take adequate amounts of fluid. The addition of bran to hot cereals, soup, mashed potatoes, casseroles, and dishes such as meatloaf or meatballs can be beneficial in increasing the fiber content of the diet. Prune juice can be an invaluable food item from the institution's kitchen for the prevention or treatment of constipation and serves as a thicker liquid for those dysphagic patients who are unable to manage thin liquids.

Patient food preferences must be taken into account. The incorporation of modified ethnic/cultural foods into the dysphagic diet should be done as frequently as possible. As well-described disease entities and processes affect dysphagic patients in differing ways, it is imperative that management of this group of patients should be predicated on individual plans.

Evaluation

Weight is a critical clinical parameter to monitor and evaluate the patient during the period of nutritional replenishment (Kamel 1990). Hydration status also must be monitored closely, especially when thin liquids are omitted from the oral dietary regimen. Signs of dehydration include poor skin turgor, dry mucous membranes, lack of axillary sweat, and, in the elderly, mental status changes (Kamel 1990). Laboratory tests that suggest dehydration, such as increased serum osmolality and urine osmolality with an elevated blood urea nitrogen/creatinine ratio, must be monitored closely (American Dietetic Association 1984). Strict input and output sheets should be kept on all patients who are restricted in free fluid intake. Patients on thickened liquid regimens, who complain of dry mouth and thirst, require meticulous oral hygiene. The use of lemon glycerine swabs to moisten lips and oral structures and, if tolerated, frozen Popsicles and lemon ice, can bring relief to those who are unable to take fluids ad lib or for those who complain of an accumulation of stringy, oral mucus associated with the ingestion of milk and/or other dairy products.

The success of dysphagia therapy and, often, the determination of long-term management of these patients, will largely depend on the amount of nutrition the patient can safely consume by mouth on a daily basis. Therefore, a convenient and simple method has to be implemented to record how well a patient eats. The use of food intake records or calorie counts is essential during swallowing retraining, especially for patients being tapered from enteral feedings. The nursing staff is generally responsible for documenting food and fluid intake. Dietitians should conduct continuous inservice education on procedures for recording accurate calorie counts, including standard measurements of fluid containers and portion sizes specific to the institution. A small chart with these measurements, attached to calorie count and/or input and output sheets, may facilitate greater accuracy in documenting nutrient intake. Staff also should be aware of the importance of recording all food and fluid taken by the patient by mouth, including calorie-containing condiments (sugar, jelly, margarine), between meal nourishments and supplements, food or fluid given with medication, and food items brought in by visitors.

If specific dietary modifications and feeding strategies are required after transfer from acute to chronic care facilities, the receiving institution should be alerted to any special feeding or dietary needs to ensure safe oral feeding. Inservice education on dysphagia management to staff of chronic care facilities may be necessary.

If it becomes clear that the patient cannot maintain nutritional status when fed any combination of food and fluid consistencies presented orally, supplemental tube feeding may be essential. Gastrostomy tubes may satisfy some quality of life issues, since patients may only need to rely on them on sick days, when intake is poor, for fluids only, or while taking tolerable foods orally.

SUMMARY

Priorities in the management of dysphagic patients include prevention of malnutrition and/or restoration of optimal nutritional status in those who are compromised. Registered dietitians play prime roles on dysphagia treatment teams and should be instrumental in identifying patients at risk, assessing overall nutritional status, assisting in determining the appropriate oral and/or enteral diet, and monitoring the outcome of the nutritional care plan on an ongoing basis. Providing inservice education to hospital staff at all levels, patients and/or their significant others, and staff of chronic care facilities presents a challenge to the dietetic professional in ensuring quality patient care in all settings.

REFERENCES

The American Dietetic Association. Suggested guidelines for nutrition management of the critically ill patient. Process criteria for nutrition assessment and support of selected conditions. 1984.

Bahn SL. Drug-related dental destruction. Oral Surg 1972; 33:50.

Bistrian BR, Blackburn GL, Vitale J, et al. Prevalence of malnutrition in general medical patients. JAMA 1976; 235:1567–70.

Blackburn GL, Bistrian BR, Maini BS, et al. Nutritional and metabolic assessment of the hospitalized patient. JPEN 1977; 1:12–22.

Ciocon JO. Indications for tube feedings in elderly patients. Dysphagia 1990; 5:1–5.

Cluskey MM. The use of texture modified diets among the institutionalized elderly. J Nutr Elderly 1989; 9:3–17.

Dereiko M, Stout PM. Swallowing safely, swallowing nutritiously. Portland: Dereiko and Stout, 1986.

Fleming S, Weaver AW, Brown JM. The patient with cancer affecting the head and neck: problems in nutrition. J Am Diet Assoc 1977; 70:391–94.

Goodhart RS, Shils ME. Modern nutrition in health and disease. Philadelphia: Lea & Febiger, 1980; 680.

Groher ME. Bolus management and aspiration pneumonia in patients with pseudobulbar dysphagia. Dysphagia 1987; 1:215–6.

Hynak-Hankinson MT. Dysphagia evaluation and treatment: the team approach. Nutr Supp Serv 1984; 4:33–41.

Jones PL, Altschuler SL. Dysphagia teams: a specific approach to a nonspecific problem. Dysphagia 1987; 1:200–5.

Kamel PL. Nutritional assessment and requirements. Dysphagia 1990; 4:189–95.

Lang CE, Cashman MD. Nutritional status. In: Skipper A, ed. Dietitian's handbook of enteral and parenteral nutrition. Maryland: Aspen Publishers, 1989; 5–17.

Mayes C. Pureed diets "come alive" with the right food processor. J Am Health Care Assoc 1985; 11:24–28.

Miller RM. Evaluation of swallowing disorders. In: Groher ME, ed. Dysphagia: diagnosis and management. 2nd ed. Boston: Butterworth-Heinemann Publishers, 1992; 143–62.

Murray JJ, Healy MD. Drug-mineral interactions: a new responsibility for the hospital dietitian. J Am Diet Assoc 1991; 91:66–70,73.

Sitzman JV. Nutritional support of the dysphagic patient: methods, risks, and complications of therapy. JPEN 1990; 14:60–3.

Vartan KS. Perspectives in practice: understanding instant food thickeners. The role of starches and gums in hydration. Lancaster, PA: American Institutional Products, 1989.

Zeman FJ. Clinical nutrition and dietetics. Lexington, MA: D. C. Heath and Co., 1983; 23.

12

Nursing Management of Swallowing Disorders

Barbara A. Griggs

Nurses have the best opportunity to discover a patient who is having difficulty swallowing. Basic knowledge of the anatomy and physiology of normal swallowing aids in alerting nurses to the potential problems and complications of dysphagia. Initial signs and symptoms include a subtle refusal to eat, coughing, choking, drooling, and pain. Awareness of these signs is important, particularly in older, malnourished, or chronically ill patients with no previous history of a swallowing disorder. Other patients of all ages who require careful evaluation of swallowing are those who have recently been transferred from special care units. Prior endotracheal intubation, especially for prolonged periods of time, can contribute to temporary or permanent vocal cord paralysis, leading to difficulty in swallowing and subsequent aspiration (Shapiro et al. 1975). It is well established that patients with tracheostoma tubes in place have swallowing difficulties and need careful monitoring for aspiration (Cameron et al. 1973; Taylor et al. 1981). Nurses should be conscious of these possibilities as a routine part of daily patient assessment (Loustau and Lee 1985). Patients with documented mechanical or neurogenic swallowing disorders need specialized care plans with specific therapeutic goals. Proper hydration, patent airways and nutritional support are requisite areas of meticulous and comprehensive nursing care. This chapter addresses each area with emphasis on providing timely and safe nutritional support.

HYDRATION

Thirst is the physiologic mechanism that governs hydration under normal circumstances. It is important to distinguish between thirst that can be sensed by patients who can take nothing by mouth and intubated or dysphagic patients, and that caused by failure to provide sufficient intravenous or oral fluids.

The initial and most common method of hydration in these patients is intravenous administration of physiologic solutions of water, dextrose, sodium, and potassium chloride. These solutions are administered through a needle or catheter inserted into a peripheral vein. The site of needle or catheter insertion should be changed every two to three days, or more frequently if necessary

(Goldmann et al. 1973). Care of the infusion site includes routine inspection for infiltration, pain, inflammation, or infection. Application of a povidone-iodine ointment and change of dry, sterile dressing once a day is generally accepted practice. Solutions are prepared on the patient care unit or under laminar flow hoods in the pharmacy every 24 hours. Administration set tubing, however, may be changed on a 24- or 48-hour basis according to hospital policy (Buxton et al. 1979). The unit nurse hangs the solution and monitors the infusion carefully, recording the rate and volume infused on a flow chart kept at the bedside. Hourly monitoring is necessary to ascertain complete delivery of required solutions and prevent fluid overload. Twenty-four-hour intake and output totals are also recorded as part of the patient's permanent record. Most intravenous solutions are administered by an infusion-control device.

In addition to basic fluid and electrolyte balance, parenteral solutions may be needed to administer medications. The patient may not be able to swallow the medication or, in the case of certain antibiotics, intravenous infusion may be the preferred route. Many medications are irritating to the vein wall, and therefore proper dilution and frequent site monitoring are essential to prevent phlebitis and potentially serious infiltrations.

MAINTAINING CLEAR AIRWAYS

Management of secretions is one of the first concerns encountered by patients who are having difficulty swallowing. This problem may have causes unrelated to dysphagia (i.e., dental work, fractures, oral tumors, etc.). It is important to distinguish between oral incompetence (such as drooling) and dysphagia that leads to pooling of secretions in the pharynx. Some patients with obstructive tumors or strictures of the esophagus may respond to surgical or irradiation therapy with relief of the anatomic problem. Swallowing retraining may be possible for those with neurologic disorders (see Chapters 8 and 9). Patients require extra care during the time that they are unable to handle their own secretions. Ambulatory and alert patients take care of their immediate needs when provided with proper receptacles and tissues. Bedridden or partially paralyzed patients require more assistance, including a properly supplied bedside stand that is within reach, and an aware nursing staff to respond promptly to their individual needs. Frequent short visits to check on the patient and change receptacles should be routine. The patient should be kept lying on one side and be turned every two hours. A protective pad or soft towel arranged over the pillow under the patient's head will collect saliva from drooling. This should be changed as often as necessary and accompanied by routine skin care to prevent unnecessary chapping. A dental suction tip with gentle suction to remove secretions may be helpful for some patients. The tip must be properly supported and repositioned every hour to prevent pressure points and possible skin breakdown. Alert patients can be taught to use this device by themselves.

Patients with tracheostoma tubes in place require special respiratory care. Many hospitals have chest physical therapists working with such patients on a

Table 12.1 How to Suction a Tracheostoma

Procedure	*Rationale*
Prepare equipment. Prepare patient	Less traumatic for the patient.
Wash hands	Prevents spread of nosocomial organisms
Put on sterile gloves	Apply universal precautions
Attach catheter to wall outlet	
Lubricate catheter tip with sterile saline solution	Aids catheter insertion
Remove ventilator or humidifier apparatus	
Hyperoxygenate and hyperinflate the lungs with 100 percent oxygen	Prevents hypoxemia
Insert catheter quickly but evenly into the trachea WITHOUT suction	Prevents trauma to mucous membranes
Start to remove catheter before applying suction	
Gently roll catheter while smoothly withdrawing it	
Reoxygenate and reinflate the lungs and observe patient	
Rinse catheter and connecting tubing with saline noting nature of secretions	Changes of consistency, color, or odor should be documented
Repeat procedure once if necessary	Do not suction patient excessively at one time to prevent bronchospasms and hypoxemia
Suction oropharyngeal cavity	This is done after tracheal suctioning to prevent contamination (if necessary to do first, a new catheter and glove are required)
Discard catheter, gloves, and saline solution	Prevents contamination, primarily with *Pseudomonas*
Reorganize suction materials to be available at all times	

daily basis. Staff nurses, however, must be trained in tracheostoma care, including proper suctioning technique (Fuch 1984; Goodnough 1985; Crow 1986; Hoffman and Moszkiewicz 1987) (Table 12.1).

Adequate ventilation is the first consideration for patients with a tracheostomy tube whether or not they are using a respirator. Suctioning as necessary prevents mucus build-up, tracheal obstruction, and hypoxemia. Aseptic technique is the second consideration, and cannot be overemphasized. Contamination of suction catheters and other related equipment can lead to pneumonia and compromised respiratory function (Shapiro et al. 1975; Egan 1977; Causey 1981). Third is avoidance of trauma to the mucous membranes of the trachea by proper suctioning (Nielsen 1980). Providing adequate nutritional support is often overlooked or is initiated too late. Nutritional repletion and maintenance are essential to prevent breakdown of respiratory musculature and progressive inability of the patient to breathe independently (Doekel et al. 1976; Waxman and Shoemaker 1980). Finally, patient education and communication are vital. Patients who are unable to talk or call for help become anxious, which may contribute to a decrease in their ventilatory capacity. Continuous explanations of what is happening and why will help to allay their fears. A clipboard with paper and pencil and a bell or buzzer give them a way to communicate. Patients in special care areas become dependent upon the constant presence of nursing staff. Therefore, sufficient preparation must precede the transfer to a regular care unit. A private duty nurse for several days and particularly at night may ease this transition. For some patients, regular visitation by individual family members may be enough.

A significant complication of tracheostomy is the development of a tracheoesophageal (TE) fistula. This can be caused by an overinflated cuff creating a pressure point with subsequent erosion (Hedden et al. 1969; Cooper and Grillo 1977). Proper inflation and the use of a low-pressure cuff helps to minimize this possibility. Coincident use of nasogastric tubes for suction or feeding increase liability to a TE fistula. Large, 16 to 18 French polyvinylchloride nasogastric tubes should be used only for gastric suctioning; it is no longer necessary or recommended to use them for feeding. The availability of small, soft nasogastric feeding tubes has markedly decreased the risk of TE fistula (Figure 12.1).

The most frequent complication of nasogastric feedings is aspiration of formula or gastric contents. It is important to note that an inflated tracheostoma (or endotracheal) tube cuff is not a guarantee against this. Signs and symptoms of aspiration include increased respiratory rate with labored breathing, pulmo-

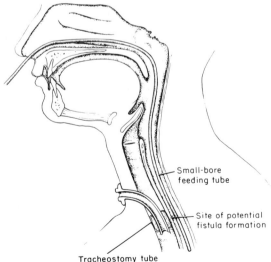

Small-bore
feeding tube

Site of potential
fistula formation

Tracheostomy tube
with cuff inflated

Figure 12.1 Site of potential tracheoesophageal fistula.

nary congestion with decreased breath sounds, cyanosis, and sweating (diaphoresis). These patients may also manifest a persistent low-grade fever. Those who are dependent on a ventilator should not be fed into the stomach because the chances of aspiration are much greater. Nasointestinal or intravenous feedings are preferred. It is probably best to wait until a patient has been weaned from the respirator before beginning nasogastric or oral feedings. Patients with dysphagia are at high risk for aspiration. Intestinal tube feedings or intravenous feedings shoud be continued until there is no evidence of reflux or aspiration through radiographic studies (Sitzmann 1990).

Guidelines for oral feeding of a patient with a tracheostoma are essentially the same as those described for the patient with a swallowing disorder in the following section. Exceptions include:

1. The tracheostoma cuff is moderately inflated prior to and for one hour following the feeding. (Patients may learn to swallow without aspiration and no longer require a cuffed tube.)
2. A test for aspiration consists of adding food coloring to a soft food such as applesauce. The tube is suctioned before the test and the patient is allowed to rest, then fed two teaspoons of the colored food. After 15 minutes, the tube is gently suctioned just beyond the end. The returns will be streaked with color if the patient has aspirated; in this circumstance feedings should be discontinued and the patient reevaluated.

NUTRITIONAL SUPPORT

Nosocomial starvation and malnutrition incident to studies and therapy have been reported in up to 50 percent of hospitalized patients (Bistrian et al. 1974, 1976; Roubenoff et al. 1987). This is especially important to note with the dysphagic patient (Groher and Bukatman 1986; Sitzmann 1990). Care givers must be aware of the rapid rate of development with which hospital-acquired malnutrition may evolve, and then do something about it by learning the current options that exist and incorporating them into daily patient therapy (Kamel 1990).

All patients should require a nutritional assessment as part of their initial physical work-up. Selected patients who are severely depleted, markedly catabolic, or who exhibit gastrointestinal symptoms require a more extensive evaluation, which is frequently done by a member of a specialized nutritional support service where available (Grant 1980). Anthropometric measurements, nitrogen balance studies, recall antigen skin testing, and oxygen consumption studies are some of the methods of nutritional assessment (Long et al. 1979; Blackburn et al. 1977). The cumulative results are then used to establish an appropriate feeding method and schedule. One must examine the cause and degree of the patients' nutritional deficit, consider the risks and benefits of each modality, and tailor immediate and long-term goals (Sitzmann and Mueller 1988; Ganger and Craig

1990). It is important to note that the evaluation of nutritional status is an ongoing process that requires reassessment as the patient's clinical condition changes.

There are two primary feeding options: enteral, using the gastrointestinal route, and parenteral, using the intravenous route. The development of parenteral hyperalimentation by Dudrick and colleagues in the late 1960s provided the means of feeding patients with nonfunctioning gastrointestinal tracts. Concurrently, elemental diets of simple protein and calorie sources that require minimal digestive capacity provided an alternate method of using the gastrointestinal tract in selected patients (Winitz et al. 1965). This heralded the beginning of specialized nutritional support as we know it today.

While parenteral hyperalimentation is an important medical advancement, patients with swallowing disorders usually have an intact gastrointestinal tract and the goal is to use this first. With special training, some patients may be able to return to oral feedings. It is important to remember that nonoral feedings should be gradually decreased, not discontinued, until the patient is able to maintain adequate oral nutrition (Logemann 1990; O'Gara 1990). For those unable to do so, there still remain two means of access to the gastrointestinal tract through noninvasive and invasive techniques; nasogastric and nasointestinal feeding tubes; percutaneous endoscopic gastrostomy and jejunostomy feeding tubes; and gastrostoma, jejunostoma, and esophagostoma feeding tubes, respectively.

FEEDINGS BY MOUTH

The oral route is the ideal way to provide required nutrients. Oral feeding is not always possible in patients with swallowing disorders, although some can be rehabilitated or trained to this method. The patient's nutritional status and the potential risk of aspiration affect the choice of feeding method. Prior to the availability of parenteral hyperalimentation, there was an urgency to have patients use the gastrointestinal tract as soon as possible, especially those who were depleted. Total parenteral nutrition may make a significant difference in the early rehabilitation of those with dysphagia, but enteral feeding remains the ultimate goal.

A formal evaluation should always precede the decision to initiate oral feedings. Once approved, the nurse's role includes proper patient preparation and supervision.

Positioning

Correct anatomic alignment will help passage of food through pharynx and esophagus with less difficulty in breathing and compromise of swallowing. Patients who can be out of bed are supported in a chair with their head and trunk flexed slightly forward. Those who remain in bed will need the head of the bed elevated and a supporting pillow at the lower back. A patient who has difficulty maintaining one position may need additional pillows on either side. A patient who slides may be stabilized by elevating the midsection of the bed or placing a pillow under the knees. A standing position is ideal for patients on circular electric beds. All patients must be relaxed and well supported in order to eat properly.

Mouth Care

Prior to the introduction of food, mouth care serves to moisten the mucous membranes of the oral cavity and stimulate salivation to prevent food sticking and possible choking. It is equally important to assist with mouth care following a meal to be sure that the oral cavity is free of small food particles that could subsequently be aspirated (Silvermann and Elfant 1979).

Suction Equipment

Suction equipment should be kept on standby for patients with a history of swallowing difficulty. It must always be available and functioning properly in case of emergency. It is best, however, to use it only when necessary because suctioning can contribute to gagging with possible regurgitation and aspiration. Patients with permanent tracheostomas requiring frequent suctioning need an organized schedule with sufficient rest time before eating to minimize this possibility.

Choice of Foods

One key to successful feeding is the choice of foods. Water is the easiest to take but the hardest to control. It goes down too fast and there is no bulk to stimulate salivation or the action of oral muscles. A semisoft solid is usually better tolerated (Hargrove 1980). (See Chapters 8 through 11 for the role of food types and their consistency.)

Close Visual Monitoring

The patient should not be left alone at mealtime. A nurse or occupational therapist should be present to assist and observe until the patient is able to swallow satisfactorily. Later the presence of an aide, a family member, or a volunteer may be sufficient. A formalized program for volunteer training and supervision can increase safety for patients during meals (Lipner et al. 1990). If not in direct attendance, nurses should be alert to potential problems and be prepared to respond quickly if called. Eating takes time and rushing a meal can be hazardous for any patient, but especially for the one with dysphagia, who may also become exhausted by the technical difficulties associated with eating. Smaller, more frequent meals may be better tolerated.

Table 12.2 Insertion Procedure for Nasogastric Feeding Tube (with Guidewire)

Procedure	Rationale
1. Prepare equipment; measure and mark feeding tube	The tube should be measured for each patient as a guide to ensure proper tip location
2. Position patient in bed at a 45 degree angle with a pillow behind the shoulders	Patients seem more secure in bed than in a chair. Bed height can be adjusted to make insertion easier
3. Have patient blow nose, and check each nostril for the side that allows for greater air passage	Nose spray may be helpful for some patients
4. Place protective drape over patient's chest, and emesis basin and tissues in patient's lap	The patient and bed area should be kept clean. Difficulties are not expected but they can arise
5. Ask patient to hold cup of water with a straw	
6. Lubricate distal end of feeding tube	Creates less friction and discomfort in nasal passage
7. Ask patient to tilt head back slightly	It is easier to insert tube in this position
8. Insert tip of tube approximately 2 inches into the nostril	See Figure 12.2
9. Ask patient to tilt head down	Closes trachea and opens esophagus
10. While advancing tube ask patient to drink water through the straw	(Figures 12.3 and 12.4). Swallowing will close epiglottis to allow passage of tube into esophagus rather than trachea
11. If there is resistance, STOP and remove feeding tube, then get assistance	To avoid nasopulmonary intubation
12. Let patient rest, then try again, following steps 6 through 10	
13. Continue advancing tube while patient swallows water until the mark is reached and feeding tube is in the body of the stomach	(Figure 12.5). Tube should go in by gravity but swallowing makes procedure easier for the patient. Water seems to work better than ice chips for most patients
	Rubbing the throat of an unconscious patient helps to stimulate swallowing
14. Loop exposed end of feeding tube, hold securely with nondominant hand approximately 3 inches from the nostril, and gently but firmly pull out guidewire with dominant hand	(Figure 12.6). Patient may feel more comfortable holding tube to keep it from partially pulling out
15. Check position of feeding tube	Tube position MUST be checked before feeding begins
Gently aspirate stomach contents with 50-mL syringe	An adapter may be needed for a more secure seal. Tubes smaller than 8

Table 12.2 Insertion Procedure for Nasogastric Feeding Tube (with Guidewire) *(continued)*

Procedure	Rationale
	French have a tendency to collapse on themselves and therefore should be used primarily when aspiration is not a factor or for supplemental feedings (this refers to nasogastric tubes)
With a stethoscope over left upper quadrant, instill 10 mL of air into feeding tube with syringe	The sound of air entering stomach can be heard. With smaller tubes, 20 mL of air may be necessary
Obtain an x-ray either routinely or if there is any question of tube position	Tubes are radiopaque to enable visualization
16. Tape feeding tube in place	Tube must be secure to prevent accidental slippage
Cleanse nose and cheek with alcohol wipe	To remove perspiration and skin oils
Pour tincture of benzoin onto sponge and wipe nose, cheek, and tube. Let air dry	To protect skin and aid with adherence of tape
Apply small piece of tape, with one split end to nose. Wrap ends in opposite directions around the tube	Too large a piece can focus patient's attention to tip of his nose. When it is necessary to avoid tape, cotton tracheostomy tape can be tied around tube and then around patient's head. Avoid pressure on nostril to prevent subsequent breakdown
Use tape to secure tube to cheek	(Figure 12.7). Alert, cooperative patients can use only cheek tape to secure feeding tube. Change tape as necessary

This is the procedure with a conscious, cooperative patient. An assistant may be necessary if patient is unconscious or uncooperative.

Education

Education of patient and family is a well-established nursing role. Careful explanations of what the nurse is doing and why relieve anxiety and fear and elicit greater cooperation and success. An explanation comes first, but time and patience must follow.

NONINVASIVE TUBE FEEDING METHODS

When a patient is unable to eat by mouth but has a functioning gastrointestinal tract, the best option is tube feeding. Nasogastric feeding tubes and enteral formulas have been in existence for many years.

Table 12.3 Modifications for Insertion of Nasointestinal Feeding Tube

Insert an additional 25 to 35 cm of tubing into stomach
Wait for tube passage into intestines:
  1 to 2 hours for ambulatory patients
  24 hours or more for bedridden patients
  If tube does not pass spontaneously, manual passage by fluoroscopy or endoscopy
    may be necessary
Document exact position of feeding tube prior to initiation of tube feeding (Figure
  12.8)

Nasogastric/Intestinal Feeding Tube

The decision to use a nasogastric or a nasointestinal feeding tube is, in part, based upon the presence or absence of a gag reflex and the risk of aspiration. Patients with some reflex, who are awake and alert, can be fed nasogastrically. For those with absent gag reflexes and a history or incidence of aspiration, the safest method is nasointestinally (Rombeau and Barot 1981). The difference between these tubes is primarily the size of the weighted tip and the length of tube that is inserted. Most nasogastric tubes have small tungsten weights that are the same, or slightly larger, in diameter than the rest of the tube. Nasointestinal tubes usually have larger bolus weights, also of tungsten, at their tips to help with their spontaneous passage through the pylorus into the small intestine. The number of tubes that pass spontaneously within 48 hours varies depending on the patient's position, ambulatory versus bedridden, and the presence of decreased gastric motility. Metoclopramide has been used successfully to aid intestinal passage when given prior to tube insertion (Whatley et al. 1984). Fluoroscopic (Grant et al. 1983) and endoscopic placement of nasointestinal feeding tubes has become common when immediate nutritional intervention is required. The regular insertion procedure is approximately the same for both. This is outlined step by step in Table 12.2 and Figures 12.2 and 12.3. Modifications for a nasointestinal tube insertion are given in Table 12.3.

Administration

There are two methods of tube feeding, continuous or intermittent. The continuous method is necessary for intestinal feedings or when the patient can tolerate only small volumes of formula at one time. For some patients, continuous feedings are better absorbed, thus increasing the number of calories provided on a daily basis. Continuous feeding implies 24 hours per day. Some patients, however, are able to tolerate larger volumes per hour, with feedings running 8 to 16 continuous hours, either during the day and evening or during the night (Bloch 1987). Intermittent feedings are given hourly or every three to four hours. They are generally initiated on an hourly basis, and graduated in schedule toward less frequent, larger-volume feedings. This becomes especially important if the patient will be continuing tube feedings on hospital discharge.

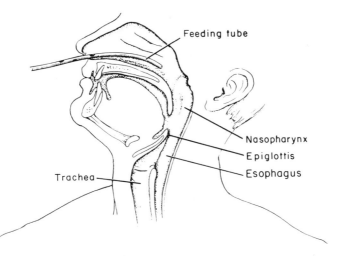

Figure 12.2 Insertion of feeding tube into the nostril.

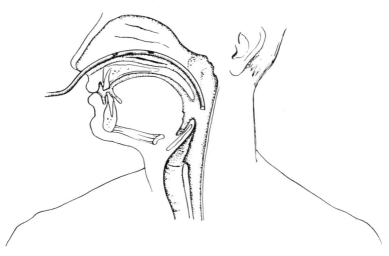

Figure 12.3 The feeding tube is guided into the nasopharynx.

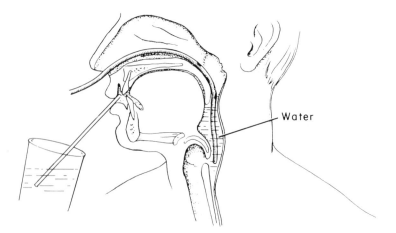

Figure 12.4   Advancement of the feeding tube with the water bolus.

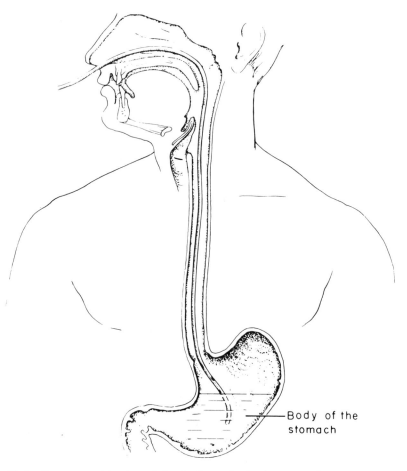

Figure 12.5   Correct positioning of the feeding tube in the stomach.

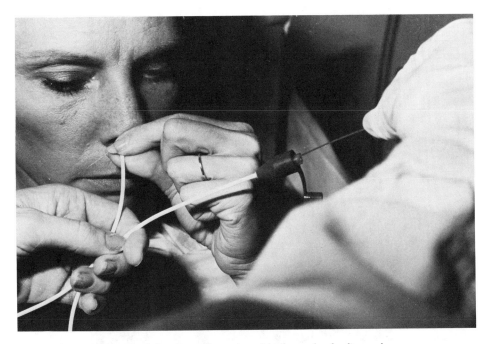

Figure 12.6 Removal of the monofilament guide from the feeding tube.

Tube feedings had been routinely administered by gravity drip; however, with the development of enteral hyperalimentation, enteral feeding pumps are predominantly used today for continuous feedings (gravity drip is more common for intermittent feedings). These pumps are less complicated than intravenous infusion devices and also less expensive (Figure 12.9). They enable more accurate administration of continuous feedings and save nursing time.

Whether tube feedings are administered continuously or intermittently, by gravity drip or by enteral pump, they all should start slowly with small volumes. Hypertonic formulas should be initially diluted; however, it is not necessary to dilute isotonic formulas. The amount is then increased every day, as tolerated, until the patient's caloric requirement has been met. This may take several days depending on formula osmolality and patient tolerance. When the maintenance rate has been achieved, adjustments can be made in the frequency and total volume of each feeding. The average adult 70-kg male, nonstressed patient will need 30 to 35 kcal per kg, or a range of 2,100 to 2,400 calories per day. Surgery and sepsis increase patient requirements to 40 to 45 kcal per kg (Walters and Freeman 1981).

Complications

The two main complications associated with tube feeding administration are aspiration and diarrhea. Decreased incidence or prevention of both can be accomplished by adhering to the following guidelines:

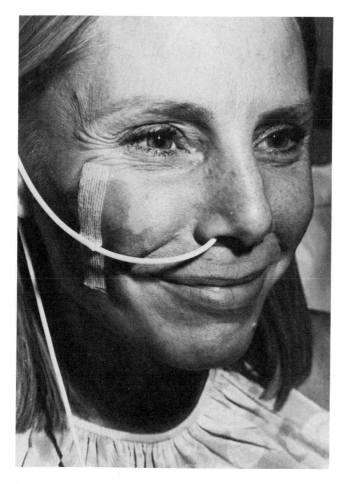

Figure 12.7 Steri-strip taping of the feeding tube.

1. Elevate the head of the bed at least 30 degrees during continuous feeding and prior to and one hour after intermittent feeding.
2. Aspirate the feeding tube routinely to check for absorption of the formula. Progressively increasing residual volumes, nausea, abdominal distention, and discomfort should alert the nurse to hold the feeding and notify the physician to re-evaluate the patient. Residual volumes to 150 to 200 mL should be questioned.
3. Administer intermittent feedings by slow, gravity drip rather than as a bolus.
4. Coordinate with the dietitian the most appropriate formula for the patient.
5. Administer antidiarrheal preparations as necessary.
6. Monitor fluid and electrolyte balance daily.

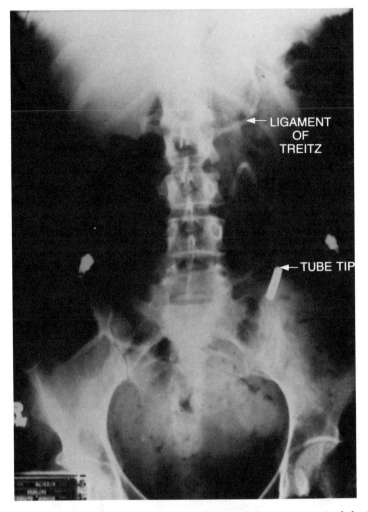

Figure 12.8 Radiographic documentation of the tip of the nasointestinal feeding tube must take place before feedings begin.

SURGICAL GASTROSTOMY, JEJUNOSTOMY, AND ESOPHAGOSTOMY

Patients who require tube feedings for prolonged or indefinite periods of time can be considered candidates for a surgically placed gastrostomy, jejunostomy, or esophagostomy. Surgical insertion of feeding tubes into the stomach, intestine, or esophagus is a sterile procedure that may necessitate general anesthesia. It may be a relatively short, minor procedure or a more extensive, major one depending upon the choice of procedure and the patient's condition. Occasionally, procedures are performed under local anesthesia in selected patients

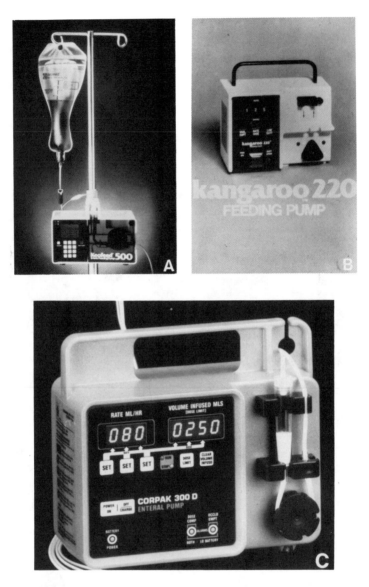

Figure 12.9 Examples of infusion-control devices specific for enteral formulations. (A) Keofeed 500 enteric feeding pump (Keofeed is a registered trademark of IVAC Corporation), (B) Kangaroo 220 feeding pump (Kangaroo is a registered trademark of Sherwood Medical), (C) Corpak 300D Enteral Pump (courtesy of Corpak, Inc.).

when general anesthesia is risky or contraindicated. Development of the needle-catheter jejunostomy has increased the use of this access route (Delaney 1973; Delaney et al. 1977). (For a detailed explanation of these surgical procedures see Chapter 13.)

The nursing care of a patient with an ostomy tube includes keeping the tube intact and patent, preventing local skin irritation, providing accurate infusions, and monitoring for potential complications.

Procedures for keeping the tube intact and patent depend on the type of tube that is inserted. All tubes are sutured in place at least initially, but inadvertent tension primarily from the administration tubing and connector can contribute to its dislodgment. Many tubes used for gastrostomies are large, 16 to 18 French, and therefore need to be taped more securely. The tape should be pinched completely around the tube, leaving about one to one and a half inches of tape on either side for adherence. Jejunostoma tubes are smaller, 5 to 8 French, but longer. The additional tubing should be coiled and taped securely, with a protective gauze covering, until the site is healed and when not in use. Esophagostoma tubes vary from red rubber catheters to smaller, soft, weighted tubes. The tubes may be sutured until a tract is formed. For some patients, the tube can be removed and be reinserted for each feeding. Unlike the noninvasive feeding tubes, gastrostoma/jejunostoma or new esophagostoma feeding tubes require surgical replacement if accidentally pulled out.

Skin cleansing and the application of a skin adherent, such as tincture of benzoin, help to prevent tissue breakdown. Changing the tape as necessary and moving the tube to alternate sides will also help to maintain skin integrity. The ostomy tube exit site is protected by a dry, sterile dressing. When gastrostoma tubes are used for intermittent feedings, the end of the tube must be clamped and covered with a gauze sponge between feedings to prevent backflow of gastric contents, which are extremely irritating. The area around eosphagostoma tubes requires more frequent skin care because of the possibility of saliva draining through the opening.

The administration of ostomy tube feedings is essentially the same as for noninvasive tube feedings, with two exceptions. First, patients with esophagostomies rarely have difficulty tolerating larger volumes of formula (350 to 500 mL) administered by gravity drip every three to four hours. We should always be aware, however, that the patients can aspirate. Second, needle-catheter jejunostomies with a 16-gauge catheter require an elemental diet and an infusion control device to guarantee consistent flow (Freeman et al. 1976).

The complications for ostomy tube feedings include postoperative edema, bleeding, tube dislodgment, and peritonitis as well as aspiration and diarrhea. The surgical procedure is short and nontraumatic for most patients. However, any incision and tissue manipulation can result in edema and bleeding. Small pressure dressings are applied in the operating room and remain in place at least overnight. Proper taping to secure the feeding tube has been previously stressed. Dislodgment could lead to leakage of gastrointestinal secretions into the peritoneal cavity and the possibility of peritonitis (Torosian and Rombeau 1980).

Patients with esophagostomas must also be closely monitored for tracheal obstruction in the early postoperative period.

PERCUTANEOUS ENDOSCOPIC GASTROSTOMY AND JEJUNOSTOMY

Another category of invasive feeding tubes includes those that are placed percutaneously. Since first described (Gauderer et al. 1980), the percutaneous endoscopic gastrostomy (PEG) has become a routine procedure in many hospitals. The primary advantage is that the procedure can be performed under local anesthesia in an endoscopy suite. Percutaneously placed gastrostomies require less time to perform and, in general, have fewer complications when compared with surgical procedures.

There are two predominant placement techniques, the Ponsky-Gauderer pull technique (Ponsky et al. 1985) and the Sachs-Vine push technique (Hogan et al. 1986). The technique selected appears to be based on physician preference. A 20 or 22 French tube is the most common size for adult patients. Less frequently used is the Russell technique (Russell et al. 1984), which uses a 14 French Foley catheter. The same formulas are used for nutritional support as those used with small-bore feeding tubes. PEG tubes have the additional advantage of a larger size, consequently formulas and medications, when applicable, are easily administered, with a decreased risk of clogging. Formulas may be administered by enteral feeding pump or gravity drip, continuously or intermittently. Feedings are usually initiated the day following the procedure.

The care of the PEG exit site is less involved than a surgical gastrostomy. There are fewer complications related to wound dehiscence, gastrointestinal bleeding, and leakage of gastric contents. Povidone-iodine ointment is generally applied at the exit site for 24 to 48 hours. Frequently no dressing is applied during the postinsertion period nor is one recommended for long-term maintenance. Daily soap and water cleansing, along with exit site inspection, comprises routine care. PEG tubes come with a variety of exit site stabilization devices. Most also require taping the tube to alleviate tension and potential irritation. Exit site complications are managed similarly to surgical gastrostomies.

Initially the complication rate for PEG tubes was low (Ponsky et al. 1983). As this procedure has gained in popularity, and higher risk patients have been selected, the complication rate has increased. It does, however, remain a well-accepted, simple procedure, with a relatively low complication rate (Kirby et al. 1986; Weg and Miskovitz 1987). In general, a patient who requires long-term tube feedings should be considered a candidate for a PEG.

The risk of aspiration in the compromised patient is the same for a PEG tube as for a nasogastric tube. Consequently an 8 or 10 French feeding tube is passed through the PEG tube into the intestines in these patients. When indicated, gastric decompression can be accomplished along with the formula administra-

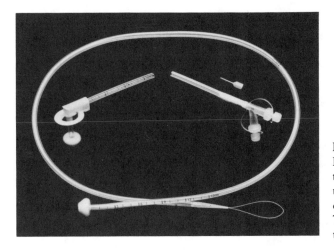

Figure 12.10 The Bower® PEG System with polyurethane retention balloon, unique fixation device, and combination Luer lock and Twoomey Y-adaptor (courtesy of Corpak, Inc.).

tion. This has been described as a percutaneous endoscopic jejunostomy (PEJ) (Ponsky and Aszodi 1984; Gottfried and Plumser 1984).

PARENTERAL NUTRITIONAL SUPPORT

The original indication for total parenteral nutrition (TPN) was for the patient with a nonfunctioning gastrointestinal tract. There are additional indications when adequate oral intake is inappropriate or even hazardous. These include patients who are malnourished or severely depleted and those who have obstructions or inflammation of the central nervous system or upper gastrointestinal tract. For example, a patient who has had a recent cerebrovascular accident and has no protective reflexes is at risk of aspiration. Similarly, a patient receiving irradiation therapy to the oral cavity or esophagus who cannot swallow. These patients can benefit from parenteral nutritional support until their conditions stabilize and a long-range nutritional plan is made. There are two methods of providing parenteral hyperalimentation: central, or total parenteral nutrition (TPN), and peripheral parenteral nutrition (PPN).

Total Parenteral Nutrition

Total parenteral nutrition is the administration of a complete metabolic diet through a central venous route. The components are carbohydrates as hypertonic dextrose, protein as synthetic amino acids, plus essential electrolytes, trace minerals, and vitamins (Dudrick et al. 1969; Shils 1972). Fat as either soybean or safflower oil is provided separately (Hansen et al. 1976; Pelham 1981). A typical TPN dextrose/amino acid solution contains approximately 25 percent dextrose and 50 g amino acids in one liter and is equivalent to 1 calorie per mL. The average patient receives 1,800 to 2,400 mL per day. When used as a caloric source, fat comprises one-third of the daily required calories (Meguid et al. 1982). Intravenous fat emulsion may be administered daily as 3-in-1 solution, combined with the dextrose and amino acids or given twice a week to prevent essential fatty acid deficiency (Riela et al. 1975; Faulkner and Flint 1977).

Hypertonic solution is irritating to peripheral veins and for this reason central venous access is necessary. A subclavian or internal jugular vein is most commonly used as an entry point for the catheter. This is a sterile procedure performed at the bedside for most patients. The catheter is threaded to its correct position in the superior vena cava; its position is documented by x-ray. The solution is ordered by the physician and prepared daily in the pharmacy under a laminar flow hood. The nurse administers the solution by an infusion-control device to ensure accuracy. In addition, the patient is closely monitored through vital signs, weight, intake and output record, urine spot tests, and routine blood tests of electrolytes, glucose, renal and liver function plus selected other values based on the individual's condition.

The complications of TPN therapy can be significant, and require awareness and professional skill to minimize or prevent their occurrence. Pneumothorax is the most common major complication associated with central venous catheterization (Mitchell and Clark 1979). Proper patient preparation and physician training will markedly decrease this possibility. The TPN catheter provides direct access to the central bloodstream and the average length of therapy for most acutely ill patients is four to six weeks. Therefore meticulous catheter care is essential. Catheter dressings are changed approximately three times a week based on hospital policy and the type of dressing material that is used. The dressing change is a sterile procedure requiring mask and gloves. A defatting agent may be used initially, then a form of povidone-iodine (solution and/or ointment) is applied (Figure 12.11). Small gauze dressings are sufficient to protect the catheter exit site because there is no drainage (Figure 12.12). A skin adhesive is recommended and finally the area is occlusively taped by one of the many tapes currently available (Figure 12.13).

The tubing used to administer TPN solution, including pump cassette, is changed every 24 hours (Goldmann and Maki 1973). This can become a routine procedure with the first container of each day. Care in handling the solution and tubing is necessary to prevent contamination and possible infection. Proper taping of the tubing will prevent separation at the catheter hub and leakage of solution, blood, or air. A wet dressing increases the chance of infection. Blood back-up can cause the catheter to clot and abrupt cessation of the solution flow, leading to a hypoglycemic episode and catheter replacement. Finally, air leakage may mean an air embolism. All three of these potential complications are avoidable through proper attention to details of care.

The most common metabolic complication of TPN is hyperglycemia because of the high concentrations of dextrose that are infused. To prevent this, one should first start at a low infusion rate, about 30 to 40 mL per hour, and gradually increase the rate over several days while closely monitoring levels of blood and urine sugar. Second, it is important to be aware of those patients who

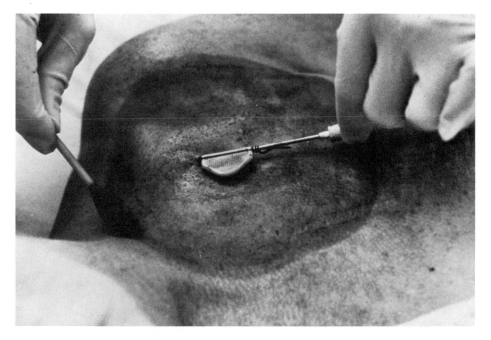

Figure 12.11 Application of povidone-iodine solution.

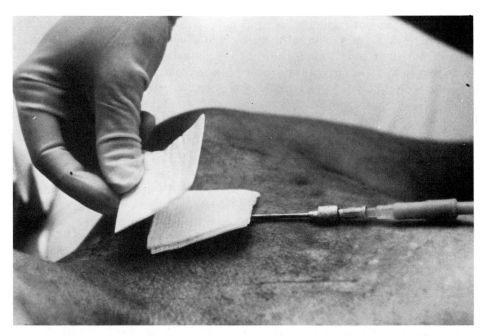

12.12 Gauze dressings are used to protect the catheter exit site.

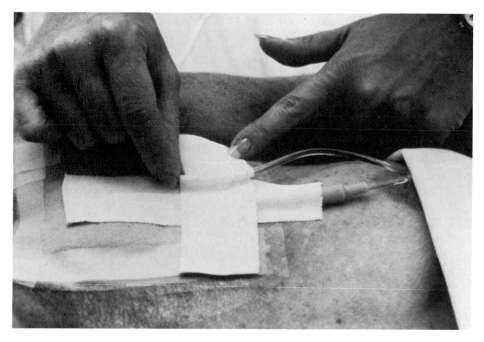

Figure 12.13 The final occlusive dressing.

are susceptible to glucose intolerance and add regular insulin to the TPN solution as necessary to avoid glucosuria and keep blood glucose levels within normal range (Dudrick et al. 1972). Other metabolic imbalances occur due to the patient's depleted or disease state and can be controlled by additions to or deletions from the TPN solution as determined by regularly scheduled laboratory monitoring. Deficiencies of essential fatty acids and trace minerals were a problem before safe intravenous fat emulsions and trace mineral preparations became available for routine administration.

Peripheral Parenteral Nutrition

Patients who need only short-term parenteral therapy, for example, seven to ten days, before starting oral or tube feedings may be able to benefit from PPN. It is made up of the same components as TPN; however, the dextrose/amino acid solution is less concentrated and comprises only half of the total therapy volume. The other half is administered as fat. Consequently, it takes one to one and a half liters of dextrose/amino acids and one to one and a half liters of 10 percent fat emulsion to provide approximately 1,400 to 2,000 calories per day (Dietel and Kaminsky 1974; Freeman 1978). The advantage of PPN solutions is that they can be administered by peripheral vein. Disadvantges are unavailability of peripheral veins and the patient's inability to tolerate the total volume of fluid and fat (Walters and Freeman 1981). Patients with cardiac or renal disorders, severe liver disease, pulmonary disease, or blood coagulation disorders are rarely candidates for this therapy (Silberman et al. 1977). Unless contraindicated, PPN may be used for the dysphagic patient who is undergoing a feeding trial. This provides sufficient calories without interference of a nasogastric or nasointestinal feeding tube.

A peripheral catheter or needle is inserted under sterile conditions and changed every 48 to 72 hours (Goldmann et al. 1973). The site is inspected hourly for signs of inflammation or infiltration. Solutions are prepared in the pharmacy on a daily basis. They are usually administered by infusion-control devices, with changes of intravenous tubing every 24 hours. A dry, sterile dressing is changed daily, with similar skin care as with central catheters, although mask and gloves are not worn. Patient monitoring is the same for both TPN and PPN.

Complications of PPN relate mainly to the infusion site. Irritation of the vein wall with painful phlebitis or infiltration is common (Gazitua et al. 1979; Massar et al. 1982). Local infection with bacteremias is rare, but does occur. Too rapid administration may lead to fluid overload and respiratory distress. Each of these complications is preventable with careful and frequent patient observations.

SUMMARY

It is important for all nurses to be familiar with the pathology of swallowing disorders, including the differences between those of neurologic, mechanical, and psychiatric origin. The specific signs and symptoms and the current treatment modalities affect daily and long-term care plans for each patient. The nursing mangement of dysphagic patients requires knowledge, skill, and patience. Attention to proper hydration and clear airways should be followed by early nutritional intervention. There is no question today that nutritional support should be a consideration for each patient. Enteral and parenteral feeding methods are available and provide options, through one or a combination of therapies, to meet the needs of all of our patients.

REFERENCES

Bistrian B, Blackburn G, Hallowell E, Heddle M. Protein status of general surgical patients. JAMA 1974; 230:858–60.

Bistrian B, Blackburn G, Vitale J, Cochran D, Naylor J. Prevalence of malnutrition in general medical patients. JAMA 1976; 235:1567–70.

Blackburn G, Bistrian B, Maini B, Schlamm H, Smith M. Nutritional and metabolic assessment of the hospitalized patient. J Parent Ent Nutr 1977; 1:11–22.

Bloch A. Nocturnal tube feedings. Dysphagia 1987; 2:3–7.

Buxton A, Highsmith A, Garner J, et al. Contamination of intravenous infusion fluid; effects of changing administration sets. Ann Intern Med 1979; 90:764–68.

Cameron J, Reynolds J, Zuidema G. Aspiration in patients with tracheostomies. Surg Gynecol Obstet 1973; 136:68–70.

Causey W. Infections complicating mechanical ventilation. In: Rattenborg C, Via-Reque E, eds. Clinical use of mechanical ventilation. Chicago, London: Yearbook Medical Publishers, 1981; 26:280–91.

Cooper J, Grillo H. Analysis of problems related to cuffs in intratracheal tubes. In: Rogers R, ed. Respiratory intensive care. Springfield, IL.: Charles C Thomas, 1977; 245–60.

Crow S. Tips for successful respiratory suctioning. RN 1986; 31–33.

Deitel M, Kaminsky V. Total nutrition by peripheral vein—the lipid system. Can Med Assoc J 1974; 111:152–54.

Delaney H, Carnevale N, Garvey J. Jejunostomy by a needle-catheter technique. Surgery 1973; 73:786–90.

Delaney H, Carnevale N, Garvey J, Moss C. Postoperative nutritional support using needle-catheter-feeding jejunostomy. Ann Surg 1977; 186:165–70.

Doekel R, Zwillich C, Scoggin C, Kryger M, Weil J. Clinical semi-starvation; depression of hypoxic ventilatory response. N Engl J Med 1976; 295:358–61.

Dudrick S, Macfadyen B, VanBuren C, Ruberg R, Maynard A. Parenteral hyperalimentation; metabolic problems and solutions. Ann Surg 1972; 176:259–62.

Dudrick S, Wilmore D, Vars H, Rhoads J. Long-term total parenteral nutrition with growth development and positive nitrogen balance. Surgery 1968; 64:134–42.

Dudrick S, Wilmore D, Vars H, Rhoads J. Can intravenous feeding as the sole means of nutrition support growth in the child and restore weight loss in an adult? Ann Surg 1969; 169:974–84.

Egan D. Fundamentals of respiratory therapy. St. Louis: C V Mosby, 1977.

Faulkner W, Flint L. Essential fatty acid deficiency associated with total parenteral nutrition. Surg Gynecol Obstet 1977; 144:665–67.

Freeman J. Peripheral parenteral nutrition. Can J Surg 1978; 21:489–92.

Freeman J, Egan M, Millis B. The elemental diet. Surg Gynecol Obstet 1976; 142: 925–32.

Fuch P. Streamlining your suctioning techniques, part 3, tracheostomy suctioning. Nursing 1984; 39–43.

Ganger D, Craig R. Swallowing disorders and nutritional support. Dysphagia 1990; 4:213–19.

Gauderer M, Ponsky J, Izant R. Gastrostomy without laparotomy: A percutaneous endoscopic technique. J Pediatr Surg 1980; 15:872–75.

Gazitua R, Wilson K, Bistrian B, Blackburn G. Factors determining peripheral vein tolerance to amino acid infusions. Arch Surg 1979; 114:897–900.

Goldmann D, Maki D. Infection control in total parenteral nutrition. JAMA 1973; 223:1360–64.

Goldmann D, Maki D, Rhame F, Kaiser A, Tenney J, Bennett J. Guidelines for infection control in intravenous therapy. Ann Intern Med 1973; 79:848–50.

Goodnough S. The effects of oxygen and hyperinflation on arterial oxygen tension after endotracheal suctioning. Heart Lung 1985; 14:11–17.

Gottsfried E, Plumser A. Endoscopic gastrojejunostomy: a technique to establish small bowel feeding without laparotomy. Gastrointest Endosc 1984; 30:355–59.

Grant J. A team approach: handbook of total parenteral nutrition. Philadelphia: WB Saunders, 1980.

Grant J, Curtas M, Kelvin F. Fluoroscopic placement of nasojejunal feeding tubes with immediate feeding using a nonelemental diet. JPEN 1983; 3:299–303.

Groher M, Bukatman R. The prevalence of swallowing disorders in two teaching hospitals. Dysphagia 1986; 1:3–6.

Hansen L, Hardie B, Hildalgo J. Fat emulsion for intravenous administration: clinical experience with Intralipid 10%. Ann Surg 1976; 184:80–88.

Hargrove R. Feeding the severely dysphagic patient. J Neurosurg Nurs 1980; 12:102–7.

Hedden M, Ersoz C, Safar P. Tracheoesophageal fistulas following prolonged artificial ventilation via cuffed tracheostomy tubes. Anesthesiology 1969; 31:281–89.

Hoffman L, Moszkiewicz R. Airway management for the critically ill patient. AJN 1987; 39–53.

Hogan R, DeMarco D, Hamilton J, et al. Percutaneous endoscopic gastrostomy—to push or pull. Gastroinvest Endosc 1986; 32:253–58.

Lipner H, Bosler J, Giles G. Volunteer participation in feeding residents: training and supervision in a long-term care facility. Dysphagia 1990; 5:89–95.

Logemann J. Factors affecting ability to resume oral nutrition in the oropharyngeal dysphagic individual. Dysphagia 1990; 4:202–8.

Long C, Schaffel N, Geiger J, Schiller N, Blakemore W. Metabolic response to injury and illness: the establishment of energy and protein needs from indirect calorimetry and nitrogen balance. J Parent Ent Nutr 1979; 3:452–56.

Loustau A, Lee K. Dealing with the dangers of dysphagia. Nursing 1985; 47–50.

Kamel P. Nutritional assessment and requirements. Dysphagia 1990; 4:189–95.

Kirby D, Craig R, Tsang T-K, et al. Percutaneous endoscopic gastrostomies: A prospective evaluation and review of the literature. JPEN 1986; 10:155–59.

Massar E, Daly J, Copeland E, Johnson D, et al. Peripheral vein complications in patients receiving amino acid/dextrose solutions. J Parent Ent Nutr 1982; 7:159–62.

Meguid M, Schimmel E, Johnson W, et al. Reduced metabolic complications in total parenteral nutrition: pilot study using fat to replace one-third of glucose calories. J Parent Ent Nutr 1982; 6:304–7.

Mitchell S, Clark R. Complications of central venous catheterization. Am J Roentgenol 1979; 133:467–76.

Nielsen L. Potential problems of mechanical ventilation. Am J Nurs 1980; 80:2206–13.

O'Gara J. Dietary adjustments and nutritional therapy during treatment for oral-pharyngeal dysphagia. Dysphagia 1990; 4:209–12.

Pelham, L. Rational use of intravenous fat emulsions. Am J Hosp Pharm 1981; 38:198–208.

Ponsky J, Gauderer M, Stellato T. Percutaneous endoscopic gastrostomy: Review of 150 cases. Arch Surg 1983; 118:913–14.

Ponsky J, Aszodi A. Percutaneous endoscopic jejunostomy. Am J Gastroenterol 1984; 79:113–16.

Ponsky J, Gauderer M, Stellato T, et al. Percutaneous approaches to enteral alimentation. Am J Surg 1985; 149:102–5.

Riela M, Broviac J, Wells M, Scribner B. Essential fatty acid deficiency in human adults during total parenteral nutrition. Ann Intern Med 1975; 83:786–89.

Rombeau J, Barot L. Enteral nutrition therapy. In: Mullen J, Crosby L, Rombeau J, eds. The surgical clinics of North America: symposium on surgical nutrition. Philadelphia: WB Saunders 1981; 610–11.

Roubenoff R, Preto J, Balke C. Malnutrition among hospitalized patients. A problem of physician awareness. Arch Intern Med 1987; 147:1462–65.

Russell T, Brotman M, Norris F. Percutaneous gastrostomy. A new simplified and cost-effective technique. Am J Surg 1984; 189:132–37.

Shapiro S, Harrison R, Trout C. Maintenance of artificial airways of extubation. In: Shapiro S et al., eds. Clinical application of respiratory care. Chicago: Yearbook Medical Publishers, 1975; 16:254–9.

Shils M. Guidelines for total parenteral nutrition. JAMA 1972; 220:1921–29.

Silberman H, Freehauf M, Fong G, Rosenblatt N. Parenteral nutrition with lipids. JAMA 1977; 238:1380–82.

Silverman E, Elfant I. Dysphagia: an evaluation and treatment program for the adult. Am J Occup Ther 1979; 33:382–92.

Sitzmann J, Mueller B. Enteral and parenteral feeding in the dysphagic patient. Dysphagia 1988; 3:38–45.

Sitzmann J. Nutritional support of the dysphagic patient: methods, risks, and complications of therapy. JPEN 1990; 1:60–63.

Taylor H, Mhoon E, Matz G. Complications due to tracheostomy and endotracheal tubes.

In: Rattenberg C, Via-Reque E, eds. Clinical use of mechanical ventilation. Chicago, London: Yearbook Medical Publishers, 1981; 25:273–75.

Torosian M, Rombeau J. Feeding by tube enterostomy. Surg Gynecol Obstet 1980; 150:918–27.

Walters J, Freeman J. Parenteral nutrition by peripheral vein. In: Mullen J, Crosby L, Rombeau J, eds. The surgical clinics of North America: symposium on surgical nutrition. Philadelphia: WB Saunders, 1981; 593–4.

Waxman K, Shoemaker W. Management of postoperative and posttraumatic respiratory failure in the ICU. In: Bartlett R, ed. The surgical clinics of North America: symposium on respiratory care in surgery. Philadelphia: WB Saunders, 1980; 1424–25.

Weg A, Miskovitz P. Percutaneous endoscopic gastrostomy (PEG): a critical appraisal. Dysphagia 1987; 1:227–31.

Whatley K, Turner W, Dey M, et al. When does metoclopramide facilitate transpyloric intubation? JPEN 1984; 6:679–81.

Winitz M, Graff J, Gallagher N. Evaluation of chemical diets as nutrition for man-in-space. Nature 1965; 205:741–43.

13

Surgical Intervention in Dysphagia

Gregory F. Hulka
Harold C. Pillsbury III

Surgical intervention in patients with dysphagia is directed toward reestablishing normal physiology or bypassing known lesions and abnormalities of the upper digestive tract. A thorough understanding of the normal anatomy and physiology of this region is therefore necessary to plan surgical therapy for patients with dysphagia. From an evolutionary point of view, the primary function of the larynx is sphincteric protection of the airway, and therefore management of disorders of deglutition must preserve this important function of the upper airway. As a complete discussion of the anatomy and physiology of the upper aerodigestive tract is given elsewhere in this text, only a brief overview is given here. The major sites of surgically treatable dysphagia are discussed, along with methods of intervention.

FUNCTIONAL ANATOMY

The act of swallowing can be broken into three stages (see Chapter 1): oral, pharyngeal, and esophageal. The first stage is voluntary, consisting of mastication, following which the muscles of the mouth and tongue mold the food bolus and push it back toward the posterior wall of the oropharynx. As the bolus moves posteriorly, the pharyngeal stage of swallowing begins as a combination of voluntary and involuntary actions. Contraction of the velopharyngeal muscles of the soft palate and the superior constrictor function to close off the nasopharynx from the oropharynx. The tongue continues to project the food bolus into the oropharynx, and this dorsal projection bends the epiglottis horizontally to cover the aditus of the larynx. Simultaneous contraction of the stylopharyngeus muscle to elevate the larynx and relaxation of the hypopharynx allow the bolus to descend downward toward the esophageal inlet.

The final stage of swallowing begins with the temporary relaxation of the upper esophageal sphincter (classically described as the cricopharyngeus muscle), located approximately at the level of C6–C7. This allows passage of the bolus into the esophagus, initiating involuntary peristalsis. The upper sphincter then resumes its normal resting tone, the larynx descends, and the epiglottis projects back into its normal upright position.

The Oral Stage

Fortunately, dysphagia during this stage of swallowing is least common because surgical treatment is limited. Hypoglossal paralysis, whether following stroke or surgery is treated with limited success. Some authors describe techniques of cross-innervation for hypoglossal paralysis. Using a midline Z-plasty incision, a portion of the tongue mucosa and underlying muscle from the unaffected side is sewn into the affected side, reintroducing innervation to the paralyzed half of the tongue. This technique is most successful when performed soon after the onset of the paralysis, as the motor end-plates have a limited lifespan following deinnervation.

Patients also may suffer from dysphagia in this stage of deglutition because of mechanical reasons. Inflammatory disease, foreign bodies, benign and malignant tumors, and structural abnormalities may all lead toward limitations in the swallowing mechanism. Surgical treatment is aimed at the appropriate management and excision of the endoluminal or extraluminal masses. Treatment of structural abnormalities, including cleft palate and oral webs, is aimed at recreating the normal anatomy of the oral cavity. The variety of techniques for their repair is beyond the scope of this chapter.

The Pharyngeal Stage

As in the oral stage, extrinsic and intrinsic compression of the lumen are more amenable to surgical correction than neurogenic lesions. It is also at this level that laryngeal function plays an important role, and, therefore, requires consideration when treatment plans are determined. Infection and trauma can both result in dysphagia in the pharyngeal stage, with extrinsic compression of the lumen through abscess, hematoma, or traumatic cervical projection into the retropharyngeal or parapharyngeal spaces.

Malignant disease must be seriously considered in any patient presenting with dysphagia in the pharyngeal stage. Although squamous cell carcinoma is the most common type of intrinsic cancer of the oropharynx and hypopharynx, extrinsic compression from parapharyngeal space tumors also needs to be considered. The Mayo Clinic series of parapharyngeal space tumors revealed the following distribution: mixed tumor, 43 percent; malignant lymphoma, 25 percent; schwannoma, 16 percent; paraganglioma, 12 percent; hemangiopericytoma, 2 percent; hemangioendothelioma, 1 percent; and lipoma, 1 percent. Sarcomas and glomus tumors also may arise in this space (Heeneman et al. 1980). Any of these parapharyngeal tumors can have dysphagia as a presenting symptom. Surgical management aims at appropriate surgical excision of the tumor.

CERVICAL OSTEOPHYTES

Cervical osteophyte formation occurs in 20 to 30 percent of the population and in some individuals results in dysphagia through either mechanical compression of the pharynx or paraesophageal inflammation caused by motion over the osteophytes (Sobol and Ringual 1984; Papadopoulos et al. 1989). Diffuse idiopathic skeletal hyperostosis, characterized by excessive bone growth at the site of attachment of a ligament or tendon to bone, has been reported by several authors (Kibel and Johnson 1987; Fahrer and Markwalder 1988; and Shergy et al. 1989) to present with dysphagia. Other conditions, including ankylosing spondolytis, infectious spondolytis, previous surgical fusion of cervical vertebrae, and local trauma (Welsh et al. 1987) all can lead to the development of large osteophytes. While the osteophytes may form throughout the spine, it is typically osteophytes located at C3 through C6 that cause dysphagia.

Treatment of osteophytes is controversial. Nonsteroidal anti-inflammatory agents and oral steroids often are recommended for nonprogressive dysphagia secondary to osteophytes. However, in the case of progressive dysphagia or dysphagia unresponsive to conservative therapy, surgical excision of the osteophytes is recommended.

The surgical approach begins with a transverse incision across the middle of the thyroid cartilage crossing the anterior border of the sternocleidomastoid muscle. The left side of the neck is traditionally chosen because it has a lower incidence of a nonrecurrent laryngeal nerve. The incision is taken down through the platysma, exposing the anterior border of the sternocleidomastoid muscle. Sharp dissection inferiorly along the anterior border of the sternocleidomastoid muscle exposes the carotid sheath and its contents. As these are retracted laterally, the prevertebral fascia can be seen. Structures that may require division to maximize exposure include the superior thyroid artery, the middle thyroid vein, and the omohyoid tendon and muscle. Care must be taken not to divide the external laryngeal nerve. Grasping the midportion of the thyroid ala and rotating it medially exposes the retropharyngeal space. Dissection of this space is carried out from superior to inferior along the midline, being careful to avoid injury to the recurrent laryngeal nerve. If access below C6 is necessary, the thyroid gland also must be medialized, and the sternocleidomastoid muscle may require division. Identification of the longus coli muscles to each side of midline helps maintain correct midline position. At this point the cervical osteophyte should be apparent. A vertical incision is made through the prevertebral fascia and periostium, and subperiostial dissection allows for exposure of the osteophytes. A cutting burr is used for removal of the bulk of the mass, and a diamond burr is used to smooth and round off all edges. Closure of the periosteum over the bone is the first layer, followed by reapproximation of all divided deep muscles. A deep drain is inserted, the platysma is closed, and the skin is closed. Patients without intraoperative complications are typically permitted peroral intake the evening of surgery.

CRICOPHARYNGEAL DYSFUNCTION
The Cricopharyngeus Muscle

A common site for dysfunction resulting in dysphagia is the cricopharyngeus muscle. It has been studied extensively and is generally considered to be the

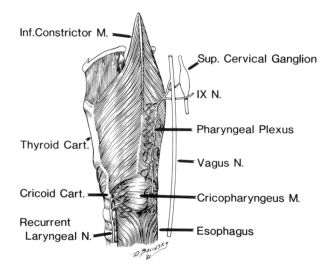

Inf.Constrictor M.

Sup. Cervical Ganglion

IX N.

Pharyngeal Plexus

Thyroid Cart.

Vagus N.

Cricoid Cart.

Cricopharyngeus M.

Recurrent
Laryngeal N.

Esophagus

Figure 13.1 Posterior view of the nerve supply to the cricopharyngeal and pharyngeal musculature. (Drawing by David Bolinsky.)

superior esophageal sphincter (Asherson 1950; Kirchner 1958; Lund 1968; Ellis 1971). Inferior to the oblique fibers of the inferior constrictor muscle, the cricopharyngeus muscle forms a sling around the pharyngoesophageal segment from anterolateral attachments to the cricoid cartilage. Inferiorly, the cricopharyngeus is generally continuous with the superior circular fibers of the esophagus (Hollinshead 1968). Manometric measurements reveal a sphincter approximately 3 cm in length and having a resting pressure of about 40 cm above atmospheric pressure (English 1980). Innervation of the cricopharyngeus (Figure 13.1) in humans remains controversial. In the dog model, Kirchner (1958) demonstrated the motor supply to the cricopharyngeus muscle to be a pharyngeal branch of the vagus nerve. In humans, it is generally considered to be innervated by the pharyngeal nerve plexus, consisting of contributions from the glossopharyngeus, vagus, and superior sympathetic ganglion (Blakley et al. 1968).

Functioning as the superior esophageal sphincter, its relaxation is considered the terminal event in the pharyngeal stage of deglutition, and abnormalities in its function can contribute significantly to dysphagia. The cricopharyngeus has been studied extensively by manometric measurements; in the pathologic state it may be in spasm (Calcaterra et al. 1975; Chodosh 1975), contract prematurely, be delayed in contraction (Ellis et al. 1969), and contribute significantly to the formation of pharyngoesophageal diverticula (Zenker's diverticulum) (Dohlman and Mattson 1960; Lund 1968; Weaver and Fleming 1978). In some diseases involving deglutition, resistance of a normally functioning superior sphincter is too great for weakened pharyngeal constrictor muscles to overcome, resulting in dysphagia (Blakley et al. 1968).

Prior to surgical intervention for dysphagia, an extensive evaluation of the upper aerodigestive tract must be completed. In addition to identifying a functional disorder, intrinsic or extrinsic masses must be eliminated as possible causes of dysphagia. The most effective preoperative evaluation includes a cine-esophageal barium swallow, esophagoscopy, and manometric measurements (Orringer 1980). The barium swallow often reveals a prominent cricopharyngeal sphincter, a prominent posterior cricopharyngeal "bar" on lateral cervical views, and Zenker's diverticulum.

Cricopharyngeal Myotomy

The most widely practiced surgical management of cricopharyngeal dysfunction has been cricopharyngeal myotomy (Blakley et al. 1968; Chodosh 1975; Mills 1975; Zuckerbraum and Bahma 1979; Ellis 1980; Black 1981; Lindgren and Ekberg 1990) or an extended myotomy (Figure 13.2). Depending on the patient's physical condition, this procedure can be performed under local or general anesthesia (Henderson et al. 1989). Either an oblique incision anterior to the sternocleidomastoid muscle or a horizontal incision at the level of the cricoid cartilage is made. The left side is preferred by most surgeons, because of the decreased likelihood of a nonrecurrent laryngeal nerve. Following sharp dissection through the subcutaneous tissues and the platysma, the larynx is exposed by separating the strap muscles. The larynx is retracted medially, while the carotid sheath and contents are retracted laterally (Calcaterra et al. 1975; Ellis 1980). The middle thyroid vein often must be cut to facilitate exposure. The recurrent laryngeal nerve must be identified and protected. Critical to the success of the myotomy is identification and division of all the cricopharyngeal

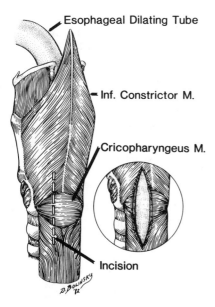

Esophageal Dilating Tube

Inf. Constrictor M.

Cricopharyngeus M.

Incision

Figure 13.2 Incision for the cricopharyngeal myotomy. The inset shows the mucosa bulging through the excised musculature. (Drawing by David Bolinsky.)

muscle fibers. To accomplish this, a bougie (weighted rubber tube) can be placed through the mouth into the esophagus, thus distending the sphincter and allowing all the fibers to be identified and cut, exposing the underlying mucosal membrane (Skolnik et al. 1966). As an additional precaution to prevent recurrent laryngeal nerve injury, the myotomy is performed in the midline on the posterior surface of the esophagus.

Zenker's diverticula are often present in association with cricopharyngeal dysfunction. The base of the diverticulum is located superior to the sling-like band of cricopharyngeus muscle and is inferior to the oblique fibers of the inferior constrictor. Diverticula range from 1 to 8 cm in length. There is evidence from clinical experience that the size of the diverticulum does not correlate with the degree of dysphagia (Orringer 1980). Subsequently, an adequate myotomy alone may resolve the symptoms of dysphagia when diverticula are present. Many surgeons have demonstrated their disappearance by postoperative esophageal swallow in patients having myotomy alone for small diverticula. For large diverticula, however, surgical resection with two-layer closure in addition to myotomy is indicated (Ellis 1969).

The complications of cricopharyngeal myotomy are few, primarily incomplete division of the cricopharyngeus muscle resulting in persistent dysphagia, damage to the recurrent laryngeal nerve, and fistula formation from unrecognized perforation of the mucous membrane. Because of these complications and the typically poor systemic condition of the patients, some advocate endoscopic resection of the common wall between a diverticulum and the esophagus by coagulating diathermy current (Dohlman and Mattson 1960). This procedure opens the diverticulum and at the same time divides the cricopharyngeus muscle. The procedure has received only modest acceptance because of limited surgical exposure, a high rate of fistulization, and a lower success rate due to the inability to detect when the cricopharyngeus has been completely divided.

Postoperative evaluation of patients having a cricopharyngeal myotomy for dysphagia reveals elimination of dysphagia or only an occasional episode of mild dysphagia in 85 percent of patients studied (Black 1981). In addition, manometric measurements demonstrate an approximately 50 percent decrease in the resting pressure of the superior sphincter. Patients who have premature contraction of the sphincter prior to myotomy continue to have it postoperatively (Ellis 1969), although they will typically have less dysphagia. Patients with multiple cranial nerve dysfunctions, especially if these include the hypoglossal nerve, or those who have significant ballooning of the pharyngeal constrictor muscles preoperatively, achieve only a modest improvement in dysphagia after cricopharyngeal myotomy (Lebo et al. 1976).

Dilatation of the superior esophageal sphincter using bougie dilators has been advocated as an alternative treatment in patients with idiopathic spasm or achalasia of the superior esophageal sphincter (Calcaterra et al. 1975). This treatment is recommended in systemically debilitated patients who cannot tolerate a more involved surgical procedure. Management of superior esophageal achalasia by dilatation is limited in effectiveness because the procedure must be repeated and relief is only short-term, although a few select patients can be taught self-dilation. Multiple dilatation of the superior esophagus can result in significant risk of esophageal perforation. Because of the necessity for repeated procedures and the significant morbidity and mortality associated with esophageal perforation, superior esophageal sphincter dilatation for dysphagia is only indicated in a select, small group of patients, such as younger persons who are not debilitated but who demonstrate mild-to-moderate narrowing. Those who do not respond readily to this treatment should not be considered for long-term repeated dilatation.

Following laryngeal surgery for carcinoma, pharyngeal structure and function are altered, and often these patients require weeks to months of practice to relearn the neuromuscular sequence for effective swallowing. By cine-esophageal swallow and manometric pressure measurements, the pharyngeal musculature has been demonstrated to be ineffective in propelling a bolus or secretions through the cricopharyngeal sphincter. Cricopharyngeal myotomy is therefore advocated (Thawley and Ogura 1978) in patients undergoing conservative surgery of the larynx, including hemilaryngectomy and unilateral and bilateral supraglottic laryngectomy. This myotomy is performed by some surgeons at the time of conservative laryngeal surgery (Nicks 1976). Some recommend myotomy in all patients undergoing supraglottic laryngectomy because there is a tendency for the cricopharyngeus to fail to relax properly following the procedure, and aspiration becomes a significant postoperative problem.

ESOPHAGEAL DYSFUNCTION

Dysfunction of the esophageal stage of deglutition also must be considered in patients with dysphagia and aspiration (see Chapter 4). To evaluate esophageal function, the following studies should be considered: cine-esophageal barium swallow, esophageal manometric measurements, pH testing (as subtle acid reflux may not be apparent on manometrics), and endoscopy. Extrinsic or intrinsic structural obstruction of the esophagus must be identified. Neuromuscular dysfunction of the esophagus may result in diffuse esophageal spasm, megaesophagus, lower esophageal achalasia, or hypotensive lower esophageal sphincter with esophageal reflux (Ellis 1980). By precise manometric measurements in patients with spasm of the esophageal body, functional obstruction can be identified at the point of highest resistance. This evaluation can guide the surgical intervention and limit an otherwise overextensive esophageal myotomy.

Typically, surgery is reserved for patients in whom dysphagia is severe and medical treatment has been unsuccessful. The esophagus is approached through a left thoracotomy incision. As in the cricopharyngeus myotomy, the circular fibers of the esophageal musculature are identified and divided longitudinally over the area of dysfunction. Megaesophagus resulting from increased resting tension of the lower esophageal sphincter and lower esophageal achalasia are treated effectively by surgical intervention using the modified Heller procedure (Asherson 1950). A myotomy is performed at the level of the gastroesophageal junction either transthoracically or transabdominally, depending on the necessity for a combined procedure. In cases of megaesophagus in which significant dilatation of the esophagus has been demonstrated preoperatively, partial resection of the esophagus is indicated (Negus 1962; Nicks 1976). Evaluation of patients following myotomy reveals an 18 to 34 percent incidence of gastroesophageal reflux (Henderson 1989). Complications from esophageal reflux include esophagitis with stricture formation, profound discomfort, and reflex upper esophageal sphincter achalasia (Ellis 1980; Vantrappen and Hellemans 1980). The mechanism of increased upper esophageal sphincter tension in esophageal reflux is attributed to chronic irritation of the esophagus, followed by a reflex tightening of the sphincter (Henderson and Marryatt 1977). Because of the high incidence of morbidity associated with reflux following a cardiomyotomy, Mansour et al. (1976) advocate a combined procedure, including a reflux-retarding procedure at the time of myotomy. Additionally, patients who have primary esophageal reflux from a hypotensive lower esophageal sphincter may benefit from an antireflux procedure. Several types of antireflux procedures are commonly practiced, including the Belsey Mark IV transthoracic reconstruction of the cardia, the Nisson fundoplication, and the Hill procedure.

In the medically compromised patient with lower esophageal achalasia, dilatation of the cardia may be an effective alternative. A forceful dilation of the sphincter is necessary, using either the Starck dilator, which consists of a balloon of fixed diameter, or the Sippy pneumatic dilator bag (Vantrappen and Hellemans 1980). Following repeated dilatations, patients experience improvement in dysphagia in 75 percent of cases, with significant reflux occurring only 1 percent of the time (Vantrappen and Hellemans 1980). The factor limiting the wider use of dilatation techniques is the relatively high incidence (5 percent) of esophageal perforation. Dilatation of the lower esophageal sphincter is effective and should be performed in patients suffering from severe dysphagia who are not candidates for a major operative procedure.

AORTIC ARCH ANOMALIES

There are multiple anomalies of the aortic arch that lead to dysphagia (Adkins et al. 1986). Bayford (1794) reported compression of the esophagus by an aberrant right subclavian artery originating in the left side of the mediastinum as the most distal branch of the aortic arch and then coursing posterior to the esophagus, leading to dysphagia. Bayford named the syndrome dysphagia "lusoria," or "jest of nature." While this anomaly occurs in 0.5 to 1.8 percent of the population, it only occasionally results in dysphagia. The original technique described for the treatment of dysphagia lusoria was simple division of the aberrant artery through a left thoracotomy (Gross 1946). Bailey et al. (1965) modified the technique to include reimplantation of the artery into the aortic arch to avoid arm ischemia. Thoracotomy has traditionally been the approach used for either simple division (Van Son et al. 1989); however, some authors (Orvald et al. 1972; Valentine et al. 1987) have described extrathoracic approaches to the aberrant arteries because they often course high in the mediastinum. Through a supraclavicular incision, the aberrant artery can be divided and reimplanted into the right carotid artery.

The double aortic arch is the most common vascular ring in infants. If the right and left arches coexist and are of equivalent size, a tight vascular ring will form around the trachea and esophagus, resulting in both breathing and swallowing difficulties. Surgical correction depends on which arch is dominant. In patients with a dominant right posterior arch, division of the left anterior arch between the left common carotid and left subclavian artery is performed (Richardson et al. 1981). When the left anterior arch is dominant, division of the posterior arch as well as the ligamentum arteriosum is performed (Richardson et al. 1981). In these patients, both recurrent laryngeal nerves are long, with the nerves looping around the arch, except on the side of the ligamentum (Nikaido et al. 1972).

Two types of right aortic arch anomalies exist. One type consists of mirror image branching of the great vessels and is typically associated with a cardiac defect involving the origin of the aorta of the pulmonary artery. In the second type, an aberrant left subclavian artery and left ductus are found. In the child, both airway and esophageal symptoms usually are present, while dysphagia is more often the complaint in the adult (Drucker and Symbas 1980). Most authors agree that for appropriate surgical management, division of the left ligamentum arteriosum and freeing of the esophagus and trachea are imperative. When an aberrant left subclavian artery is present, some authors recommend division of this subclavian artery (Hallman and Cooley 1964; Jung et al. 1978). Disagreement exists as to the importance of reanastamosis of the subclavian artery. Those who choose to reimplant the left subclavian usually implant the artery into the arch or left carotid artery (Wychulis et al. 1971; Jung et al. 1978).

LASER PALLIATION FOR MALIGNANT DYSPHAGIA

Until recently, dysphagia due to unresectable esophageal carcinoma with occlusion of the esophageal lumen has been treated with placement of a feeding gastrostomy. Multiple authors (Krasner et al. 1987; Bown et al. 1987; Ahlquist et al. 1987; Barr et al. 1990) have recently described palliative laser procedures for malignant dysphagia. Following endoscopy under local anesthesia with intravenous sedation, an Nd-YAG laser is used to reestablish an esophageal lumen through excision of tumor. The procedure is not intended to completely excise the lesion, but rather provide palliative relief to the patient. Symptomatic relief, as measured by subjective improvement in swallowing, was achieved in 80 percent (Ahlquist et al. 1987) to 85 percent (Bown et al. 1987) of patients. Endoscopic esophageal intubation following laser therapy did not seem to influence the patient's quality of life (Barr et al. 1990). Mortality due to the procedure is between 0 and 5 percent (Ahlquist et al. 1987; Krasner et al. 1987, respectively).

SURGICAL INTERVENTION IN PERSISTENT DYSPHAGIA

When the upper aerodigestive tract fails to perform its role of providing both protected ventilation of the lungs and a passageway for alimentation, separation of these functions by surgical intervention may be required for the patient's survival. A nasogastric tube is an effective temporary means to provide adequate nutrition in the debilitated or unconscious patient who has significant aspiration. Long-term use of the nasogastric tube is limited by discomfort, bleeding, and irritation along the course of the tube, resulting in increased mucous membrane secretions, regurgitation of feedings, and impairment of pharyngeal swallow (Acquarelli et al. 1972). Surgical intervention to provide adequate feedings without associated aspiration include pharyngoesophagostomy, flap esophagostomy, gastrostomy, and jejunostomy (Table 13.1).

Esophagostomy

The pharyngoesophagostomy is an effective means of long-term tube feeding, and in some patients provides control of secretions in the pharynx that are difficult to manage (Skolnik et al. 1966; Dobie et al. 1979). A fistula is created from the hypopharynx to the skin anterior to the sternocleidomastoid muscle. A Levin tube or similar feeding tube is placed through the fistula tract into the stomach (Figure 13.3). If secretions in the pharynx pose a life-threatening condition because of recurrent aspiration, the fistula tract can be constructed using a skin flap, providing a more permanent fistula and allowing the feeding tube to be removed for short periods of time. Graham and Royster (1967) described a surgical technique that allows placement of a pharyngotomy tube into the

Table 13.1 Surgical Routes for Tube Feeding

Procedure	Advantages	Disadvantages
Esophagostomy	Minimal skin care, tube out between meals, feedings taken upright; reversible as office procedure	Contraindicated in esophageal obstruction, irradiated neck, superior vena cava syndrome
Gastrostomy	Standard procedure; preferable in children	Skin care often troublesome; patient must disrobe for feeding
Jejunostomy	Minimizes gastroesophageal reflux	Increased diarrhea
Pharyngotomy	Local anesthesia, minimal risk	Stoma high in neck, tube changing often difficult

Reprinted by permission of the publisher, from Doby, *American Family Physician,* 1978.

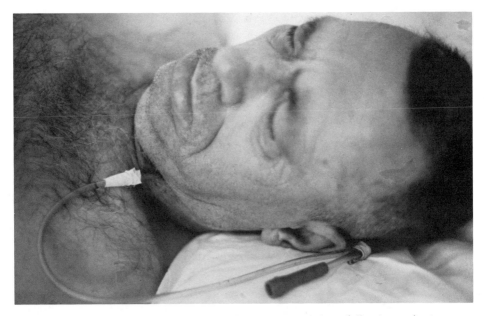

Figure 13.3 Patient with a cervical esophagostoma in place following a brain stem cerebrovascular accident. Note the marked bilateral facial weakness.

piriform sinus. This procedure, performed under local anesthesia at the bedside, is ideal for the compromised patient who requires urgent placement of a feeding tube and cannot tolerate general anesthesia or abdominal placement.

Advantages of the esophagostoma over the gastrostoma tube are avoidance of an abdominal procedure, use of local anesthesia, the ability to feed the patient in the sitting rather than the supine position, and the ability to begin feedings immediately following the procedure. There are several disadvantages of an esophagostomy tube. In addition to local irritation to skin, there is a general contraindication in patients with tumor or severe venous congestion in the neck, esophageal obstruction or significant reflux, significant lower respiratory disease and/or dyspnea or frequent cough, and frequent emesis or extensive gastro-esophageal reflux.

Gastrostomy

The most common surgical approach for placement of a feeding tube is gastrostomy. The popularity of the feeding gastrostomy is best explained by mentioning some of its advantages. The feeding tube is away from the head and neck and therefore can be placed in patients with a head and neck or esophageal tumor. A gastrostomy is technically a straightforward procedure that can be done under local anesthesia. Peristomal irritation is less significant than that in the head and neck region.

In patients with significant esophageal reflux, the gastrostomy, pharyngoe-sophagostomy, and nasogastric feeding tube should be avoided, as they increase the likelihood of postprandial reflux and aspiration. An exception is the new soft, Silastic pediatric feeding tubes that have proved quite valuable in providing enteral nutrition.

Jejunostomy

When esophageal reflux and associated aspiration are strongly suspected by history or demonstrated by attempted feeding with a nasogastric tube, a feeding jejunostoma tube is indicated. As with gastrostomy, placement of the jejunostoma tube requires an abdominal procedure, but differs in that a general anesthesia usually is required (Liffman and Randall 1972). The advantage of this type of feeding tube is its placement distal to the duodenum, therefore minimizing the potential of reflux. Early selection of the appropriate mode of tube placement in the patient with severe dysphagia is a necessity to prevent starvation and aspiration pneumonia associated with attempted feedings.

LARYNGEAL PARALYSIS

In severe dysfunction of the upper aerodigestive tract, a more immediate problem than establishing a mode for feedings is protection of the airway from life-threatening aspiration. The primary function of the larynx is to act as a sphincter for the airway, preventing the aspiration of secretions and food. To provide normal function, the supraglottic mucous membrane, which is innervated by the internal branch of the superior laryngeal nerve, must respond to the presence of foreign material or secretions by initiating glottic closure (this is also accomplished by direct stimulation of the trachea). To complete the sphincter-like action, the intrinsic musculature of the larynx that is innervated by the recurrent laryngeal nerve approximates the vocal cords, thus tightly closing the glottis. Surgical intervention to manage partial or total laryngeal paralysis must be selective, based on the degree and level of paralysis present.

Unilateral low vagal paralysis below the level of the nodose ganglion results initially in paramedian-positioned vocal cords, producing hoarseness and minimal aspiration (Figure 13.4). In the later stages of paralysis the vocal cord moves to the abducted position as the ipsilateral muscles slowly atrophy (Sasaki 1980). In this position the patient may experience mild aspiration and marked hoarseness.

Vocal Cord Injection

Several different materials have been used for vocal cord injection. The three best studied materials are Teflon, Gelfoam, and collagen. By injecting Teflon into a paralyzed cord (Rontal et al. 1976), partial closure of the glottic space can be achieved, resulting in improved voice and decreased aspiration. Using the

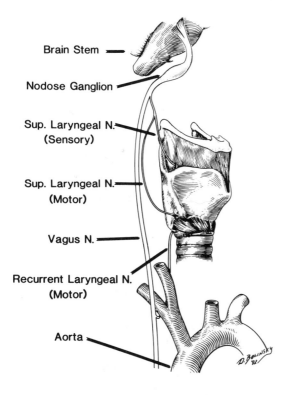

Brain Stem

Nodose Ganglion

Sup. Laryngeal N.
(Sensory)

Sup. Laryngeal N.
(Motor)

Vagus N.

Recurrent Laryngeal N.
(Motor)

Aorta

Figure 13.4 Branches of the vagus (superior and recurrent laryngeal nerves) that innervate the sensory and motor aspects of the larynx. Loss of sensory and motor innervation above and below the level of the nodose ganglion produces different pathology. (Drawing by David Bolinsky.)

Arnold-Breuning syringe, approximately 0.25 mL of Teflon paste is injected into the paralyzed vocal cord at two points: (1) the middle third of the cord, and (2) immediately above the vocal process of the arytenoid (Figure 13.5). The procedure is typically performed under local anesthesia, with visualization of the vocal cords obtained by suspension laryngoscopy. By moving the paralyzed cord to the median position, voice quality is markedly improved and aspiration may be decreased.

Prior to injecting Teflon, the surgeon may elect to inject absorbable gelatin sponge (Gelfoam) into the paralyzed vocal cord to anticipate the more permanent effects of Teflon. Gelfoam injections usually are made with patients who are expected to have return of function or when there is a quesiton as to the efficacy of Teflon. Teflon often is preferred in patients with carcinoma and generalized neurologic deficits because it is a quick, easy procedure, and it may not be prudent to do more than one procedure on patients in this group due to the increased morbidity.

More recently, collagen (Ford and Bless 1984) has been used to inject vocal cords. It is injected in a similar fashion to Teflon, and studies thus far indicate it maintains its volume in the cord without absorption in 3- to 4-year follow-up (Remacle et al. 1989). Thus far this relatively new material has not been used for treatment of aspiration; however, it seems like a reasonable alternative.

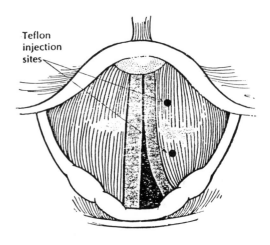

Figure 13.5 Superior view of the vocal cords illustrating the Teflon injection sites on the paralyzed vocal cord. (Reprinted by permission of the publisher, from Doby, *American Family Physician,* 1978.)

Arytenoid Adduction

There are multiple techniques described for arytenoid adduction (Morrison 1948; Montgomery 1966; Isshiki et al. 1978). The basis of these procedures is the surgical repositioning of the paralyzed cord toward the midline. Morrison (1948) describes a "reverse King operation" to displace the arytenoid toward the midline. Using a stainless steel pin, Montgomery (1975) fixes the arytenoid and cricoid cartilages in a new position to medialize the paralyzed cord.

Multiple procedures are attributed to Isshiki et al. (1978). One of the first described was the medialization of the cord by rotating the vocal process of the arytenoid cartilage in a posteromedial fashion and suturing its muscular process through the thyroid cartilage for fixation. This is primarily indicated in the presence of a wide glottic chink and a difference in the height of the two vocal cords. Also described is the placement of a small block of silicone through a window in the thyroid cartilage at the level of the paralyzed vocal cord, thus medially displacing the vocal ligament. One of the advantages of this procedure is the relative ease of its reversal.

While these procedures are not classically indicated for aspiration alone, they should all be considered for patients with dysphagia when medialization of the vocal cord is required.

Nerve-to-Muscle Pedicle

In bilateral low vagal paralysis, deglutition is rarely impaired, and aspiration is often a minimal problem as the vocal cords tend to be in the median position and sensation of the hypopharynx remains intact.

Initial therapy involves providing an adequate airway and protecting against aspiration by the placement of a cuffed tracheostomy tube. Improved respiration may be accomplished by fixed lateralization of one of the paralyzed cords; however, by permanently widening the glottic space for increased respiration, aspiration will increase and may pose a difficult management problem. An alternative surgical approach that has achieved some popularity is the use of a nerve-to-muscle pedicle transferred from the omohyoid muscle to the paralyzed posterior cricoarytenoid (Tucker 1976). Inspiratory activity of the omohyoideus mediated by the ansa hypoglossi results in phasic vocal cord abduction, which may be adequate to allow increased ventilation and at the same time protect the airway against aspiration.

Tympanic Neurectomy

High unilateral vagus paralysis above the nodose ganglion results in vocal cord and pharyngeal paralysis that produces significant dysphagia and aspiration of stagnated material retained in the hypopharynx (Figure 13.5). Surgical intervention in these cases requires a combination of procedures to facilitate deglutition and protect the airway from aspiration. Initially, a cuffed tracheostomy tube is placed, followed by the insertion of a feeding tube, Teflon injection of the paralyzed vocal cord, and cricopharyngeal myotomy (Glenn et al. 1980). If persistent aspiration of secretions in the pharynx continues, bilateral chorda tympani and tympanic nerve sections may be performed by a transtympanic approach under local anesthesia (Townsend et al. 1973; Mills 1975). By sectioning the chorda tympani and tympanic nerve, the parasympathetic innervation of the submandibular and parotid glands is interrupted, markedly decreasing the oral secretions (Figure 13.6). These nerve sections often are effective in controlling secretions, but approximately 30 percent of patients have a recurrence of symptoms within the first 6 months following the operation.

Laryngeal Closure

In high bilateral vagal nerve paralysis, immediate airway control is required to maintain life. As soon as is practical, a cuffed tracheostomy tube and a feeding tube (usually gastrostoma) are placed. In the past, this condition and cases in which the ninth, tenth, eleventh, and twelfth cranial nerves are involved required laryngectomy to prevent recurrent aspiration, pneumonia, and death. There are now alternative procedures, including diversion of the larynx (Lindeman 1975), an epiglottic flap (sewing the epiglottis over the false cords and into the arytenoids) (Habal and Murray 1972), and laryngeal closure (Sasaki et al. 1980). The most practical and effective approach is the laryngeal closure described by Montgomery (1975) and modified by Sasaki (1980). Both procedures close the larynx and are reversible if there is significant neurologic improvement.

Following placement of a permanent tracheostoma, a horizontal skin incision over the cricoid is made to approach the larynx. The larynx is entered by a vertical midline thyrotomy. Mucous membrane between the free edges of the vocal and vestibular folds is resected. The glottis is then closed, beginning su-

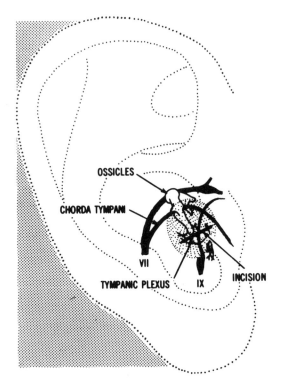

Figure 13.6 Diagram of the parasympathetic nerve supply to the major salivary glands and their accessibility within the middle ear. Tympanic neurectomy is performed within the tympanic plexus. (Reprinted by permission of the publisher, from DeLisa et al., *American Family Physician*, 1979.)

periorly by approximating the denuded edges of the vestibular folds. A superior-based sternohyoid muscle pedicle is then passed through the thyroid notch and sutured to the interarytenoideus muscle at the posterior commissure. The vocal folds are then approximated, followed by closure of the thyrotomy and the skin incision. By the placement of the sternohyoid muscle pedicle, the dead space between the vocal and vestibular folds is eliminated, and the larynx is closed in three layers. The major advantage of laryngeal closure is the protection of the respiratory tract from aspiration while allowing the upper aerodigestive tract to be used for alimentation.

SUMMARY

The goals of surgical intervention in patients with dysphagia should be the reestablishment of normal physiology or the bypassing of known lesions and abnormalities of the upper digestive tract. It is crucial to separate the airway from the passage of secretions and feedings. Appropriate surgical management requires an extensive knowledge of the normal anatomy and physiology of the upper aerodigestive tract in addition to an understanding of the methods of evaluation of dysphagia.

REFERENCES

Acquarelli MJ, Fenno G, Ward PH. Cervical esophagostomy (an improved technique for alimentation of the debilitated patient). Arch Otolaryngol 1972; 96:453–56.

Adkins RB, Maples MD, Graham BS, et al. Dysphagia associated with aortic arch anomaly in adults. Am Surg 1986; 52:238–45.

Ahlquist DA, Gostout CJ, Viggiano TR, et al. Endoscopic laser palliation of malignant dysphagia: a prospective study. Mayo Clin Proc 1987; 62:867–74.

Asherson N. Achalasia of the cricopharyngeal sphincter: record of cases, with profile pharyngograms. J Laryngol Otol 1950; 64:747–58.

Bailey CP, Hirose T, Alba J. Re-establishment of the continuity of the anomalous right subclavian artery after operation for dysphagia lusoria. Angiology 1965; 16:509–13.

Barr H, Krasner N, Raouf A, et al. Prospective randomized trial of laser therapy only and laser therapy followed by endoscopic intubation for the palliation of malignant dysphagia. Gut 1990; 31:252–8.

Bayford D. An account of a singular case of obstructed deglutition. Mem Med Soc Lond 1794; 2:275–86.

Black RJ. Cricopharyngeal myotomy. J Otolaryngol 1981; 10:145–8.

Blakley WR, Garety EJ, Smith DE. Section of the cricopharyngeus muscle for dysphagia. Arch Surg 1968; 96:745–60.

Bown SG, Hawes R, Matthewson K, et al. Endoscopic laser palliation for advanced malignant dysphagia. Gut 1987; 28:799–807.

Calcaterra JC, Kadell BM, Ward PH. Dysphagia secondary to cricopharyngeal muscle dysfunction. Arch Otolaryngol 1975; 101:726–9.

Chodosh PL. Cricopharyngeal myotomy in the treatment of dysphagia. Laryngoscope 1975; 85:1862–73.

Delisa JA, Mikulic MA, Miller RM, et al. Amyotrophic lateral sclerosis: comprehensive management. Am Fam Physician 1979; 19:137–42.

Dobie RA, Cox KW, Larsen GL. Skin flap esophagostomy: a new procedure. Arch Otolaryngol 1979; 105:200–2.

Doby RA: Rehabilitation of swallowing disorders. Am Fam Physician 1978; 17:84–95.

Dohlman G, Mattson O. The endoscopic operation of hypopharyngeal diverticula: a roentgenocinematographic study. Arch Otolaryngol 1960; 71:744–52.

Drucker MH, Symbas PN. Right aortic arch with aberrant left subclavian artery: symptomatic in adulthood. Am J Surg 1980; 139:432–5.

Ellis FH Jr, Schlegel JF, Lynch VP, et al. Cricopharyngeal myotomy for pharyngo-esophageal diverticulum. Ann Surg 1969; 170:340–9.

Ellis FH. Upper esophageal sphincter in health and disease. Surg Clin North Am 1971; 51:553–65.

Ellis FH. Surgical management of esophageal motility disturbances. Am J Surg 1980; 139:752–9.

English GM. Otolaryngology. New York: Harper and Row, 1980.

Fahrer H, Markwalder T. Dysphagia caused by diffuse idiopathic skeletal hyperostosis. Clin Rheumatol 1988; 7:117–21.

Ford CN, Bless DM. Clinical experience with injectable collagen for vocal cord augmentation. Laryngoscope 1986; 96:863–9.

Glenn WWL, Hoak B, Sasaki C, et al. Characteristics and surgical management of respiratory complications accompanying pathologic lesions of the brainstem. Ann Surg 1980; 191:655–63.

Graham W, Royster HP. Simplified cervical esophagostomy for long-term extraoral feeding. Surg Gynecol Obstet 1967; 125:127–8.

Gross RE. Surgical treatment for dysphagia lusoria. Ann Surg 1946; 124:532–4.

Habal MB, Murray JE. Surgical treatment of life endangering chronic aspiration pneumonia. Plast Reconstr Surg 1972; 49:305–11.

Hallman GL, Cooley DA. Congenital aortic vascular ring. Surgical considerations. Arch Surg (Chicago) 1964; 88:666–74.

Heeneman H, Gilbert JJ, Rood SR. Paralaryngeal space: anatomy and pathologic conditions with emphasis on neurogenous tumors—a self instructional package. American Academy of Otolaryngology, Rochester, NY, 1980.

Henderson RD, Hanna WM, Henderson RF, et al. Myotomy for reflux induced cricopharyngeal dysphagia. Five year review. J Thorac Cardiovasc Surg 1989; 98:428–33.

Henderson RD, Marryatt G. Cricopharyngeal myotomy as a method of treating cricopharyngeal dysphagia secondary to gastroesophageal reflux. J Thorac Cardiovasc Surg 1977; 74:721–5.

Hollinshead WH. Anatomy for surgeons. New York: Harper & Row, 1968.

Isshiki N, Tanabe M, Sawada M. Arytenoid adduction for unilateral vocal cord paralysis. Arch Otolaryngol 1978; 104:555–8.

Jung JY, Almond CH, Saab SB, et al. Surgical repair of right aortic arch and aberrant left subclavian artery and left ligamentum arteriosum. J Thorac Cardiovasc Surg 1978; 75:237–43.

Kibel SM, Johnson PM. Surgery for osteophyte-induced dysphagia. J Laryngol Otol 1987; 101:1291–6.

Kirchner JA. The motor activity of the cricopharyngeus muscle. Laryngoscope 1958; 68:1119–59.

Krasner N, Barr H, Skidmore C, et al. Palliative laser therapy for malignant dysphagia. Gut 1987; 28:792–8.

Lebo CP, Kwei SU, Norris PH. Cricopharyngeal myotomy in amyotrophic lateral sclerosis. Laryngoscope 1976; 86:862–8.

Liffmann KE, Randall HT. A modified technique for creating a jejunostomy. Surg Gynecol Obstet 1972; 134:663–4.

Lindeman RC. Overting the paralyzed larynx: a reversible procedure for intractable aspiration. Laryngoscope 1975; 85:157–80.

Lindgren S, Ekberg O. Cricopharyngeal myotomy in the treatment of dysphagia. Clin Otolaryngol 1990; 15:221–7.

Lund WS. The cricopharyngeal sphincter: its relationship to the relief of pharyngeal paralysis and the surgical treatment of early pharyngeal pouch. J Laryngol 1968; 82:353–67.

Mansour KA, Symbas P, Ellis J, et al. A combined surgical approach in the management of achalasia of the esophagus. Ann Surg 1976; 42:192–5.

Mills CP. Cricopharyngeal sphincterotomy and bilateral division of the chorda tympani in bulbar palsy. Proc R Soc Med 1975; 68:644–6.

Montgomery WW. Cricoarytenoid arthrodesis. Ann Otol Rhinol Laryngol 1966; 75:380–91.

Montgomery WW. Surgery to prevent aspiration. Arch Otolaryngol 1975; 101:679–82.

Morrison L. The "reverse King operation." Ann Otol Rhinol Laryngol 1948; 57:945–56.

Negus VE. Comparative anatomy and physiology of the larynx. New York: Hafner, 1962.

Nicks GR. Webs, dysrhythmias and diverticulae of the esophagus. NZ Med J 1976; 84:179–83.

Nikaido H, Riker WL, Idriss FS. Surgical management of "vascular rings." Arch Surg 1972; 105:327–33.

Orringer MB. Extended cervical esophagomyotomy for cricopharyngeal dysfunction. J Thorac Cardiovasc Surg 1980; 30:669–78.

Orvald TO, Scheerer R, Jude JR. A single cervical approach to aberrant right subclavian artery. Surgery 1972; 71:227–30.

Papadopoulos SM, Chen JC, Feldenzer JA, et al. Anterior cervical osteophytes as a cause of progressive dysphagia. Acta Neurochir 1989; 101:63–5.

Pome G, Vitali E, Mantovani A, et al. Surgical treatment of the aberrant retroesophageal right subclavian artery in adults (dysphagia lusoria). Report of two new cases and review of the literature. J Cardiovasc Surg (Torino) 1987; 28:405–12.

Remacle M, Marbaix E, Hamoir M, et al. Initial long-term results of collagen injection for vocal and laryngeal rehabilitation. Arch Otorhinolaryngol 1989; 246:403–6.

Richardson JV, Doby DB, Rossi NP, et al. Operation for aortic arch anomalies. Ann Thorac Surg 1981; 31:426–32.

Rontal E, Rontal M, Morse G, et al. Vocal cord injection in the treatment of acute and chronic aspiration. Laryngoscope 1976; 86:625–34.

Sasaki CT. Paralysis of the larynx and pharynx. Surg Clin North Am 1980; 60:1079–92.

Sasaki CT, Milmoe G, Yanagisawa E, et al. Surgical closure of the larynx for intractable aspiration. Arch Otolaryngol 1980; 106:422–3.

Shergy WJ, Nunley JA, Caldwell DS. Dysphagia due to diffuse idiopathic skeletal hyperostosis. Am Fam Physician 1989; 39:149–52.

Skolnik EM, Tenta LT, Massair FS. Pharyngo-esophagostomy. Arch Otolaryngol 1966; 84:534–7.

Sobol SM, Rigual NR. Anterolateral extrapharyngeal approach for cervical osteophyte-induced dysphagia. Ann Otol Rhinol Laryngol 1984; 93:498–503.

Thawley SE, Ogura JH. Cricopharyngeal myotomy. Laryngoscope 1978; 88:872–4.

Townsend G, Morimoto AM, Kralemann H. Management of sialorrhea by transtympanic neurectomy. Mayo Clin Proc 1973; 48:776–9.

Tucker HM. Human laryngeal reinnervation. Laryngoscope 1976; 86:769–79.

Valentine RJ, Carter DJ, Clagett GP. A modified extrathoracic approach to the treatment of dysphagia lusoria. J Vasc Surg 1987; 5:498–500.

Van Son JA, Vincent JG, van Oort A, et al. Translocation of aberrant right subclavian artery in dysphagia lusoria in children through a right thoracotomy. Thorac Cardiovasc Surg 1989; 37:52–4.

Vantrappen G, Hellemans J. Treatment of achalasia and related motor disorders. Gastroenterology 1980; 79:144–54.

Weaver AW, Fleming SM. Partial laryngectomy: analysis of associated swallowing disorders. Am J Surg 1978; 136:486–9.

Welsh LW, Welsh JJ, Chinnici JC. Dysphagia due to cervical spine surgery. Ann Otol Rhinol Laryngol 1987; 96:112–5.

Wychulis AG, Kincard OW, Weidman WH, et al. Congenital vascular ring: surgical considerations and results of operation. Mayo Clin Proc 1971; 46:182–8.

Zuckerbraum L, Bahma MS. Cricopharyngeus myotomy as the only treatment for Zenker's diverticulum. Ann Otol 1979; 88:798–803.

14

Establishing a Swallowing Program

Michael E. Groher

It may seem somewhat ironic that this book ends with a discussion devoted to beginning a swallowing program. The preceding chapters help to provide the clinician with the basic theoretical and technical knowledge needed to evaluate and treat swallowing disorders. A thorough and working understanding of the issues and topics discussed is the first step in developing a program. It is necessary to become familiar with the literature and professional staff involved, and with the evaluation and treatment procedures recommended. All can serve as important resources when problems and questions arise.

Putting this knowledge into place in a clinical setting may be the greatest challenge of all. This chapter focuses directly on organizing and developing a dysphagia program. Clinicians who have had direct experience in managing swallowing disorders on a regular basis would agree that there are certain key organizational steps that must be taken. By accepting the fact that good dysphagia programs do not evolve overnight one can adjust to the potential psychologic disappointments that may be frequent in the initial stages. Most programs take three full years before becoming a variable and recognized part of the hospital's life. Others have taken longer.

ESTABLISHING GOALS

There are many kinds of programs that can be established. Each of the contributors to this book has had a different experience, whether in a hospital-wide, multidisciplinary dysphagia clinic, or as a single therapist incorporating the techniques into a personal schedule of rehabilitation treatment. The size and type of patient population, attitudes of the staff toward rehabilitation, available personnel, the real opportunity for program development, and most important, individual interest in dysphagia are essential considerations in defining a program suitable to a particular setting. Some settings will not have the laboratory (videoradiography, scintigraphy) or consultive (gastroenterology, neurology) support that may be necessary in diagnosis. In this circumstance, treatment will be more conservative, emphasizing correct feeding postures during enteral and oral intake and monitoring intake in an effort to avoid medical complications secondary to malnutrition. Jones and Altshuler (1987) found that an absence of videoradiographic studies would not impede a functional approach to treatment if the clinicians were skilled in those physical signs and symptoms that predispose one to aspiration (see Chapter 6). The type of program ultimately established will depend on the goals defined. Three goals should be universal to all dysphagia programs: (1) identification of the patient who may be at risk for aspiration, (2) prevention of aspiration, and (3) prevention of malnutrition. The minimal requirement of the staff to achieve these goals is careful evaluation and reevaluation of the patient to determine the extent to which oral foods are tolerated. It can be argued that the additional goal of improvement of swallowing behavior be included whenever possible.

Ideally, the patient should achieve a nutritionally complete oral diet. If this is not possible, nonoral supplements or total feedings should be recommended. The rudiments of a successful dysphagia program can be established based on evaluation and careful monitoring to achieve the first three goals. Following the diagnostic evaluation described earlier, it is preferable to attempt the active intervention described in the treatment chapters where potential for improvement has not been ruled out.

Depending upon the capabilities of the staff and the extent to which the dysphagia program is incorporated into general rehabilitation, other goals may be expressed, for example, increasing the patient's independence in eating (or in self-administration of tube feedings) and assisting the family to care for the patient's special nutritional needs at home. Some centers have established outpatient clinics and/or a system of outpatient follow-up to provide continuing care to their dysphagic patients.

ASSEMBLING A TEAM

The contributors to this book are representatives of diverse fields of health care management, all with a common interest in swallowing disorders. Those in other disciplines such as psychiatry, dental, social service, general surgery, respiratory therapy, and physical therapy also have an interest. Dysphagia management will be maximized if each participate, either directly and on a daily basis or by periodic consultations. An organizational chart of the potential participants in both clinical and research contributions is presented in Figure 14.1. If possible, an individual or individuals from each service can be identified who have a particular interest in dysphagia and who can serve as direct resource persons for consultations or in-service training. For a section head or supervisor to give tacit approval for the department as a whole to participate is not as useful as specifically designating an individual to be an active representative.

The continuity of care and specialization of knowledge needed to manage dysphagic patients is facilitated if one individual assumes direct responsibility and it is clear to the rest of the team who that individual is. This individual should be familiar with each participating discipline's potential for interaction with the dysphagic patient. This person will be the most visible member and therefore the one to whom consultations will be directed. The team leader

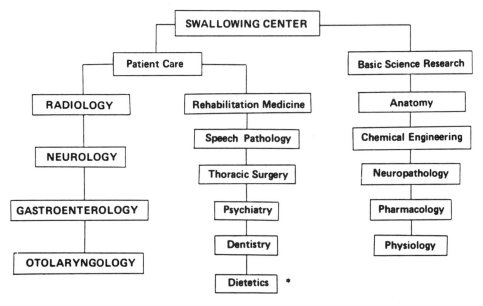

Figure 14.1 Proposed interdisciplinary organization of a swallowing center. (Reprinted with permission of Springer-Verlag from Ravich WJ, Donner MW, Kashima H, et al. The swallowing center: concepts and procedures. Gastrointest Radiol 1985; 10:255–61.)

probably will be the prime participator in dysphagia management on a daily basis. In increasingly large numbers, this role has been assumed by the speech pathologist. Responsibilities usually include accepting consultations, completing the evaluation with appropriate recommendations, coordinating the necessary rehabilitation or further diagnostic tests, and providing some direct feeding training. The team leader will eventually have to devote 35 to 45 percent of total working hours to dysphagia management if employed in a hospital or rehabilitation center setting.

The role played by each member of the dysphagia management team may differ from clinic to clinic; however, most contributions are established as part of traditional roles. A specialized interest or demonstrated expertise in dysphagia management may lead to some overlapping of responsibilities. This should not be viewed by other team members as encroachment, but as a way to complement and verify information that will result in improved care. Mody and Nagai (1990) present a model for patient allocation when similar competencies and roles for care overlap. Some dysphagia rehabilitation programs have failed to sustain themselves because of the failure of team members to define and accept their roles. The following may help to serve as useful guidelines.

Nursing Staff

The nurses, through physician orders, have the direct responsibility of monitoring the patient's medical and nutritional status. In many institutions, they coordinate dysphagia consultations and as such serve as a dysphagia team leaders. Overall responsibilities usually include administration and care of nonoral feeding including hyperalimentation and tube feedings, recording oral and non-oral intake (particularly of fluids), care and suctioning of tracheostoma tubes, maintaining good oral hygiene, and assigning nursing staff or volunteers to assist with feeding at mealtimes. Nurses should be responsible, in part, for reporting successes and failures during oral feedings. These impressions are recorded in the progress notes. The patients' intake and output (I and O) usually are recorded on a separate sheet at the bedside.

Occupational Therapist

Concern for manual feeding skills has been a traditional part of an occupational therapist's involvement in improving the patient's daily living skills. Experience in training patients with motor weakness or loss of function to adapt to new feeding techniques has often led the occupational therapist to coordinate dysphagic rehabilitation. This therapist is a specialist in suggesting which types of adaptive equipment would be best suited for the patient's needs and in providing specific technical assistance at mealtimes in addition to being well trained in general physical rehabilitation techniques (see Chapter 9). In conjunction with the physical therapist, the occupational therapist may provide preliminary therapy to reduce muscle spasticity, improve muscle strength and coordination, and prevent primitive reflex patterns from interfering with swallowing.

Dietitian

The dietitian monitors the patient's overall nutritional status, ensuring that the patient's intake of fluids and nutrients meets the requirements as appropriate to the medical condition (see Chapter 11). The dietitian coordinates special diet orders with the kitchen, assists in obtaining a dysphagia evaluation tray, takes a dietary history when possible, and makes specific recommendations relating to food textures and nutritional values (Curran and Groher 1990). If the patient is receiving tube feedings, the dietitian can make recommendations about the type, adequacy, and regulation of the feedings. The dietitian also is a consultant on the visual presentation of food items, including the environment in which food is served (Hotaling 1990).

The dietitian is the most important resource when treatment involves provision of specialized nutritional and food technological requirements. An example might be to combine foods that provide high-caloric or low-salt content with gelatin to facilitate swallowing, together with some special spices to appeal to the patient's taste. This person who serves as the liaison between the team and the kitchen may find it useful to develop a specialized dysphagia diet that facilitates swallowing while maintaining nutritional integrity (Clusky 1989; Curran and Groher 1990).

Speech Pathologist

Many patients with swallowing difficulty also have accompanying disorders of speech production (Martin and Corlew 1990). It follows that the speech pathologist would become directly involved with both the diagnosis and management of dysphagic patients. Many times the patient's swallowing disorder must be managed before speech rehabilitation can begin. The speech pathologist is expert in muscle reeducation of the oral and laryngeal structures. In many institutions the speech pathologist is the team leader. The knowledge and skills necessary for the speech pathologist to assume this role have been documented (Erlichman 1989; ASHA 1990). Speech pathologists have taken an active role in both clinical and basic research in establishing diagnostic and treatment protocols for patients with swallowing impairments (Groher 1992).

Neurologist

The neurologist is one of the primary diagnosticians on the swallowing management team (Bass 1991). It is this person's responsibility to help differentiate neurologic from mechanical and psychogenic swallowing disorders. The neurologist combines the results of physical examination with those of radiography, electromyography, electroneurography, and muscle and nerve biopsy to arrive at an etiologic diagnosis. Recommendations for special techniques may be combined with prescribing medications that assist in swallowing management by modification of the neurologic disease.

Otolaryngologist/Head and Neck Surgeon

The otolaryngologist/head and neck surgeon has a special interest in the differential diagnosis of mechanical swallowing disorders. Usually he is the most familiar with the sensory and motor abnormalities of the pharynx and larynx. This includes surgical management of the majority of head and neck cancers and post-surgical swallowing disorders and subsequent nutritional status. The otolaryngologist may perform specialized surgical procedures such as cricopharyngeal myotomy or esophagostomy to manage persistent dysphagia (see Chapter 13). Their use of fiberoptic endoscopy is a valuable tool in evaluating the patient's ability to protect the airway during swallow (Langmore et al. 1988).

Gastroenterologist

The gastroenterologist serves as a diagnostician and surgical consultant for patients with suspected dysphagia related to the esophagus and/or gastrointestinal tract (see Chapter 4). While usually not directly involved in daily dysphagia behavioral treatment, an interested gastroenterologist can be an important member of the swallowing management team. The gastroenterologist provides direct visualization of the esophagus and stomach, recommending surgical evaluation and providing medical management, which may include dilatation or drug therapy regimens. The gastroenterologist is consulted for percutaneous endoscopic placement of gastrostoma tubes (PEG) (Weg and Miscovitz 1987).

Pulmonologist/Respiratory Therapist

The pulmonologist or respiratory therapist is not usually directly involved on the dysphagia team, but does provide valuable information relating to patients with respiratory disorders and tracheostoma tubes. This includes monitoring pulmonary toilet and assisting the physician by making recommendations for removal of the tracheostoma tube. Often this therapist will provide expert consultation on the choice of tracheostoma tube and how it should be used during feedings. Some are important resources in developing strategies for feeding patients who need ventilator support, and can provide valuable insights into the consequences of aspiration (Elpern, Jacobs, and Bone 1987; Terry and Fuller 1989).

Attending Physician

Although each patient's attending or primary physician is not necessarily an active member of the dysphagia team, all communications must include this person. The physician as coordinator of the patient's total medical and surgical management must order the original consultation to the dysphagia team or medical specialist. Within each facility, it is imperative for orders to be written clearly. The dysphagia evaluation should be prescribed specifically. If the patient is a candidate for oral intake, the orders should reflect the physician's concurrence because of the potential risks of aspiration and subsequent illness. Any changes in dietary management should also be accompanied by written orders. Sometimes these orders are privileged to the dysphagia team leader to facilitate care. The question of liability is often the first issue to be raised when a dysphagia program is introduced in a new setting. The primary care physician must be in agreement with each step involved in the patient's dysphagia management, since they ultimately carry the responsibility for that patient's care.

TIME ASSESSMENT

The amount of time needed to serve as team leader may appear excessive, especially for the individual who is already fully involved in specialized patient care. The team leader should first try to free this amount of time through direct reassignment of responsibilities within the hospital or clinic. The attainment of this goal is facilitated by presenting rationales for the position, through data describing dysphagia incidence, by comparisons of successful programs in similar settings, and by obtaining support from other team members.

The major activity in a dysphagia rehabilitation program is feeding patients at mealtimes. Although this should be overseen by the team leader, feeding training sessions may be carried out by assigned (trained) nursing or therapy personnel. Volunteers and, when possible, family members should be so assigned only after a patient has demonstrated repeated success at swallowing and requires no more than standby assistance. The time expended by staff who are involved in training volunteers or directly involved in feeding at mealtimes may be exorbitant, especially in the initial stages of program development. However, the net result of this initial time expenditure is to reduce the time needed to manage dysphagic patients. Weekends and holidays are the most difficult times for program coordination and implementation. Therefore, the need arises to develop a dependable corps of trained volunteers or family members who can be instructed to follow a prescribed feeding program without direct assistance. Lipner et al. (1990) have described the use of volunteers to meet this need.

Team members also must make some personal commitments to changes in their work schedules. The hours of eight to four and nine to five with an hour off for lunch are incompatible with care of dysphagia patients. Most in-patient settings serve meals at 7 A.M., noon, and 5 P.M. Therefore if one is to assist in feeding, consideration must be given to rearrangement of working hours.

IDENTIFYING THE POPULATION

A dysphagia team may wish to limit the scope of its initial efforts to a small segment or service of the hospital population; for example, rehabilitation, neurology, and otolaryngology/head and neck service. The team might decide to run a demonstration diagnostic and treatment dysphagia program on one of these services in an effort to evaluate the efficacy of beginning such a program and to eliminate some of the problems that can arise as it is established before offering the service to the entire hospital.

As the program develops, the need for diagnostic and swallowing treatment services will become apparent. One new consultation a week will quickly turn into five and perhaps ten, as word of its existence spreads. Dysphagia programs in the initial stages will usually treat 12 to 15 patients per week. The number of dysphagic patients in a given institution may vary depending on the setting and patient population. In an acute care setting, one-third may be dysphagic (Groher and Bukatman 1986). In chronic care settings these percentages range from 59 (Siebens et al. 1986) to 66 percent (Layne et al. 1989). In those with single hemispheric stroke, one can expect nearly one-third to be dysphagic (Veis and Logemann 1985; Barer 1989; Young and Durant-Jones 1990). In those with dysphagia following trauma, nearly one-third will require remediation (Winstein 1983; Field and Weiss 1989).

Growth of the program depends upon available staff time and efficient coordination of team effort. Team members who can spend only a limited amount of time per day with dysphagic patients normally will limit their efforts to those who can benefit the most. The same principle holds true for those very active programs that attempt to provide services to more patients than their resources can support.

Some centers have found it necessary to provide outpatient clinics for patients who continue to have episodes of dysphagia following hospital discharge, and for those who do not need hospitalization but who complain specifically of swallowing difficulty. Such clinics require additional space and staff time, both of which must be carefully budgeted. Clinics are usually formed only after the dysphagia program has become well recognized both in the hospital and in the immediate community.

OUTLINING THE PROGRAM AND PROCEDURES

At this point it should be possible to outline the structure of the dysphagia program in terms of who will participate, how much they will participate, where they will participate, and finally, the rationale for beginning such an effort. This information is usually passed through the hospital's appropriate chain of command for final approval. A statement of procedures is a useful attachment to the program outline. The following are questions for consideration:

1. How will dysphagic patients be identified?
2. To whom will consultations and follow-up orders be directed?
3. What is the process for constructing and ordering a swallowing evaluation diet?
4. Will the need to have dysphagic patients eat smaller portions more times per day require procedural changes between the dietary service and the kitchen?
5. Who will be responsible for monitoring the results of dysphagia rehabilitation?
6. How are the results to be documented?
7. What medical precautions must be taken when dysphagia therapy is initiated?

Following administrative approval, a policy memorandum or directive authorizing the team's activities may need to be developed. A sample policy memorandum is presented in Appendix 14.A. Question number 7 requires some elaboration. As pointed out in Chapter 6, one can minimize risks of aspiration after introducing food orally by completing a thorough evaluation of the patient's neuromuscular and cortical potentials before beginning. Patients can and do aspirate during trial periods of swallowing rehabilitation, and the dysphagia team must delineate the types of precautions to be taken. This includes knowledge of suctioning and emergency medical procedures and, of course, clearance from the attending physician. Some centers begin by having the attending physician or registered nurse present during all first-time attempts at oral feeding; as the feeder becomes more experienced, this support may not be as necessary. The therapist who provides feeding training should receive special clinical privileges from the hospital's chief of staff before independent first-time feedings begin.

Finally, a pilot study might be initiated at this stage with permission from the appropriate medical or research committee. When the program has been outlined and the dysphagia team has become familiar with the procedures, such a study may facilitate final acceptance of the program. A small sample of patients should be drawn from those who are identified as being most in need of the team's services. Physicians who support the program may be enlisted to refer candidates from among their patients. For example, a neurologist may refer a patient who has recently had a cerebrovascular accident. By carefully documenting evaluation and treatment results, the team will be able to make a preliminary assessment of the success of the program. Prior to the formal recognition of their dysphagic team, Martens et al. (1990) sought to gather appropriate incidence data and conduct a prospective study to ascertain the effects of the team on caloric intake, body weight, instances of aspiration pneumonia, and feeding independence.

INITIATING THE PROGRAM

After final approval has been given, announcements should be sent to each service director and ward physician briefly describing the program's intent and consultation procedures.

At this point, training should begin, focusing on the types of services the team will offer and their importance to the patient's medical recovery. Training should be offered first to staff physicians and nurses. It is best accomplished if the physician and nursing members of the dysphagia team teach their peers; however, to enhance collaboration and improve the visibility of the program, the team leader should be included in all educational sessions. Members from the allied health sector (dietetics, speech pathology, rehabilitation) can provide training to their own peers and can assist in training volunteers to serve as feeders. Publicity should be ongoing to alert nonrelated hospital staff and consumers that such a specialized program exists. This may be especially important in active medical centers with constant changes of house staff assignments. Grand rounds presentations and hospital newsletter articles can communicate achievements as well as assist in gaining wider acceptance of the program.

Volunteer training should focus on the basics of the swallowing act and the importance of strictly adhering to the prescription for feeding designed by the rehabilitation team. Such prescriptions should be clearly posted at bedside with a copy in the nursing files to facilitate communication among day, evening, and night shifts. Each prescription should be clearly signed and provide an appropriate telephone or call number of a person to contact for additional assistance. An example of such a prescription is as follows:

1. Make sure patient is sitting upright during and one-half hour after eating.
2. Pull curtains around bed to minimize distractions.
3. Let the patient feed himself making sure he takes one bite and swallows before taking another. He will require reminders to do so.

4. Do not talk with the patient while he is eating as this serves as a distraction and interferes with swallowing.

For more information call: R. Y., Ex. 212

Beeper: 303

When appropriate, the prescription should also include the types of foods and liquids that are and are not permitted. This helps to eliminate confusion that may result from a patient receiving the wrong food tray. These prescriptions greatly facilitate the passing of information from shift to shift and from volunteer to volunteer, as most volunteers do not come each day, nor do they always feed the same patients.

The team leader should monitor any changes needed in diets and/or procedures for feeding. Ideally, one member from the dysphagia team makes rounds with the ward physicians to report progress in dysphagia rehabilitation and to keep informed of changes in the patient's medical status that may preclude oral feeding or dictate different nutritional requirements. The importance of passing clear and relevant information from the team leader to the nursing staff and volunteers cannot be overestimated. Dysphagia rehabilitation efforts can change from day to day, and unless requests and orders are easily translated and implemented, they can be hampered and lead to undue frustration.

MAINTAINING RECORDS

Daily notes are generally kept by physicians and therapists, while nurses record progress notes for each shift. The team leader should ensure that progress is addressed at least once a day or as often as each meal. An immediate notation should be made on any occurrence or suspicion of significant aspiration, including which staff member was notified and the action taken. Immediate notation should also be made after diet changes, either to add a newly tolerated food or to delete an item that is not well tolerated. A change in the patient's alertness, physical appearance, metabolism, or mental status, as well as new evaluative findings such as the return or absence of swallowing reflexes should be reported as soon as they are observed.

Routine daily notes should review the gains and/or losses achieved by dysphagia rehabilitation. They should indicate both the training techniques employed and the success or failure of the prescribed diet. The nursing staff and dietitian are usually responsible for recording fluid intake and output. In addition, a daily record of food intake can be charted, identifying the exact quantity of each item actually consumed as closely as can be estimated. Allowance should be made for spillage or drooling, as this may significantly alter estimates made from leftovers on the tray.

Close examination of these charts often shows patterns of food intake that might otherwise have gone unnoticed. For instance, it may become clear that a patient seems to swallow best when macaroni rather than ground meat is on the menu. Another patient may swallow better at the noon meal, related to the level of alertness at that particular time, or to the diet or therapist. This specific information can prove useful for supporting changes in diet or modifications of training techniques.

Charting food consumption will give a good picture of the patient's progress in eating as well as of daily nutritional intake in the absence of a calorie count. In the event a calorie count is ordered, the dietitian keeps a careful record of the daily calorie intake, usually done over a period of several days (see Chapter 11).

MEASURING RESULTS

If a pilot study is completed before the program begins, a follow-up study should be done to measure the effectiveness of the program in progress. It is essential to determine the program's success in achieving its objectives, such as reducing the incidence of aspiration pneumonias, reducing dependence on tube feedings (measured by days of use or incidence), shortening total dysphagia recovery time, and promoting a normal oral diet (measured by the diet achieved at the conclusion of the program or at discharge). The efficacy of instituting a dysphagia team on a 26-bed neurology/neurosurgery unit was studied prospectively by Martens and her colleagues (1990). They divided their patients into those who received a team evaluation and those who were managed without a team approach. In those who had the team management there was a significant improvement in weight gain and caloric intake. Presumably this would have positively affected the patient's nutritional status although this was not measured due to administrative restrictions. Using the reduction in the occurrence of aspiration pneumonia as an outcome measure, Kasprisin and her colleagues (1989) found that their team approach effected a significant reduction in the incidence of aspiration pneumonia even for patients with moderate-to-severe dysphagia. In a retrospective review of their dysphagia teams, Jones and Altschuler (1987) discussed the following findings after comparing the records of patients before and after an interdisciplinary management approach. They included (1) increased and earlier use of feeding tubes (to prevent malnutrition), (2) a decrease in pulmonary aspiration, (3) increased intradepartmental cooperation, (4) earlier documentation of the problem, and (5) improved oral intake.

The dysphagia team must keep careful records on each patient who is referred for evaluation. Maintaining separate files can facilitate data collection for future use. Data should be organized so that they specifically describe the patient population, including age, cause of dysphagia, and significant contributing medical history. Evaluation techniques and results should be coded for each patient. These basic data eventually can be compared with the goals that were originally set. They can also serve as a program evaluation tool, as the basis for scientific investigation, or as a part of a quality assurance program. The use of a quality assurance audit to establish the need for services and the demonstration of intervention with dysphagia patients in a chronic care setting is described by Musson and her colleagues (1990).

The study might seek to evaluate treatment techniques, such as the effects manipulation of diet might bring versus only cognitive training without diet manipulation. Unfortunately, some experimental designs of this nature involve depriving a control group of selected intervention. One way to avoid this ethical dilemma is to use the chart audit procedure now routinely performed in many institutions. By establishing outcome criteria for the chart review, a sample can be selected and charts collected from a specific, predetermined time period. A matched group of charts then can be drawn for comparison from a previous time period (prior to initiation of the program, but recent enough to ensure similar medical management). This step is not essential to the chart audit, as the first sample is intended to be measured only against its own criteria. Even if chart audit fails, it provides a valuable tool for identifying and correcting problems that surface during the review. A subsequent reaudit should succeed if the program is, in fact, effective.

Finally, administrators and colleagues must be informed of both the positive and negative results of the studies, as they can be important for keeping the program visible and viable.

ETHICAL CONSIDERATIONS

As the dysphagia management team develops, they often become involved in issues relating to the ethics of providing or withholding nutrition. For these reasons it is important that the dysphagia team interface with their medical center's ethics committee. It is important that each medical center develop policy that directs the medical personnel in situations in which the patient refuses to be fed, when the family wishes that the patient not be fed, or when the risks of providing nutrition outweigh the benefits (Quill 1989; Groher 1990).

SUMMARY

The diagnosis and management of dysphagic patients has become a subspecialty for many professions. There is general agreement that a multidisciplinary approach in their management will provide the care necessary to justify the resources needed to achieve a favorable impact. The number of centers developing teams that interact in behalf of the dysphagic patient has grown steadily. In the Department of Veterans Affairs in 1986, 17 of 172 medical centers had established teams. In 1990 the number grew to 97. There is a growing scientific base for understanding the mechanisms of swallow that has provided the dysphagia team with improved rationales for treatment. The efficacy of treatment approaches in controlled studies remains to be established.

REFERENCES

Barer DH. The natural history and functional consequences of dysphagia after hemispheric stroke. J Neurol Neurosurg Psychiat 1989; 52:236–41.
Clusky MM. The use of pureed diets among the elderly. Diet Curr 1989; 16:17–20.

Curran J, Groher ME. Development and dissemination of an aspiration risk reduction diet. Dysphagia 1990; 5:6–12.

Elpern EH, Jacobs ER, Bone RC. Incidence of aspiration in tracheally intubated adults. Heart Lung 1987; 16:527–31.

Erlichman M. The role of speech pathologists in the management of dysphagia. National Center for Health Services, Research and Health Care Technology Assessment, U.S. Department of Health and Human Services, 1989; 1:1–10.

Field LH, Weiss CJ. Dysphagia with head injury. Brain Injury 1989; 3:19–26.

Groher ME. Ethical dilemmas in providing nutrition. Dysphagia 1990; 5:102–9.

Groher ME. The role of the speech-language pathologist in the evaluation and care of oral and pharyngeal dysphagia. J Neuro Rehab 1992; 3:5–8.

Groher ME, Bukatman R. The prevalence of swallowing in two teaching hospitals. Dysphagia 1986; 1:3–6.

Groher ME, Gonzalez EE. Swallowing treatment outcomes in patients following head/neck surgery. Quality Assurance Report, Department of Veterans Affairs Medical Center, New York, 1989.

Hotaling DL. Adapting the mealtime environment: setting the stage for eating. Dysphagia 1990; 5:77–83.

Jones PL, Altschuler SL. Dysphagia teams: a specific approach to a nonspecific problem. Dysphagia 1987; 1:200–5.

Kasprisin AT, Clumeck H, Nino-Murcia M. The efficacy of rehabilitation management of dysphagia. Dysphagia 1989; 4:48–52.

Layne KA, Losinski DS, Zenner PM, et al. Using the Fleming index of dysphagia to establish prevalence. Dysphagia 1989; 4:39–42.

Langmore SE, Schatz K, Olsen N. Fiberoptic endoscopic examination of swallowing safety: a new procedure. Dysphagia 1988; 2:216–9.

Lipner HS, Bosler J, Giles G. Volunteer participation in feeding residents: training and supervision in a long-term care facility. Dysphagia 1990; 5:89–95.

Martens L, Cameron T, Simonsen M. Effects of a multidisciplinary management program on neurologically impaired patients with dysphagia. Dysphagia 1990; 5:147–51.

Martin BJ, Corlew MM. The incidence of communication disorders in dysphagic patients. J Speech Hear Disord 1990; 55:28–32.

Mody M, Nagai J. A multidisciplinary approach to the development of competency standards and appropriate allocation for patients with dysphagia. Am J Occup Ther 1990; 44:369–72.

Musson ND, Kinkaid J, Ryan P et al. Nature, nurture, nutrition: interdisciplinary programs to address the prevention of malnutrition and dehydration. Dysphagia 1990; 5:96–101.

Quill TE. Nasogastric feeding tubes in a group of chronically ill elderly patients in a community hospital. Arch Intern Med 1989; 149:1937–41.

Siebens H, Trupe E, Siebens A et al. Correlates and consequences of eating dependency in institutionalized elderly. J Am Geriatr Soc 1986; 34:192–8.

Skills needed by speech-language pathologists providing services to dysphagic patients/clients. ASHA 1990; 32(suppl 2):7–12.

Terry PB, Fuller SD. Pulmonary consequences of aspiration. Dysphagia 1989; 3:179–83.

Veis S, Logemann JA. Swallowing disorders in persons with cerebrovascular accident. Arch Phys Med 1985; 66:372–5.

Weg AL, Miskovitz PF. Percutaneous endoscopic gastrostomy (PEG): a critical appraisal. Dysphagia 1987; 1:227–31.

Winstein CJ. Neurogenic dysphagia: frequency, progression, and outcome in adults following head injury. Phys Ther 1983; 63:1992–7.

Young EC, Durant-Jones L. Developing a dysphagia program in an acute care hospital: a needs assessment. Dysphagia 1990; 5:159–65.

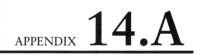

Sample Policy

DYSPHAGIA TEAM

1. **PURPOSE.** To define the organization and functions of an interdisciplinary Dysphagia Team for the management of patients with swallowing disorders. The intent of this Dysphagia Team is to implement protocol and procedures for the identification, assessment, and treatment of patients with dysphagia in order to optimize nutrition, promote feeding independence of the patients, minimize the need for feeding tubes, and to reduce the incidence of complications of dysphagia (e.g., aspiration pneumonia, dehydration, and/or malnutrition).

2. **POLICY.** To provide diagnostic and rehabilitative services to all eligible inpatients and outpatients with dysphagia (swallowing problems). It is necessary that these patients be identified and treated in a coordinated manner by the appropriate clinical services.

3. **DEFINITION.** Dysphagia is difficulty in one or more stages of deglutition from placement of food in the mouth, oral motor manipulation and control of the bolus, triggering of the swallowing action and pharyngeal peristalsis, through relaxation of the cricopharyngeal sphincter which allows the bolus to pass into the esophagus. Etiologies of such disturbances include varied neuropathologies, head and neck disease, in addition to other medical and psychological problems which may affect oral nutritional intake.

4. **RESPONSIBILITIES.**

   A. Team membership shall include representation from the following services/sections:

   > Speech-Language Pathology
   > Physician
   > Dietetics
   > Nursing

   Other disciplines may participate on an as-needed basis (e.g., Gastroenterology, Digestive Diseases and Nutrition Section, Radiology, Surgery, Social Work, Hospital Based Home Care, Oncology, Pulmonary, etc.)

   B. Team Responsibilities.

   (1) Facilitate identification of patients with swallowing problems.

(2) Recommend, implement, and modify dysphagia management plans in cooperation with the primary care physician.

(3) Hold regularly scheduled patient care staff meetings for purposes of reviewing patients referred and developing, recommending, and monitoring the interdisciplinary patient care plans for further evaluation and/or treatment.

(4) Request consultation as needed of other services.

(5) Document clinical activities.
   (a) Response to consultation request
   (b) Flowsheet data on each team referral
   (c) Progress notes by individual team members

(6) Educate medical center personnel about Dysphagia Team purpose and increase their awareness of dysphagia as a patient problem.

(7) Promote continuing education of team members.

(8) Propose and generate research where issues of dysphagia are unclear.

C. Specific responsibilities of team members.

(1) Speech-Language Pathologist. Serves as coordinator of the Dysphagia Team. The speech-language pathologist obtains a history and description of the problem, and performs the initial screening of the patient in order to determine his candidacy for further evaluation of the dysphagia problem by the Team. The initial screening and further evaluation of the dysphagia by the speech-language pathologist may include evaluation of oral motor function, and integrity of the components of the swallowing process (as observed on physical examination as well as via videofluoroscopic study in conjunction with the radiologist). Treatment activities of the speech-language pathologist may include direct activities such as oromuscular strengthening, thermal stimulation to improve the swallowing mechanism, and exercises to increase adduction of the vocal folds. Direct treatment activities may include recommendations re: compensatory adjustments (e.g., posture, protective swallow techniques, and prostheses) as well as participation in the determination of appropriate food consistencies for the dysphagic patient.

(2) Physician. To participate in patient examination with the speech pathologist to relate findings to patient's general medical condition and to act as liaison with patient's attending physician.

(3) Dietitian. Coordinates the nutritional assessment, recommendations, and documentation of plans with the ward dietitian to accomplish nutritional goals. Serves as liaison between the

team, patient, and food service personnel to assure that diet order and food served are consistent with patient's nutritional needs. Participates in the determination and provision of texture/consistency needs to optimize oral intake and monitors nutrient intake as needed to insure adequacy and/or tolerance of texture. Recommends enteral/parenteral feeding modalities as appropriate. Provides education to the patient and/or care giver on diet modification, weight gain/loss, etc. prior to discharge. Arranges follow up visit with the outpatient dietitian if needed.

    (4) Nurse. Integrates the dysphagia program into the total patient needs. Participates during the evaluation process by providing nursing assessments of the patient in the following areas: cognitive, functional, sensory, communicative, learning ability and social support. The nurse member will communicate the recommendations of the Team to the nursing staff caring for the patient. Will also be available for consultation for the nursing staff, the patient, and/or patient's care giver.

5. PROCEDURES.

    A. Authorized medical staff will send a Consultation Request (SF 513) to: Dysphagia Team Speech Pathology, Mail Code 126.

    B. The Speech-Language Pathologist will contact Dysphagia Team members following the initial review of the problem.

    C. Dysphagia Team members will perform their respective assessments and document same on progress notes, as delineated in the Responsibilities Section.

    D. The findings of the Dysphagia Team and recommendations for management will be discussed at the next scheduled patient care meeting. The patient's primary physician and charge nurse will be informed of the recommendations. Recommendations for management may include:

    (1) Oral vs. non-oral feeding; oral feeding with assistance.

    (2) Head, neck, and body posture and positioning.

    (3) Food textures and consistencies.

    (4) Food placement.

    (5) Adaptive equipment.

    (6) Oral-motor facilitation techniques.

    (7) Reflex sensitization techniques.

Index